Melancholy and the Care of the Soul

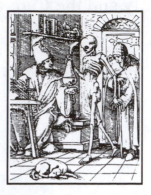

The History of Medicine in Context

Series Editors: Andrew Cunningham and Ole Peter Grell

Department of History and Philosophy of Science
University of Cambridge

Department of History
The Open University

Titles in this series include:

The Making of Addiction
The 'Use and Abuse' of Opium in Nineteenth-Century Britain
Louise Foxcroft

Hospital Care and the British Standing Army, 1660–1714
Eric Gruber von Arni

Health Care and Poor Relief in 18th and 19th Century Southern Europe
Edited by Ole Peter Grell, Andrew Cunningham and Bernd Roeck

*Health, Sickness, Medicine and the Friars in the Thirteenth
and Fourteenth Centuries*
Angela Montford

The Rise of Causal Concepts of Disease
Case Histories
K. Codell Carter

Melancholy and the Care of the Soul

Religion, Moral Philosophy and Madness
in Early Modern England

JEREMY SCHMIDT

ASHGATE

Published by
Ashgate Publishing Limited
Gower House
Croft Road
Aldershot
Hampshire GU11 3HR
England

Ashgate Publishing Company
Suite 420
101 Cherry Street
Burlington, VT 05401-4405
USA

BT32.4
.S36
2007

0701224(7

Ashgate website: http://www.ashgate.com

British Library Cataloguing in Publication Data
Schmidt, Jeremy, 1977-
  Melancholy and the care of the soul: religion, moral philosophy and madness in early modern England. – (The history of medicine in context)
1.Depression, Mental – England – History – 16th century 2.Depression, Mental – England – History – 17th century 3.Depression, Mental – England – History – 18th century 4.Melancholy in literature
  I.Title
  616.8'527'00942'0903

Library of Congress Cataloging-in-Publication Data
Schmidt, Jeremy, 1977-
 Melancholy and the care of the soul: religion, moral philosophy and madness in early modern England / Jeremy Schmidt.
    p. cm. – (The history of medicine in context)
 Includes bibliographical references.
 ISBN-13: 978-0-7546-5748-4 (alk. paper)
 ISBN-10: 0-7546-5748-5 (alk. paper)
  1. Melancholy–Religious aspects–Christianity. 2. Melancholy–England–History. 3. Depression, Mental–Religious aspects–Christianity. 4. Depression, Mental–England–History. 5. Spiritual healing. I. Title.
  BT732.4.S36 2007
  152.4–dc22

                                                                                        2006018494

ISBN-13: 978-0-7546-5748-4

Printed on acid-free paper

Printed and bound in Great Britain by MPG Books Ltd, Bodmin, Cornwall.

Contents

Acknowledgments

The research for this book was enabled by fellowships from the History Department at the Johns Hopkins University, from the Henry E. Huntington Library, and from the Mellon Foundation. My very warm thanks to (in no particular order) Anthony Pagden, Mary Fissell, Mordechai Feingold, Alan Hall, Matthew Bell, Andrew Solomon, Angus Gowland, and members of the Mellon Summer Seminar in Intellectual History held at the California Institute for Technology in 2004 for reading and commenting on various parts of this project as it took shape as a Ph.D. dissertation and afterwards. I would especially like to thank John Marshall, who was an exceptionally attentive reader and generous supervisor throughout my tenure as a graduate student at the Johns Hopkins University. David Bell and Sean Greenberg also read the whole of the Ph.D. thesis, and provided some very insightful direction and criticism, and I benefited further from a discussion with Anita Guerrini about George Cheyne and the project more generally.

I am deeply indebted to my parents for their generous support throughout some rather trying years, and also to my former teachers at the University of British Columbia, many of whom have read and commented on parts of this work: Ed Hundert, Ernie Hamm, Allen Sinel, Evan Kreider, and the late Stephen Straker. Their kind encouragement and interest has been most welcome, and I continue to learn from the classes I took with them years ago. Many thanks as well to my colleagues at the University of King's College for their conversation and support, and to the Early Modern Studies Programme at King's for the opportunity to give a talk on my work which helped in clarifying some of my ideas.

My greatest thanks is to my friend and partner, Krista Voth, who has been a continual source of consolation, courage and hope, and without whom the completion of this project would be a melancholy affair indeed.

Introduction: Melancholy, Language, and Madness

Jean Starobinski writes that "the Renaissance is the golden age of melancholy."[1] The intense interest in melancholy we find in this period is due partly to the revival and popularization in the Florentine Renaissance of the ancient association of melancholy with genius found in the Aristotelian *Problemata* 30.1.[2] Fed by the Florentine tradition and by aristocratic pretensions to refined sensibility, melancholy also became fashionable as a sign of nobility of mind. (Jacques in William Shakespeare's *As you like it* exhibits such refined, and self-indulgent, melancholy, claiming to be able to "suck melancholy out of a song as a weasel sucks eggs"[3]). Melancholy was the "crest of courtiers' arms," as a character in John Lyly's *Midas* (1592) puts it.[4] And it was, as a crest, *displayed* in both behavior and dress. Hamlet, himself one of the more famous Elizabethan figures of melancholy, gives an eloquent catalog of the "forms, moods, shapes" of fashionable melancholy in one of the opening scenes of the play: "customary suits of solemn black," windy suspiration of forced breath," "the fruitful river of the eye," "the dejected haviour of the visage."[5]

In describing the appearance of the melancholic personality, Hamlet himself insists that while these "indeed might seem / For they are the actions that a man might play / ... I have that within which passes show."[6] His own melancholy is thus not to be understood as fashionable aristocratic affectation. Nor can it be interpreted

---

1   Jean Starobinski, *A History of the Treatment of Melancholy from Earliest Times to 1900* (Basle: Geigy, 1962), 38.

2   On the idea of melancholy and genius in the Florentine Renaissance and beyond, see Raymond Kiblansky, Erwin Panofsky, and Fritz Saxl, *Saturn and Melancholy: Studies in the History of Natural Philosophy, Religion, and Art* (London: Nelson, 1964). The entire text of *Problemata* 30.1 is reproduced in *Saturn and Melancholy*, 15–41.

3   Shakespeare, *As You Like It*, II, ii, 13.

4   Lyly, *Midas* (London: Thomas Scarlet for I[ohn] B[roome], 1592), 5, ii. On the fashionableness of melancholy, see Lawrence E. Babb, *The Elizabethan Malady: A Study of Melancholia in English Literature from 1580–1642* (East Lansing, MI: Michigan State College Press, 1951); Bridget Gellert Lyons, *Voices of Melancholy: Studies in Literary Treatments of Melancholy in Renaissance England* (London: Routledge & Kegan Paul, 1971); Michael MacDonald, *Mystical Bedlam: Madness, Anxiety and Healing in Seventeenth-century England* (Cambridge: Cambridge University Press, 1981), 150–60; M.A. Screech, *Montaigne & Melancholy: The Wisdom of the Essays* (Selinsgrove, PA: Susquehanna University Press, 1983), 22–41.

5   William Shakespeare, *Hamlet, Prince of Denmark*, ed. Philip Edwards, New Cambridge Shakespeare (Cambridge: Cambridge University Press, 1985), I, ii, 78–82.

6   Ibid., I, ii, 83–5.

simply as a medical condition involving a basically physical pathology, in spite of centuries of medically minded interpretations of *Hamlet*.[7] It is true that by the end of the sixteenth century the ancient medical concept of melancholy had become widely available as a mode of understanding the emotions and trouble of mind. Besides Florentine celebrations of melancholic genius, the other major catalyst of the Renaissance interest in melancholy was the increased humanist scrutiny of ancient medical texts on the subject, most of which analyze melancholy not as a privileged philosophical temperament, but as a form of madness and disease caused by the excess of black bile (*melankolia* in Greek), or by the burning of one of the other three postulated constituent fluids of the body (choler, or yellow bile, phlegm, and blood).[8] Throughout Acts II and III of *Hamlet*, there is some question as to whether Hamlet has indeed gone mad, and Hamlet himself mentions the melancholic weakness of his body.[9] King Claudius concludes worriedly, however, that Hamlet has not been put "so much from the understanding of himself" simply because of a diseased brain. Rather, "there's something in his soul / O'er which his melancholy sits on brood," a "something-settled matter in his heart / Whereon his brains still beating puts him thus / From fashion of himself."[10]

There are, of course, many ways of understanding the something in his soul over which Hamlet broods throughout the play. Initially, it is his moral outrage at his mother's hasty marriage to his uncle Claudius after the death of her husband. After the first encounter with his father's ghost, his despairing and self-loathing soliloquies seem to be driven both by his encounter with the moral rot of the world and by his own inability to rectify this dissolution by acting on his oath to avenge his father's murder. But what Claudius' formulation of Hamlet's melancholy captures so well is the general approach to thinking about and treating the melancholic condition in the late sixteenth and seventeenth centuries. Melancholy was seen by many of Shakespeare's contemporaries as a pattern of thought, mood, and behavior the precise severity, nature, and prognosis of which was determined not only by the condition of the body, but also by the state of the soul. It was thus thought to require equally the attention of the physician of the body and the physician of the soul. In England of the seventeenth and eighteenth centuries, the disciplines of psychiatry and clinical psychology had yet to be fully born. The idea of the health of the soul was articulated in early modern Europe in terms of ancient philosophical and early Christian discussions of the good and of human happiness, and the concepts and

---

7   See William F. Bynum and Michael Neve, "Hamlet on the Couch", in W.F. Bynum, Roy Porter, and Michael Shepherd, eds., *The Anatomy of Madness: Essays in the History of Psychiatry, Volume 1: People and Ideas* (London and New York: Tavistock Publications, 1985), 289–304.

8   See H.C. Erik Midelfort, *A History of Madness in Sixteenth-century Germany* (Stanford, CA: Stanford University Press, 1999), 140–63. For a discussion of the various analyses of melancholy in ancient thought, see Kiblansky, Panofsky, and Saxl, *Saturn and Melancholy*, 3–66.

9   Shakespeare, *Hamlet*, II, ii, 118; II, iii, 1–9; III, i, 551–6; III, i, 158–69.

10   Ibid., III, i, 158–9; III, i, 167–9.

techniques elaborated in these discussions were fashioned by early modern writers as therapeutic languages for the melancholic condition.

The spiritual and moral analysis of melancholy continued to be articulated after the Renaissance and into the late seventeenth and early eighteenth centuries, which have been singled out as constituting yet another "Age of Melancholy."[11] Eighteenth-century literature is indeed filled with reflections on the melancholic condition, but it would be more correct to call it the age of *hypochondriac* melancholy. The term needs some explaining in the twenty-first century. In one of the earliest popular English works on melancholy, the physician Timothy Bright had noted how melancholy could be accompanied by "shortness of breathing," "an unnaturall boyling of heate, with wyndines under the left side," and a "palpitation of the heart."[12] Other writers separated out such melancholic symptoms as cases of hypochondriac melancholy, which affected both the mind and the vital and digestive organs of the body.[13] Eighteenth-century medical theorists ran the hypochondria diagnosis together with the hysteria diagnosis, previously understood as an affliction caused in some way by the womb, and both were taken to be disorders of the nerves which erupted into a variety of physical symptoms as well as melancholic fear and sorrow. The language of hypochondria and hysteria became quite widespread in the eighteenth century, and eighteenth-century observers referred to them as "fashionable" diseases; but whereas Hamlet had indexed melancholy in terms of its conspicuous shows of emotion, hypochondriac and hysteric individuals in the eighteenth century displayed their condition by complaining of their bodily ailments and by perfuming themselves with asafœtida, a type of medication with a rather malodorous scent.[14] This seemed to remove the condition from the jurisdiction of the priest and philosopher. But when James Boswell commented late in the eighteenth century that hypochondria could be considered to be "a disorder in the mind itself, which neither the most potent medicines nor most violent exercise can remove," he was echoing a series of late seventeenth and early eighteenth-century writers who had asserted that hypochondriac melancholy and hysteria were conditions produced by an interaction of moral character, spiritual discipline, and bodily disposition.[15]

This dimension of the early modern discourse on melancholy has been largely overlooked by historians. In the large scholarly literature on early modern English melancholy, analysis has concentrated on either medical theories of melancholy, or

---

11   Cecil A. Moore, *Backgrounds of English Literature 1700–1760* (Minneapolis, MN: University of Minnesota Press, 1953), 179–238.

12   Bright, *A Treatise of Melancholie* (London: Thomas Vautrollier, 1586), 125.

13   See Robert Burton, *The Anatomy of Melancholy*, ed. A.R. Shilleto (New York: AMS Press, 1973), I.i.III.iv: 199–202.

14   Moore, *Backgrounds*, 192; Jean Bernard Le Blanc, *Letters on the English and French Nations* (London: J. Brindley, 1747), Letter 27, 130–40. This was a translation of *Lettres d'un François* (Le Haye: J. Neaulme, 1745).

15   Boswell, "On Hypochondria," no. 63, Dec. 1782, in *The Hypochondriack*, ed. Margery Bailey (Stanford, CA: Stanford University Press, 1928), 2: 236, 238.

on literary representations and expressions of melancholy.[16] Studies of Elizabethan intellectual history often discuss melancholy as a feature of commonplace humoral models of psychology, according to which a given balance of the bodily humors was thought to produce certain mental dispositions and characteristics.[17] In literary studies of Elizabethan culture, there is, perhaps quite naturally, a tendency to approach melancholy as an artefact of the artistic vision elaborated within the context of a given literary work. On this level of analysis, melancholy comes to be seen as a thematic, a trope, a character type, or again as a kind of *Weltanschauung*. What drops from the picture is the problem of melancholic suffering among early modern men and women at large, which demanded consolation and cure at the same time that it elicited literary comment and expression; and religion and moral philosophy as therapeutic languages of melancholy, if they are treated of at all, have so far been relegated to a discussion of the "background" of literature.[18] Thus, aside from some limited discussions of Robert Burton's famous work *The Anatomy of Melancholy* (1621), the use of moral philosophical techniques and approaches in several of the key seventeenth-century texts on melancholy has been largely unexplored.[19] And while the treatment of melancholy by clerics has been noted by scholars of seventeenth-century English history, little attention has been given to the many pastoral works on the affliction of conscience and the consolation of sorrow that dealt extensively with melancholy. Several important texts have been ignored entirely, and historians have only cursorily examined others.[20]

16　Stanley W. Jackson, *Melancholia and Depression: From Hippocratic to Modern Times* (Hartford, CT: Yale University Press, 1992); "Melancholia and Mechanical Explanation in Eighteenth-century Medicine," *Journal of the History of Medicine and Allied Sciences* 38 (1983): 298–319; "Melancholia and Partial Insanity," *Journal of the History of Behavioural Sciences* 19 (1983): 173–84; "Melancholy and the Waning of the Humoural Theory," *Journal of the History of Medicine and Allied Sciences* 33 (1978): 367–76; T.H. Jobe, "Medical Theories of Melancholia in the Seventeenth and Early Eighteenth Centuries," *Clio Medica* 11 (1976): 217–32; Carol Falvo Heffernan, *The Melancholy Muse: Chaucer, Shakespeare and Early Medicine* (Pittsburgh, PA: Duquesne University Press, 1995), 1–33.

17　See in particular Babb, *Elizabethan Malady*; and Ruth Leila Anderson, *Elizabethan Psychology and Shakespeare's Plays*, 2nd edn. (New York: Russell & Russell, 1966).

18　See Lyons, *Voices of Melancholy*; Moore, *Backgrounds*.

19　On Burton, see Stanley W. Jackson's essay "Robert Burton and Psychological Healing," *Journal of the History of Medicine and Allied Sciences* 44 (1989): 160–178, as well as his more recent *Care of the Psyche: A History of Psychological Healing* (London and New Haven, CT: Yale University Press, 1999); cf. the important critical comments on the approach to Elizabethan "psychology" via medical theory in Judith Kegan Gardiner, "Elizabethan Psychology and Burton's *Anatomy of Melancholy*," *Journal of the History of Ideas* 38 (1977): 373–88.

20　See Michael MacDonald, *Mystical Bedlam*, 217–31, and his "Religion, Social Change and Psychological Healing in England, 1600–1800," in W.J. Sheils, ed., *The Church and Healing* (Oxford: Basil Blackwell, 1982), 101–26. See also the ambitious but confusing attempt at analysis in John Owen King, *The Iron of Melancholy: Structures of Spiritual*

Something similar can be said of the scholarship on eighteenth-century hypochondria and hysteria. G.S. Rousseau pointed out some years ago that the history of hypochondria and hysteria in the eighteenth century has for the most part been told as a chapter in the history of medical science and theory, without discussions of the social, cultural, or political context.[21] The sustained level of criticism of both hypochondriacs and their medical theorists throughout the eighteenth century has often been noted, but for the most part, discussions of the eighteenth-century discourse on nervous disorder do not progress beyond dividing English culture into believers and skeptics, providing little in the way of a more substantive analysis of what made believers believe and skeptics skeptical.[22] The hypochondriac melancholic cases of key eighteenth-century literary figures such as Samuel Johnson, James Boswell, and Thomas Gray have received attention, but here the approach has most often been oriented around biographical explanation or literary explication.[23] Anita Guerrini's recent study of Dr. George Cheyne, one of the most important eighteenth-century physicians specializing in nervous disorders and a sufferer himself, is an exception in its careful contextual approach to Cheyne's writing, and Guerrini's biography is invaluable for illuminating the religious, philosophical and social concerns which shaped Cheyne's treatment of melancholy.[24] I follow a similar contextual approach here in discussing the history of hypochondria and hysteria in the early eighteenth century, exploring some of the cultural conditions which led to the initial popularization of the language of nervous disorder, as well as analyzing medical and non-medical texts in relation to the broader social, moral, and political worries in terms of which they were often framed.

One of the things which a contextual approach to the history of melancholy shows is that the question of the proper conceptualization and treatment of melancholy is not simply a static "psychiatric" problem posed throughout the early modern period, but one which rather occurs and reoccurs as a feature of broader currents and

---

Conversion in America from the Puritan Conscience to Victorian Neurosis (Middletown, CT: Wesleyan University Press, 1983), Ch. 1.

21   G.S. Rousseau, "Psychology," in *The Ferment of Knowledge: Studies in the Historiography of Eighteenth-century Science*, ed. G.S. Rousseau and Roy Porter (Cambridge: Cambridge University Press, 1980), 205. See, for example, Moore, *Backgrounds*, 209–10.

22   Important exceptions are: John Mullan, "Hypochondria and Hysteria: Sensibility and the Physicians," *Eighteenth Century: Theory and Interpretation* 25 (1983): 141–74; his *Sentiment and Sociability: The Language of Feeling in the Eighteenth Century* (Oxford: Oxford University Press, 1988), and Roy Porter, "The Rage of Party: A Glorious Revolution in English Psychiatry?" *Medical History* 27 (1983): 35–50.

23   Allan Ingram, *Boswell's Creative Gloom: A Study of Imagery and Melancholy in the Writings of James Boswell* (London: Macmillan, 1982); Roy Porter, "'The Hunger of the Imagination': Approaching Samuel Johnson's Melancholy," in Bynum, Porter, and Shepherd, *Anatomy of Madness*, 1: 63–88; Robert L. Snyder, "The Epistolary Melancholy of Thomas Gray," *Biography* 2 (1979): 125–40.

24   Anita Guerrini, *Obesity and Depression in the Enlightenment: The Life and Times of George Cheyne* (Norman, OK: University of Oklahoma Press, 2000).

problems. In some cases it is indeed quite central to wider debates about religion and society. In the late sixteenth and early seventeenth centuries, many ministers among the more evangelical wing of the Elizabethan Church urged that cases of melancholy which issued in religious worries about salvation, as well as cases of non-religious melancholy, should be treated spiritually, and this approach to melancholy received the level of articulation it did in part precisely because of the Reformed Protestant concern to evangelize the English nation and provide attentive pastoral care for the concerns of parishioners (see Chapter 3). The theology which informed the pastoral efforts of these self-styled "godly" churchmen – called the "Puritans" by their detractors – became increasingly controversial as the seventeenth century wore on, and after the English Civil War and the Interregnum especially, the "Puritan" approach to the care of melancholy came under severe criticism (see Chapter 4). A specifically "Anglican" style of consoling melancholy developed out of this criticism, which tended to place more emphasis than late sixteenth and early seventeenth-century pastoral works had on the use of reason and will to combat melancholic feelings; and while older "Puritan" approaches survived among some Dissenting congregations, the heightened emotional rhetoric that was integral to this consolatory idiom seems to have fallen out of favor among those caught up in the concern among England's elite ranks with polished and refined self-presentation (see Chapters 5 and 6). Furthermore, the expression of melancholy as spiritual trouble of mind was to some extent displaced by the popularized medical language of hypochondria and hysteria and its articulation of a range of bodily symptoms and complaints (see Chapter 6). But eighteenth-century writers continued to use a moral philosophical idiom to insist that hypochondriac melancholy was a disease of the mind, and indeed the perceived epidemic of cases of hysteria and hypochondria was taken by some as an indication of contemporary moral and political degeneration. Returning full circle, George Cheyne, one of the most famous eighteenth-century medical specialists in hypochondriac and hysteric disorders, argued that the "epidemic" was in fact punishment for sinful material excesses, a somatized form of the affliction of conscience which late sixteenth and early seventeenth-century ministers had sought both to cultivate and treat in their evangelization efforts (see Chapter 7).

The history of the treatment of melancholy is thus in many ways a history of English culture more broadly, and it offers a window into, *inter alia*, the nature of Elizabethan "Puritan" movement, Restoration and early eighteenth-century Dissenting sensibilities, the eighteenth-century culture of politeness, and the early modern debate about luxury. The history of the treatment of melancholy confirms the view that, in terms of practical divinity, the "Puritans" and "Anglicans" of the Elizabethan and early Jacobean Church shared a great deal in terms their intellectual framework and vocabulary, at least up to the middle of the seventeenth century; and it reveals a certain uneasiness among some post-Restoration Dissenters about their "affectionate" style of piety, which is sometimes taken to be the hallmark of Dissenting religion. Melancholy was also a concept long discussed by early modern demonologists, and as I suggest in Chapter 6, changes in styles of piety may help to explain the waning of demonology as a therapeutic and experiential language.

In addition, the history of the treatment of melancholy is an important feature of the history of women in early modern England. Running through the following chapters is a thread which traces how certain therapeutic languages altered and enabled certain perceptions of gender. Late sixteenth and early seventeenth-century evangelical therapies saw in women's melancholic spiritual suffering the potential for a heightened spiritual sensitivity and saintliness, whereas Restoration pastoral writers emphasized the link between melancholy and female weakness and sinfulness. In the eighteenth century, female hysteria was analyzed by some as intentionally subversive and disorderly, while others argued that the "epidemic" of hysteric and hypochondriac symptoms in the early eighteenth century signaled the growing effeminacy of the English nation.

Michel de Certeau has pointed to a central ambiguity in the role of the modern historian. The historian has been provided a place among academic disciplines by the social powers which organize knowledge with the mandate to order the fragments of the past into an understandable form. The historian thus orders these fragments according to modern models and practices of power, playing the role of power in a virtual world of the past: "historians will be teaching lessons of government without knowing either its responsibilities or its risks. They reflect on the power that they lack. Their analysis is ... deployed 'next to' the present time, in a staging of the past."[25] The same holds true for the historian of "psychiatry" and madness as for the political or social historian. The history of madness is now a defined subgenre of the historical discipline, rather than a past owned by the psychiatric profession. Yet no matter how naïve the professional historian poses, they inevitably play the role of the psychiatrist, hospital administrator, or bureaucrat in a staging of past scenes of madness. This is evident in the very existence of the area of specialization, as well as in the collection of demographic material, measurements of therapeutic efficacy, categorizations of illnesses, and in comparisons of past understandings of "mental illness" with contemporary theories and enquiries into the theoretical and institutional origins of the present. Many studies in the history of madness and psychiatry have indeed been explicitly framed as lessons written to current concerns, taking sides on contentious political and theoretical issues in the contemporary care of mental health, often against the dominant models of the psychiatric profession.[26]

---

25   Michel de Certeau, *The Writing of History*, trans. Tom Conley (New York: Columbia University Press, 1988), 8.

26   The most famous is probably Michel Foucault's *Histoire de la folie à l'âge classique* (1961), translated in abridged form as *Madness and Civilization: A History of Insanity in the Age of Reason* (New York: Vintage Books, 1965). See also Andrew Scull, *The Most Solitary of Afflictions: Madness and Society in Britain, 1700–1900* (London and New Haven, CT: Yale University Press, 1993), 1–10; Gerald Grob, *Mental Institutions in America: Social Policy to 1875* (New York: Free Press, 1973); Leonard D. Smith, *'Cure, Comfort and Safe Custody': Public Lunatic Asylums in Early Nineteenth-century England* (London and New York:

The present historical study is self-conscious of its peculiar modern site of production, and is motivated as much by the concerns of the professional historian and engagement with the academic literature as it is by contemporary discussions and controversy surrounding the depression diagnosis. But where some are comfortable as psychiatrists of the past and advisors to the present, I have remained distinctly uncomfortable assuming this role, which I nevertheless regard to be constitutive of the writing of the history of madness – it is in fact what makes researching and writing the history of madness worthwhile and interesting. But, importantly, the historian is not merely an amateur psychiatrist taking sides on an issue defined by contemporary discourse; they are also bound to the recovering of voices that have been excluded in order to constitute the present. The attempt to do so takes place as part of the fundamental tension Michel de Certeau has explored at length, for "the discourse destined to express what is *other* remains *their* discourse and the mirror of their own labors."[27] This is, as Certeau insists, a tension and not an opposition; it is a position which opens a space to view the modern world in more complex ways. I will sketch here what I see as one of the perspectives to which the present study may give rise in working between the past and the present.

It must be stated at the outset that early modern melancholy is not exactly depression. The psychiatrist, pharmacological researcher, and historian David Healy points out that well into the nineteenth century, "any state that could lead to underactivity or inactivity, for one reason or the other, was diagnosed as melancholia."[28] Indeed, when the Oxford don Robert Burton attempted in his encyclopedic *The Anatomy of Melancholy* to compile an exhaustive list of melancholic symptoms, culled from ancient and modern medical sources, he concluded that "the Tower of *Babel* never yielded such confusion of tongues, as this Chaos of Melancholy doth variety of symptoms."[29] To avoid contributing to this "confusion of tongues," I have throughout avoided anachronistic diagnostic language in describing early modern cases of melancholy, which today might elicit quite a different diagnosis than depression. On the other hand, Burton also noted that melancholy was taken in common early modern usage to be "*a kind of dotage without fever, having for his ordinary companions fear and sadness, without any apparent occasion,*" which definition, he asserted, was also approved by most medical authorities.[30] This definition would not qualify as a diagnostic test for depression along the lines of the American Psychology Association's current *Diagnostic and Statistical Manual of Mental Disorders* (*DSM-IV*), but it easy to see that such a usage corresponds very broadly with our own use of the term "depression." And it is in part because of this

---

Leicester University Press, 1999). See also Michael MacDonald's now infamous evaluation of eighteenth-century therapies for the insane in MacDonald, *Mystical Bedlam*, 232.

27 See *The Writing of History*, quote at 36.

28 Healy, *The Antidepressant Era* (Cambridge, MA: Harvard University Press, 1997), 30.

29 Burton, *Anatomy*, II.iii.I.i: 440; I.iii.I.ii: 442, 456.

30 Ibid., I.i.II.i: 193–4.

similarity between melancholy and depression that the study of the discourse on early modern melancholy is of particular interest, for there are, I believe, important moments of insight into the melancholic condition in the early modern period.

It may come as a surprise that many of these insights are found in the works of moralists and clerics. In today's popular media, depression is often casually referred to as a biochemical imbalance, and there is strong resistance among many in the medical community to admit the need for any kind of non-medical perspective in the analysis and treatment of melancholy.[31] Healy argues that this is largely the result of the pharmacological revolution in the 1950s and 1960s, during which a range of relatively effective pharmaceuticals became available. These drugs now depend for governmental approval and marketing success on being prescribable for a specific medically defined condition – thus the push to conceptualize depression as an organic disease best treated through medication.[32] But another way to view the pharmacological revolution in the treatment of depression is as the latest and most complete move to overcome the tendency throughout Western history to spiritualize and moralize mental illnesses. On this view, the use of moral philosophical and Christian vocabularies to treat melancholy in early modern England can be interpreted as both mistaken and mystifying.[33]

Ultimately, I leave it to the reader's judgment as to whether this charge sticks for the early modern analyses of melancholy discussed here. I do not believe that it does – at least not in all cases. There are at least three points worth considering on the matter. First, some early modern writers offered an interpretation of the melancholic condition similar to a view of depression which has had various exponents throughout the twentieth century and into the twenty-first. Building on the psychopathology of Karl Jaspers and Kurt Schneider, Healy has argued that some kind of non-specific physical malaise similar to jet-lag becomes exacerbated into feelings of hopelessness and worthlessness by the confluence of its demoralizing persistence, the inability of medical examination to locate any specific pathology and the very use of the label of depression by a physician to provide an explanation for the mysterious ailment. On this view, the specifically mental symptoms which identify clinical depression are not somehow produced by a purported chemical imbalance; rather, even in its apparently delusional aspect, clinical depression consists of an illness behavior which is a reaction to a series of social and psychological situations which are themselves created by an actual physiological disturbance.

Of fundamental therapeutic importance here is the language which is used to describe and treat depression. Healy's suggestion is that current medical language is at times counter-productive rather than helpful: "exposure to the mental health services opens patients to a substantial risk of having psychological problems created where none existed before" by making available certain illness behaviors, such as

---

31   Healy, *The Suspended Revolution: Psychiatry and Psychotherapy Re-examined* (London and Boston, MA: Faber and Faber, 1990), 65–7.

32   Healy's argument is developed at length in his *The Antidepressant Era*.

33   Healy, *Suspended Revolution*, 34–8, 214–15.

suicidal ideation, as expressions of the condition the patient is said to have.[34] (Robert Burton noted that people who were predisposed to melancholy actually contracted it when studying its symptoms.[35]) The seventeenth-century Royal Chaplain and Bishop of Ely, Simon Patrick, developed a similar analysis of cases of religious melancholy, arguing that feelings of spiritual despair were the consequence of attaching a specific kind of theological language to certain kinds of bodily feelings; and the essayist Sir William Temple argued that the conditions of hypochondria and hysteria were generated when patients suffering from non-specific and vague feelings of unease appropriated a formal disease diagnosis in order to express and make sense of their condition in a legitimated fashion. Patrick and Temple provide a "psychopathological" analysis of melancholy as sensitive to the interplay of illness behavior and disease in the production of a clinical profile as Healy's analysis of depression. Depending on one's own psychiatric allegiances, Temple and Patrick could well be regarded as the heroes of this story.

Second, even where writers did not advance such a thesis about the relation between the melancholic condition and its language of expression in creating a given presentation of melancholia, many early modern clergy and moralists who offered advice on the cure and management of melancholy display a self-conscious awareness that they were applying the therapies of moral philosophy and religion to a condition which was, on their own belief, correctly understood as in part medical. Thus, not all early modern writers who articulated moral philosophical and spiritual therapies for melancholy can be said to have mystified melancholy into a condition of moral or spiritual weakness, although some did. Many attempted to provide therapeutic techniques and social settings similar to those that are available for the modern-day depressive in the form of Rational Emotive Therapy, Cognitive Therapy and Psychosocial Rehabilitation, and a host of other therapies which offer to guide the depressive into a healthier management of life and thought. Early modern writers

---

34   See ibid., 144–7, 153–9, 171–8, quotation on 178, and Healy, *The Antidepressant Era*, 2–6. On illness behavior and depression more generally, see the work of anthropologist and psychiatrist Arthur Kleinman: *Patients and Healers in the Context of Culture: An Exploration of the Borderland between Anthropology, Medicine and Psychiatry* (Berkeley, CA and Los Angeles, CA: University of California Press, 1980); *Social Origins of Distress and Disease: Depression, Neurasthenia and Pain in Modern China* (New Haven, CT and London: Yale University Press, 1986), and *The Illness Narratives: Suffering, Healing and the Human Condition* (New York: Basic Books, 1988). See also the essays in Arthur Kleinman and Byron Good, eds., *Culture and Depression: Studies in the Anthropology and Cross-cultural Psychiatry of Affect and Disorder* (Berkeley, CA, Los Angeles, CA, and London: University of California Press, 1985). The great philosopher and historian of science Ian Hacking has reflected at length on the ways in which descriptions of disorders and diagnostic criteria have a kind of feedback effect, shaping the disorders themselves: see Hacking, *Rewriting the Soul: Multiple Personality and the Sciences of Memory* (Princeton, NJ: Princeton University Press, 1995), and *The Social Construction of What?* (Cambridge, MA: Harvard University Press, 1999), 100–24.

35   Burton, *Anatomy*, I.iii.I.ii: 446.

justified their non-medical intervention in terms of the idea that the health of the soul and the health of the body are united through mutual causal influence. In the early modern period this view of the relationship of body to mind was a central theoretical and therapeutic assumption. Today, the issue of psychosomatic phenomena remains of interest, but as more of a problem than an axiom. However, most present-day experts on depression advocate a mixture of some form of psychotherapy and medication for many cases of depression, and this, practically speaking, corresponds to the early modern approach.

Third, while moral philosophical and religious therapies sometimes had the effect of attaching stigma to those melancholics who were not able obtain the good of their soul (and importantly it is at such points that the discourse on the treatment of melancholy becomes most clearly gendered), clergymen and moralists often adopted a consolatory rather than a condemnatory tone in addressing melancholics since they recognized that, to some degree, the melancholic was limited by their diseased body. And this consolatory stance implied that the melancholic was not simply sick or mad, but could also be seen as a member of the human community struggling with the same sorts of moral and spiritual temptations and dangers with which others who took seriously the good of their soul also struggled. It is thus arguable that a kind of "moral treatment" of the mad existed long before the therapeutic innovations of the Quaker Retreat at York and Philippe Pinel, a kind of treatment which, like the therapies of Pinel and the York Retreat, entailed the consolation and care of the melancholic as a human being rather than as an embodiment of "unreason" or an incomprehensible abyss of "nonbeing," the terms in which Michel Foucault famously characterized early modern perceptions of madness.[36]

Foucault argued that madness was analyzed as an assertion of illusion which used the logic and form of reason: "affirming nothing true or real, it does not affirm at all; it is ensnared in the non-being of error ... Joining vision and blindness, image and judgement, hallucination and language, sleep and waking, day and night, madness is ultimately nothing, for it unites in them all that is negative."[37] Hence the moral treatment of madness was unthinkable. Madness was in its essence *nothing* but a systematic perversion of reason, such that reason could not engage with it except in the form of a substanceless alterity, as unreason.[38] Foucault saw this conception of madness as being of a piece with the institutional confinement of the mad, which he asserted was increasingly widespread in the seventeenth and eighteenth centuries, and with the forms of physical coercion practiced in these institutions.[39]

---

36   On the Quaker retreat at York, see Anne Digby, *Madness, Morality, and Medicine: A Study of the York Retreat 1796–1914* (Cambridge: Cambridge University Press, 1985), and her "Moral treatment at the Retreat, 1796–1846," in Bynum, Porter, and Shepherd, eds., *The Anatomy of Madness*, 1: 52–72. On Pinel, see Jan Goldstein, *Console and Classify: The French Psychiatric Profession in the Nineteenth Century* (Cambridge: Cambridge University Press, 1987), 64–119.

37   Foucault, *Madness and Civilization*, 107.

38   Ibid., 107, 158, 252–3.

39   Ibid., 38–64, 115–16.

The notion of a "Great Confinement" has been all but disproved by more recent work in the history of madness.[40] Yet the larger question of whether and to what extent madness was viewed as unreason and nonbeing in the early modern period has scarcely generated any critical engagement. While I make no claims here about the general nature of the perception of madness in early modern England, I do think that the history of the care of melancholy shows that certain kinds of madness were thought to be appropriately engaged with through discourse and consolation, and that this treatment opened up the possibility of a perception of the mad individual as a human moral agent.

Against such a claim, it may be argued that these therapies were limited to milder forms of mental distraction and were not applied to madness itself. Such distinctions were indeed made in earlier modern discussions, but we should be careful not to import our own assumptions into the matter. Contemporary psychiatric categories as defined in the *DSM-IV* drive a sharp wedge between clinical, or psychotic, depression and milder forms of depression, and clinical depression is generally thought to be a medical condition for which periods of hospitalization, psychopharmaceutics, and sometimes electroconvulsive therapy (ECT) are the most appropriate forms of treatment.[41] But early modern authorities did not distinguish between cases of melancholic madness so much in terms of symptomology or severity *per se* as in terms of the length of time someone had been afflicted, for in time, it was thought, what often began as a case of affective and cognitive disturbance caused by grief, fear, or sorrow effected a change in the body through which the original mental disease became more stubbornly rooted. Thus, moral philosophy and religion were thought in many circumstances to be appropriate as early interventions in cases of severe melancholy, and in some circumstances even after, when they were combined with medicine. This approach to classifying the mad lasted well into the nineteenth century, and the early public asylums in England were intended originally to house and cure only the curable mentally ill, whose madness was relatively fresh, and thus "functional" rather than "organic."[42] The aim of religious and moral philosophical therapies on the whole was to limit and contain melancholic patterns of thought so that they did not settle into incurable insanity.

Aside from questions of severity, which in any case related primarily to definitions of insanity developed in and for particular institutional settings, it was by reason of the general pattern of thought evidenced by all melancholics that

---

40   Porter, *Mind-forg'd Manacles: A History of Madness in England from the Restoration to the Regency* (London: Athlone Press, 1987), 7–9.

41   This is in spite of the evidence that some forms of psychotherapy work for cases of both mild and clinical depression: see Healy, *Suspended Revolution*, 199–200, and *Antidepressant Era*, 238–55.

42   On the seventeenth century, see page 41 below; on the curable/incurable distinction in the context of seventeenth and eighteenth-century Bethlem, see Jonathan Andrews, "Bedlam Revisited: A History of Bethlem Hospital, *c*. 1634–*c*. 1770" (Ph.D. dissertation, London University, 1991), 453; on the nineteenth century, see Smith, *'Cure, Comfort and Safe Custody'*, 116–17.

melancholy was considered by early moderns to be a species of madness. This is clear from an example discussed at length by Foucault. The seventeenth-century Dutch physician Ijsbood van Diemerbroeck describes "an unwarranted melancholia in a man who wrongly accuses himself of having killed his son." Diemerbroeck's melancholic, whose child drowned accidentally when they had gone bathing together, considers himself damned by God and handed over to Satan. He is so possessed by these apprehensions and fears that he actually begins to inhabit the world of his damnation, imagining and conversing with the demon to whom he has been handed for his torment; he is enmeshed in "an infinitely repeated discourse apropos of the punishment God must reserve for sinners guilty of homicide."[43] Foucault argues that the melancholic's emotion and behavior is appropriate, given the beliefs he holds about his guilt and the judgment of God. That he is guilty of homicide might be considered delusory, and the necessity of his damnation is at least up for theological debate. But his melancholy makes him impervious to consider the matter from any other perspective than that which his melancholic feelings, now fixed in the image of a demonic power tormenting him, demand.

Melancholy is thus not simply a delusion accompanied by a "rational" emotional response; rather, the logic of the melancholic emotions seems to create and sustain their objects and concerns. As Foucault puts it, beyond the level of delusion in madness "we find a rigorous organization dependent on the faultless armature of a discourse. This discourse, in its logic, commands the firmest belief in itself, it advances by judgements and reasonings which connect together."[44] Where the emotions require an object that can be assessed in a certain manner, as dangerous or grievous to the individual, for example, melancholic fear and sorrow create and continually bring to mind such objects. In Diemerbroeck's example, the man considers himself responsible for his son's accidental death, since it was he who had taken the boy to bathe. Here we have sorrow and remorse, with some level of guilt. Melancholy is the movement of these emotions in successive discursive steps, each involving a heightening of sorrow and fear. Judging himself responsible in some way, the man judges himself to be guilty of homicide, and then infers his damnation and his devilish torment. At each step, his emotions are more or less culturally appropriate. Where parents are the guardians of their children, remorse and guilt might be expected in even an accidental death; the assumption of guilt raises in many Christian cultures the fear of divine punishment and of damnation. We know also from the work of the historians Michael MacDonald and Stuart Clark that demonic affliction in early modern culture was accompanied, and was sometimes even signified, by a great deal of emotional anguish, and that the perception and invocation of demons were pervasive and accepted features of early modern discourse. Demons were a category of everyday experience.[45] Yet what causes each of these steps to be taken? The links

---

43 Foucault, *Madness and Civilization*, 97.

44 Ibid., 100.

45 MacDonald, *Mystical Bedlam*, 133–4; Clark's *Thinking with Demons: The Idea of Witchcraft in Early Modern Europe* (Oxford: Oxford University Press, 1997) stresses this

may be comprehensible; but they are not necessary. They seem to be motivated by something other than the normal operation of the mind. The answer was to invoke melancholy. Melancholy was the name of the force that replicated the logic of the emotions by directing reason according to fearful and sorrowful judgments ineradicably imprinted on the mind.

Foucault uses the example of Diemerbroeck's melancholic to argue that "[*l*]angauge is the first and last structure of madness, its constituent form; on language are based all the cycles in which madness articulates its nature."[46] Yet according to Foucault's analysis of the early modern approach to madness, this language is taken to say nothing, a sign of the nonbeing of madness. Thus the apparent paradox of the mad*person*: "The paradox of this *nothing* is to *manifest* itself," he writes, "to explode in signs, in words, in gestures."[47] What Foucault nowhere recognizes, however, is that it was just such "delirious discourse" which moralists and divines as well as physicians attempted to turn back through reasoned persuasion and consolation. Engaging with the melancholic on the level of their language was an important means of breaking the links the chain of melancholic logic (logic which, as Temple and Patrick suggested, may have been reinforced by certain specific cultural mentalities). In many parts of Europe, and certainly in the context of "Puritan" England, Diemerbroeck's melancholic would have been treated as an individual suffering under severe affliction of conscience, to be healed through the application of the Gospel, and perhaps also through various forms of exorcism. The same is true for moral philosophical therapies (although admittedly there is less evidence of individuals actually practicing philosophical healing rather than simply advising it). Writers like Robert Burton attempted to limit the expanding range of melancholic fear and grief by providing a series of philosophical perspectives which were intended to restore the mind's equilibrium in judging. Perhaps Diemerbroeck's melancholic was too far gone to engage on this level. But even here, moral philosophical therapy asserted the importance of distraction, diversion, and entertainment in restoring the mind's balance.

Early modern healers thus might very well have seen more moral agency than Foucault's reified explication of early modern madness as unreason would suggest. Peter Barham writes perceptively that "Foucault entertained a curiously innocent and untamed conception of madness. There is no sense of a residual reasonableness or sociability internal to the doings and beings of mad people, the struggles of the disturbed to secure recognition for themselves as intelligible agents not entirely dispossessed of their faculties."[48] The use of moral philosophical and religious ideas to analyze and treat melancholy contributed to providing a context in which the

---

point throughout, but see the discussion on 393 in particular.

46   Foucault, *Madness and Civilization*, 100.

47   Ibid., 107.

48   Barham, "Foucault and the psychiatric practitioner," in Arthur Still and Irving Velody, eds., *Rewriting the History of Madness: Studies in Foucault's 'Histoire de la folie'* (London: Routledge, 1992), 47.

melancholy were seen less as embodiments of incorrigible unreason than as people struggling towards peace of mind, self-possession, and (not to omit the obvious) healing.[49]

From Foucault's perspective, however, the moral treatment of madness can scarcely be considered benevolent and enlightened compared with confinement; it is an alternative and in some ways even more tormenting form of confinement. Foucault assaults the "moral therapy" of William Tuke's Quaker Retreat in these terms:

> We must ... re-evaluate the meanings assigned to Tuke's work: liberation of the insane, abolition of constraint, constitution of a human milieu – these are only justifications. The real operations were different. In fact Tuke created an asylum where he substituted for the free terror of madness the stifling anguish of responsibility; fear no longer reigned on the other side of the prison gates, it now raged under the seals of conscience. Tuke now transferred the age-old terrors in which the insane had been trapped to the very heart of madness.[50]

There is indeed a tendency in Foucault to celebrate madness as a complete freedom of being from all social and moral constraints, and to condemn any attempt to demand conformity, regulation, and discipline.[51] It is paradoxically questionable if any therapy which purported to treat the mad as moral agents rather than under the category of the incomprehensible "other" would have met Foucault's approval. In any case, I would argue that the melancholic condition was not simply a territory which rationality sought to construe within its categories in order to comprehend and conquer, to tame and control; it was also a point from which many sought a return through a culture system of values and meanings they could and did apply to their own experience. And, for many early modern sufferers, religious and moral philosophical therapies offered not guilt, but consolation and comfort, allowing them to gain freedom from the terrors of melancholic emotion.

There is another theme besides the confinement of madness in Foucault's *Madness and Civilization*: that of an ongoing dialog between reason and unreason in the early modern period, in which reason was forced to confront and account for the phenomenon of madness at a point before madness came to signal "nothing more than the natural constants of a determinism" as it did with the birth of psychiatric knowledge and power in the nineteenth century.[52] In addition to the disciplining

---

49   In fact, in some contexts, melancholy's "delirious discourse" could share in both "unreason" and "reason," to some extent simultaneously. See the excellent essay by Michel de Certeau, "Surin's Melancholy," in *Heterologies: Discourse on the Other*, trans. Brian Massumi (Minneapolis, MN: University of Minnesota Press, 1986), 101–15. The original French title of the essay captures the point much better: "Mélancholique et/ou mystique: J.-J. Surin," in *Analytiques* 2 (October 1978): 35–48.

50   Foucault, *Madness and Civilization*, 247.

51   See Dominick LaCapra, "Foucault, History and Madness," in Still and Velody, *Rewriting the History of Madness*, 84.

52   Foucault, *Madness and Civilization*, 83–4.

of madness, Foucault lamented the fact that our perception of the madperson has become thoroughly medicalized under the category of mental illness. The result, he argued, was the cessation of authentic communication:

> In the serene world of mental illness, modern man no longer communicates with the madman: on one hand, the man of reason delegates the physician to madness, thereby authorizing a relation only through the abstract universality of disease; on the other, the man of madness communicates with society only by the intermediary of an equally abstract reason which is order, physical and moral constraint, the anonymous pressure of the group, the requirements of conformity. As for a common language, there is no such thing.[53]

The present study confirms that the writings of early modern ministers and moralists evidence moral constraint, the pressure of the group, and the requirements of conformity in their treatment of the melancholy. Yet at the same time, religion and moral philosophy registered the melancholic experience in terms of the shared moral and religious vocabularies of early modern culture, and at least some of those who articulated these moral philosophical and religious therapies were themselves melancholic. Melancholy was not just a medical problem as mental illness is today. Many early modern writers explicitly resisted handing melancholy over completely to the physician. Furthermore, if ministers and moralists did themselves treat melancholy as a kind of mental disease, a disease of the soul which demanded the institution of order, discipline, and reason, their treatments entailed approaching the melancholic as a person engaged in a fundamentally human struggle towards spiritual well-being.

It is good to be reminded, as Edward Shorter has recently done, that the early modern period as a whole is hardly one we would wish to call exemplary in its treatment of the mad and the insane.[54] It can be assumed that not all of the applications of moral philosophy or religious consolation yielded felicitous therapeutic results. Yet the early modern writers I discuss here recognized, as we are now in danger of ignoring, that melancholy/depression is a problem of the person, not simply of the body or of the mind, that the treatment of melancholy is the subject not simply of medical ethics, but of ethical thought construed much more broadly. They thus suggest that we think too narrowly if we think only about curing a medical condition. It was their contention that melancholy was a special and at times delicate case of the greater work of fulfilling moral and Christian duty – in other words, of becoming good. Many of them thus approached the care of the melancholic soul in the context of the whole of an individual's beliefs, conduct, and social and familial relations; they wrote about melancholy as a condition bound up in all of these features of life and personality, not as one simply incidental, and thus its treatment involved all of these dimensions. The care of the melancholic soul was, at its best, a rich mixture

---

53   Ibid., x.

54   See the comments in Edward Shorter, *A History of Psychiatry: From the Era of the Asylum to the Age of Prozac* (New York: John Wiley & Sons, 1997), 1–32.

of "comfortable speeches, exhortations, arguments [and] advice," as Robert Burton put it in *The Anatomy of Melancholy*.[55] And the aim was not simply the cure of melancholic disease, but the consolation, edification, and strengthening of the soul for the purpose of carrying out its defining tasks of moral and spiritual duty. If we have retained a few philosophical techniques in the present-day armory of psychological healing, we have all the same largely neglected the much more expansive endeavor of the care of the soul of which the care of melancholy was but a part.

---

55 Burton, *Anatomy*, III.iv.II.vi: 468.

Therapeutic Languages: Ancient Moral Philosophy and Patristic Christianity

It was something of a commonplace in Greek philosophical thought that both body and soul could be diseased and that both had their proper forms of healing: the medical art for ailments of the body and philosophy for the diseases of the mind.[1] In *The Republic*, Plato explained his conception of the just soul with an analogy to Greek medical ideas about health and disease: just as "health is produced by establishing a natural relation of control and subordination among the constituents of the body, disease by establishing an unnatural relation ... [s]o justice is produced by establishing in the mind a similar natural relation of control and subordination among its constituents, and injustice by establishing an unnatural one." Thus Plato called the subordination of the appetitive and spirited elements of the soul to the rational element "a kind of mental health."[2] And where Plato outlined the course of education needed to enable the soul to achieve justice through an apprehension of the Good, he stressed in particular the need to shape carefully the student's emotional life.[3] Aristotle likewise argued in his *Nicomachean Ethics* that "anyone who is going to be a competent student in the spheres of what is noble and what is just – in a word, politics – must be brought up well in his habits."[4] Indeed, Aristotle went on to define human good precisely in terms of these moral habits, which he argued to involve a tempering of character according to a mean between opposite emotional dispositions as well as an understanding of what feelings and actions are appropriate in a given situation and in what measure.[5] Clearly, as in Plato, rational thought was to supervene on natural human impulse in the formation of virtuous character.[6] And that this achieved the good of the soul Aristotle clarified by analogy to bodily health and disease, noting that "we must use clear examples to illustrate the unclear." Just

---

1   See Martha C. Nussbaum, *The Therapy of Desire: Theory and Practice in Hellenistic Ethics* (Princeton, NJ: Princeton University Press, 1994); see also Pedro L. Entralgo, *The Therapy of the Word in Classical Antiquity*, ed. and trans. L.J. Rather and John M. Sharp (New Haven, CT: Yale University Press, 1970).

2   Plato, *The Republic*, trans. Desmond Lee, 2nd edn. (London: Penguin Books, 2003), bk. 4, 444d–e.

3   Ibid., bk. 3, 386a–392a; 398c–399c.

4   Aristotle, *Nicomachean Ethics*, trans. and ed. Roger Crisp, *Cambridge Texts in the History of Philosophy* (Cambridge: Cambridge University Press, 2000), 2.1, 1,104a.

5   See Aristotle's discussion in *Nicomachean Ethics*, 2.5, 1,105b; 2.6, 1,106b.

6   Ibid., 2.1, 1,103a; 2.6, 1,107a.

as "too much food and drink and too little ruin one's health, while the right amount produces, increases and preserves it", in the same way, "temperance, courage and the other virtues ... are ruined by excess and deficiency, and preserved by the mean."[7]

The post-Aristotelian, Hellenistic philosophical schools in particular concentrated on the importance of controlling the emotions in the endeavor to attain the health of the soul.[8] The Stoics advocated the position that the emotions are the soul's diseases because they consist of judgments of good and evil not in accordance with reason.[9] Since the Stoics defined the good strictly in terms of the moral goods of virtue and vice, many of the common human emotional responses to events of the social and natural world – grief at the death of others, pity for human suffering, for example – were considered as diseased states of mind, incompatible with virtue and wisdom. These emotions took for real goods and evils objects which were not moral goods and moral evils.[10] The Stoics thus encouraged their students to cultivate a posture of indifference to political and natural events, but this posture was clearly only conceivable within the context of the Stoic belief that reason governed the cosmos through divine providence. Rather than becoming distressed with apparent evil, the sage accepted calmly that all which occurred in the universe was governed by divine reason.[11]

Ancient discussions of the emotions thus generally advanced the idea that they could be modified and shaped according to reason, and that doing so would contribute significantly to human happiness. But whereas the Platonists explained the conflict between reason and passion by locating the passions in the appetitive and spirited parts of the soul, "below" reason, most of the Stoics insisted that soul consisted only of a rational part which issued both rational judgments and "irrational" judgments, or passions, and that the passions could therefore, at least notionally, be eliminated

---

7   Ibid., 2.2, 1,104a.

8   Besides Nussbaum, see William V. Morris, *Restraining Rage: The Ideology of Anger Control in Classical Antiquity* (Cambridge, MA and London: Harvard University Press, 2001), 99.

9   See Josiah B. Gould, *The Philosophy of Chrysippus* (Albany, NY: State University of New York Press, 1970), 181–96; A.A. Long and D.N. Sedley, eds. and trans., *The Hellenistic Philosophers* (Cambridge: Cambridge University Press, 1987), 1: 410–23, and Galen, *On the Doctrines of Hippocrates and Plato, Books I–V*, ed. and trans. by Phillip de Lacy, 3rd edn. (Berlin: Akademie-Verlag, 1984), bk. 5, K 428–504, pp. 293–5, and K 441–2, p. 303. See also Jackie M. Pigeaud, *La maladie de l'âme: étude sur la relation de l'âme et du corps dans la tradition médico-philosophique antique* (Paris: Société d'édition "Les Belles Lettres," 1981), 265–300.

10   This is the burden of Cicero's argument in *Tusculan Disputations*, bks 3 and 4; see Cicero, *Tusculan Disputations*, trans. J.E. King, *Loeb Classical Library* 141 (Cambridge, MA: Harvard University Press, 1927). But it is a misnomer that the Stoics aimed at eliminating all emotion, although rather infamously they did argue that pity was a disease of the soul. See Long and Sedley, *Hellenistic Philosophers*, 1: 412, 420.

11   See Pierre Hadot, "Marcus Aurelius," in *Philosophy as a Way of Life*, trans. Michael Chase (Oxford: Blackwell Publishing, 1995), 179–204; Cicero, *Tusculan Disputations*, 3.xxv.60: 297.

entirely by rectifying the judgments of the soul. Against this, the Epicureans argued that feelings of pleasure and pain were to some degree natural, and could not be eliminated. But the Epicureans were as insistent as others that they, too, could provide insight into the grounds of human happiness, which they argued to consist in peace of mind and a body free from pain. Considerable human suffering could be alleviated by rationally trimming human desire to what was naturally necessary. Thus Epicurus recommended a rather spare diet, to control both the suffering of ardent appetitive longing and to keep the body in good health, and advocated withdrawal from the political sphere to avoid the over-elation and deep disappointments of public life.[12] Recognizing that grief, disappointment, and suffering were to some degree natural and inevitable, however, the Epicureans suggested turning thought to more pleasant objects and memories to alleviate emotional distress.[13]

Many of the views of these Greek philosophical schools on the emotions and the health of the soul were later taken up by Roman writers such as Seneca and Cicero, who dealt extensively with the problem that the passions posed to the cultivation of the health of the soul, and who discussed and developed the remedies that various Hellenistic philosophies had suggested.[14] Both Seneca and Cicero had certain moral philosophical commitments, mainly Stoic in nature. But because most philosophical perspectives converged on the idea that an emotional life ungoverned by reason was in conflict with happiness, which was taken by all to be conterminal with the good and with the fulfilment of human nature, moral philosophy could be viewed from a pragmatic or therapeutic point of view as a means of relieving wretchedness and suffering. In the *Tusculan Disputations*, after rehearsing the various arguments of the philosophic schools on the cure of distress (*aegritudo*), Cicero says that "in my *Consolation* I threw them all into one; ... for my soul was in a feverish state and I attempted every means of curing its condition."[15]

Such therapeutic eclecticism was in an important way not as available within the context of Christianity, which was defined by its espousal of Christ as the only true source of comfort. Many of the Patristic authorities were deeply influenced

---

12 See the selection of texts in Long and Sedley, *Hellenistic Philosophers*, 1: 112–57; see also Walter Charleton, *Epicurus' Morals, collected partly out of his own Greek Text, in Diogenes Laertius, and partly out of the Rhapsodies of Marcus Antoninus, Plutarch, Cicero and Seneca* (London: for H. Herringman, 1656).

13 Cicero discusses (and ridicules) this therapy in the *Tusculan Disputations*, 3.xviii.43: 277.

14 Cicero, *Tusculan Disputations*, 3.x.22–3; 4.v.11, x.23–xiv.33; Seneca, *De tranquilitate animi*, in *Moral Essays*, vol. 2, trans. John W. Basore, *Loeb Classical Library* 254 (Cambridge, MA: Harvard University Press/London: William Heinemann, 1935), 2.1–5: 213–14; Letter 104, *On Care of Health and Peace of Mind*, in Seneca's *Works, Volume 6: Epistles 93–124*, trans. Richard M. Gummere, *Loeb Classical Library* 77 (London and Cambridge, MA: Harvard University Press, 1920), 190–211; Letter 75, *On the Diseases of the Soul*, in *Works, Volume 5: Epistles 66–92*, trans. Richard M. Gummere, *Loeb Classical Library* 76 (London and Cambridge, MA: Harvard University Press, 1920), 137–47.

15 Cicero, *Tusculan Disputations*, 3.xxxi.75–6: 315–17.

by Greco-Roman philosophy, incorporating its concepts, ideals, and techniques into their writing and practice, but they insisted that the soul's well-being could only be achieved through the aid of divine grace.[16] In his *Confessions* (397–400), Augustine recounted his wretched state of restless and unsatisfied desire before his conversion. Importantly, it is through Neoplatonic philosophical reasoning and spiritual exercise that Augustine was at last able to envision human fulfilment and happiness through an apprehension of God, man's greatest good, in whom alone can restless human desire be satisfied. But, as Augustine later confessed to his God, "to enjoy you I was too weak." His analysis of his weakness is in fact an indictment of heathen philosophy:

> I prattled on as if I were expert, but unless I had sought your way in Christ our Saviour (Titus 1:4), I would have been not expert but expunged. I began to want to give myself airs as a wise person. I was full of my punishment, but I shed no tears of penitence … Where was the charity which builds on the foundation of humility which is Christ Jesus? When would the Platonist books have taught me that?[17]

Later, Augustine states, when "my wounds were healed by your gentle fingers, I would learn to discern and distinguish the difference between presumption and confession, between those who see what the goal is but not how to get there and those who see the way which leads to the home of bliss, not merely as an end to be perceived but as a realm to live in."[18]

This statement encapsulates the distinction between heathen philosophy and Christianity which would become commonplace in the Western tradition. The philosopher is able to define the good, but is not able to achieve it. This was more or less admitted by ancient philosophers. Pierre Hadot writes that "with the possible exception of the Epicurean school, wisdom was conceived as an ideal after which one strives without the hope of attaining it."[19] Yet the philosopher insistently strove after wisdom, and Christian thinkers took this as a manifestation of pride: the philosopher vainly attempts to heal his soul through his own effort, whereas the Christian humbly admits that he needs God to heal him. And the Christian thus does not view the practice of philosophical dialectic as important, but rather prays, repents, and confesses. The pages of the Platonist books, Augustine writes, "do not contain the face of this devotion, tears of confession, your sacrifice, a troubled spirit, a contrite and humble spirit (Psalms 50:19)."[20]

---

16   Hadot, "Ancient Spiritual Exercises and 'Christian Philosophy'", in *Philosophy as a Way of Life*, 126–44; Hadot, *What Is Ancient Philosophy?*, trans. Michael Chase (Cambridge, MA: Harvard University Press, 2002), 237.

17   Augustine, *Confessions*, trans. Henry Chadwick, *Oxford World's Classics* (Oxford: Oxford University Press, 1992), 7.xx(26): 130.

18   Ibid., 7.xx(26): 130. On the nature and importance of dialectic in ancient philosophy, see Hadot, "Spiritual Exercises," in *Philosophy as a Way of Life*, 89–93.

19   Ibid., 103.

20   Augustine, *Confessions*, 7.xxi(27): 131.

This kind of devotion created a further disjunction between Christian and philosophical models of the soul's health. As Augustine's quotation from the Psalms indicates, a state of spiritual sorrow was a well-developed *topoi* in Christianity's Old Testament, and in the second letter to the Corinthians, Paul contrasts a form of sadness which "worketh death" with a "sorrow to repentance," or "godly sorrow."[21] But the cultivation of sorrow was entirely perverse from an Epicurean perspective, and seemed equally contrary to the Stoic goal of indifference, or *apatheia*. In *The City of God against the Pagans* (426), Augustine agreed with the Stoics that the ideal of "a life without those emotions which arise contrary to reason and which disturb the mind … is clearly a good and desirable condition." But although Augustine achieved a substantial measure of peace of mind through his conversion, in *The City of God* he argued that the Stoic state of *apatheia* "does not … belong to this present life." Humans remain in a condition of sin, and rightly feel "pain for their sins," as well as pain and anxiety in their temptations to sin.[22]

Paul's "godly sorrow" is a good rather than an evil, Augustine argued against the Stoic position on emotion, because it is derived from the love of God. Augustine concluded that Christians were thus in the position of Alcibiades, whose story was recounted by Cicero in the *Tusculan Disputations*:

> He seemed to himself to be happy; but when Socrates demonstrated to him by argument how miserable he was because he was foolish, he wept. For him, then, foolishness was the cause of a useful and desirable grief: the grief of one who deplores that he is not what he ought to be.[23]

The point which Cicero had argued with the story of Alcibiades was that some forms of distress seemed appropriate. But the lesson that Augustine sought to impress was that Alcibiades' sorrow was not simply a byproduct of not being what he ought to be, but the necessary means to gain the soul's health. The soul's health required a posture of active repentance and sorrow for sin. As Augustine wrote in his exposition of Psalm 59:

> All iniquity, be it little or great, punished must needs be, either by man himself repenting, or by God avenging. For even he that repenteth punisheth himself. Therefore, brethren, let us punish our own sins, if we seek the mercy of God. God cannot have mercy on all men working iniquity as if pandering to sins, or not rooting out sins. In a word, either thou punishest, or He punisheth.[24]

---

21   2 Corinthians 8:8–10 (KJV).

22   Augustine, *The City of God against the Pagans*, trans. and ed. R.W. Dyson, *Cambridge Texts in the History of Political Thought* (Cambridge: Cambridge University Press, 1998), 14.8: 593–4.

23   Augustine, *City of God*, 14.8–9: 593–602.

24   Augustine, *Expositions on the Book of Psalms*, ed. A Cleveland Coxe, *A Select Library of the Nicene and Post-Nicene Fathers of the Christian Church*, ed. Philip Schaff, vol. 8 (New York: Charles Scribner's Sons, 1917), 239.

Augustine's own repentant punishment is recounted in Books 7 and 8 of his *Confessions*. Weighted down by sinful self-will, he found himself unable to sustain his intellectual union with the object of his deepest desire, and experienced instead a violent "gnawing at my inner self" and a profound self-hatred. "From a hidden depth a profound self-examination had dredged up a heap of all my misery and set it 'in the sight of my heart' (Psalms 18:15)," Augustine recounted. "That precipitated a vast storm bearing a massive downpour of tears," which was only finally consoled by a moment of divine grace allowing Augustine to repent and turn to God: "it was as if a light of relief from all anxiety flooded into my heart. All the shadows of doubt were dispelled."[25]

But, as Augustine indicated in *The City of God*, godly sorrow was a life-long work, and tranquility was ultimately deferred to the next life. In a homily on the Gospel of Matthew, John of Chrysostom wrote that he whom the "fire of the Spirit" has entered, "such a one abides in continual compunction, pouring forth never ceasing fountains of tears, and thence reaping fruit of great delight. For nothing so binds and unites unto God as do such tears."[26] Chrysostom went on to argue that sorrow rather than joy was to constitute the very character of the Christian, as it did in both Christ and St. Paul. Cicero had written in the *Tusculan Disputations* that while all emotional perturbation is "wretchedness, 'distress' (*aegritudo*) means being actually put upon the rack … it rends and corrodes the soul and brings it to absolute ruin."[27] In a homily on 2 Corinthians 8:8, Chrysostom echoed this idea, asking rhetorically "what is more oppressive than sorrow?" "Still," he insisted, "when it is after a godly sort, it is better than the joy in the world."[28]

Neither Augustine nor Chrysostom addressed at any length the problem of melancholic suffering in their works.[29] As for ancient moral philosophical texts, there is little suggestion that philosophical spiritual therapy was seen as directly relevant to the treatment of melancholy as the condition was defined in medical thought.[30]

---

25 Augustine, *Confessions*, 7.x(16): 123; 7.xvii(23): 127; 8.v(10): 140; 8.vii(17–18): 145; 8.xii(28–9): 152–3.

26 John Chrysostom, *Homilies on the Gospel of Saint Matthew*, trans. Sir George Prevost, *A Select Library of the Nicene and Post-Nicene Fathers of the Christian Church*, ed. Philip Schaff, vol. 10 (New York: Charles Scribner's Sons, 1908), 41.

27 Cicero, *Tusculan Disputations*, 3.xiii.27: 259.

28 Chrysostom, *Homilies on the Epistles of Paul to the Corinthians*, ed. Talbot W. Chambers, *A Select Library of the Nicene and Post-Nicene Fathers of the Christian Church*, ed. Philip Schaff, vol. 12 (New York: Charles Scribner's Sons, 1905), 351.

29 But see also Jerome, Letter 125, "To Rusticus," in *The Principal Works of St. Jerome*, trans. W.H. Fremantle, *A Select Library of the Nicene and Post-Nicene Fathers of the Christian Church*, ed. Philip Schaff, vol. 6 (New York: Charles Scribner's Sons, 1905), 249; Panofsky, Kiblansky, and Saxl, *Saturn and Melancholy*, 75–7, and Siegfried Wenzel, *The Sin of Sloth: Acedia in Medieval Thought and Literature* (Chapel Hill, NC: University of North Carolina Press, 1960).

30 The Aristotelian *Problemata* 30.1 is an important exception, but this text reinvented the idea of melancholy almost entirely, associating it not with disease but with philosophic

But both ancient moral philosophy and early Christian thought gave to the Western intellectual tradition a way of talking about the health of the soul, as well as a way of conducting spiritual therapy, that remained immensely influential down to the early modern period. And for a variety of reasons having to do with the particularities of early modern intellectual and cultural history, these forms of spiritual therapy were asserted throughout the seventeenth and eighteenth centuries as appropriate to the conceptualization and treatment of the melancholic condition. At the same time, and also for historical reasons, their precise articulation and implementation were often matters of severe contention.

---

genius and insight. See also the comments on Stoic discussions of melancholy in Kiblansky, Panofsky, and Saxl, *Saturn and Melancholy*, 43–4. The Stoics apparently affirmed that, even though his mind was impervious to folly, the sage could lose his wisdom in being overtaken by melancholy madness.

CHAPTER TWO

Melancholy among the Passions in Seventeenth-century Thought

When Claudius becomes worried about the possible political threats masked by Hamlet's apparent madness in Act III of *Hamlet*, he proposes a diplomatic journey to England for his melancholic nephew, with the hope that "Haply the seas, and countries different / With variable objects, shall expel / This something settled matter in his heart."[1] The diplomatic mission is a convenient way to dispose of the discontent and seditious prince, but the therapy Claudius suggests was entirely conventional for cases of melancholy. It can be traced back to the writings of the first-century Roman physician Aulus Cornelius Celsus.[2] Pleasurable recreation and diversion was also an Epicurean moral philosophical therapy for grief and sorrow, and it was mentioned by Seneca in his *De tranquilitate animi* as a means of treating *taedium uitae*.[3] Jackie Pigeaud has argued that the symptoms of this philosophical disease of the soul, diagnosed by Seneca and others to be brought about through an incorrect conduct of life and of the passions, are almost identical to the mental symptoms of melancholy described in the Hippocratic corpus and other ancient medical texts.[4] "Melancholy," Pigeaud concludes, "is the point of medical reflection most advanced towards philosophy, as … inversely, the philosophical literature on *euthymia* [Greek for "well-being of the soul"] is the point of philosophical reflection most advanced towards medicine."[5]

But although both the moral philosopher and the physician were interested in melancholic suffering in antiquity, they divided the phenomenon strictly into the disciplinary compartments of body and soul – thus the difference in terms to describe what Pigeaud suggests were forms of emotional suffering symptomologically identical. Indeed, the Roman philosopher Cicero resisted the conceptual implications

---

1   Shakespeare, *Hamlet*, III, i, 165–7.

2   Kiblansky, Panofsky, and Saxl, *Saturn and Melancholy*, 45–6.

3   Cicero, *Tusculan Disputations*, 3.xviii.43: 277; 3.xix.46: 281.

4   See Pigeaud, *La maladie*, 122–9, 132–3; "Prolégomenes à une histoire de la mélancholie," *Histoire, économie et société* 3 (1984), 506–7; Seneca, *De tranquilitate animi*, in *Moral Essays*, vol. 2, XVII.8–9: 283.

5   Pigeaud, *La maladie*, 124: "En somme, la mélancholie est la pointe la plus avancée de la réflexion médicale vers la philosophie, comme nous verrons qu'inversement, la littérature philosophique sur l'euthymie est la pointe la plus avancée de la réflexion philosophique vers la médicine." On the term *euthymia*, see Seneca, *De tranquilitate animi*, in *Moral Essays*, vol. 2, 2.3: 213.

of the Greek term "melancholy" to describe certain states of fury (*furor*), arguing that it suggested that in fits of heightened passion an individual was influenced "by black bile only" rather than by the opinions and beliefs embedded in the emotions, for which an individual was responsible and over which he could exercise control. The Latin language, Cicero argued, was better able to distinguish "between 'unsoundness of mind' [*insaniam*], which from its association with folly has a wider connotation, and 'frenzy' [*furore*]."[6]

It is fair to say that the strict separation of moral philosophical diseases of the soul and organic diseases of the body which affect the mind is generally current orthodoxy in the field of mental health. The notion of mental illness as a disorder of the body is indeed currently being used as leverage to create a clear distinction between mental and moral illness, between involuntary suffering and more voluntary mental disorders.[7] The success of this move is not for us to determine. But the notion that there is a clear distinction has sometimes colored perceptions of past conceptualizations of the relation between mental and moral illness. Jean Delumeau writes of a "confusion often maintained in the Renaissance epoch between vice and sickness," and attributes the predominance of a "suspicious attitude towards melancholy" to this confusion.[8] It is true that early modern writers concerned themselves with the moral analysis of melancholy. This way of approaching melancholy, however, was not rooted in conceptual confusion, but in the fact that the role of the mind in causing and sustaining the melancholic condition remained an open question in the early modern period. Pigeaud argues that a certain ambiguity was built into the ancient medical concept of melancholy, which often listed mental symptoms and physical symptoms alongside each other without reducing the illness of the mind to that of the body.[9] In the early modern context, few thinkers adopted the position of Cicero in dismissing the worth of the medical analysis of the melancholic condition entirely. Indeed, the term "melancholy" had expanded in its range of reference in late medieval literature from designating a disease and a temperament to designating sorrowful and fearful emotions and moods themselves, and the medical notion of melancholy itself had become important in the moral psychological vocabulary used to analyze the emotions.[10] The conceptualization of "normal" emotions of fear and sorrow and that of their melancholic variants came to overlap considerably, and in this context it made a great deal of sense to consider melancholy itself under the category of a moral philosophical disease of the soul.

---

6   Cicero, *Tusculan Disputations*, 3.v.11: 237; see also Cicero's influential cognitive definition of grief or distress (*aegritudo*) as "the idea of a present evil with this implication in it, that it is a duty to feel distressed" (*Tusculan Disputations*, 3.xxxi.74: 315).

7   David Healy, *Suspended Revolution*.

8   Delumeau, "L'âge d'or de la mélancolie," *L'histoire* 42 (1982), 35: "Le regard soupçonneux sur la mélancholie s'explique … par une confusion souvent maintenue à l'époque de la Renaissance entre vice et maladie."

9   Pigeaud, *La maladie*, 124–5.

10   On late medieval linguistic and conceptual innovations, see Kiblansky, Panofsky, and Saxl, *Saturn and Melancholy*, 217–28.

This is borne out in the writing of two seventeenth-century authors: Robert Burton, in his *Anatomy of Melancholy*; and the influential physician and natural philosopher Thomas Willis, in his *De anima brutorum* (1672) and in the lectures he gave as Sedleian Professor of Natural Philosophy at Oxford. Burton fully accepted the medical analysis of melancholy articulated and popularized throughout the Renaissance. But working from Galenic medical premises, he insisted that melancholy was a condition the cure of which required both physician and philosopher. Willis was a physician and medical theorist with extensive interests in moral philosophical discourse, and his analysis of both melancholy and the passions exhibits clearly the interplay of medical and moral language in the approach to melancholic emotion common in the early modern period. Burton and Willis both show that moral philosophical techniques and ideas can be considered to be central features of the treatment of melancholic madness in the early modern period, in both medical and non-medical work. Melancholy was considered to be as much a disease of the mind, understood in a broadly moral sense, as of the body.[11]

Spiritual exercises and the anatomy of melancholy

While the philosophical tradition which concerned itself with the health of the mind never disappeared in medieval Europe, worry over the dangers that the passions posed to the health of the soul intensified in the late Renaissance period. Beginning in the late sixteenth century, a series of works that explored the nature of the passions in detail and suggested remedies for these moral diseases were published in France and England.[12] The impetus for this concern was in part the sense among many intellectuals of a growing disjunction between the civic life, which demanded the fostering of self-aggrandizing passions, and the vision of the good life articulated by ancient philosophers. Some were attracted by Hellenistic ethical orientations

---

11 Cf. Akihito Suzuki's argument that until the middle of the eighteenth century, psychiatry could not conceive of madness as a disease of the mind: "Dualism and the Transformation of Psychiatric Language in the Seventeenth and Eighteenth Centuries," *History of Science* 23 (1995): 417–47, and "Anti-Lockean Enlightenment? Mind and Body in Early Eighteenth-century England" in Roy Porter, ed., *Medicine in the Enlightenment* (Amsterdam: Rodopi, 1995), 336–59. See also Porter, *Mind-forg'd Manacles*, 54.

12 See, among others, Thomas Rogers, *A Paterne of a passionate minde* (London: Thomas East, 1580); Thomas Wright, *The Passions of the minde in generall* (London: Valentine Simmes for Walter Burre, 1604); Nicolas Coeffeteau, *A Table of Humane Passions: With their Causes and Effects*, trans. Edward Grimston (London: Nicolas Okes, 1621); Edward Reynolds, *A Treatise of the Passions and Faculties of the Soule of Man* (London: R.H. for Robert Bostock, 1640); Jean François Senault, *The Use of Passions*, trans. Henry Earl of Monmouth (London: for J.L. and Humphrey Moseley, 1649); Walter Charleton, *A Natural History of the Passions* (London: T.N. for James Magnes, 1674), and William Ayloffe, *The Government of the Passions According to the Rules of Reason and Religion* (London: for J. Knapton, 1700). See also the discussion in Susan James, *Passion and Action: The Emotions in Seventeenth-century Philosophy* (Oxford: Clarendon Press, 1997), 1–15.

in the endeavor to define the good life and care for the soul, orientations which themselves had originally implied various degrees of emotional disengagement from the *vita activa*, if not disengagement from politics entirely. The Stoic ideal of *constantia* through rational self-discipline had been popularized on the Continent in the late sixteenth century by Michel de Montaigne, Justus Lipsius, and others. Many of the Continental Neostoic works were translated into English, and Stoic ideas were particularly celebrated in the social and political circle of the influential and powerful Sir Philip Sidney.[13] The result was that much ethical thought of the late sixteenth and seventeenth century took its main concern to be the taming and controlling of human desire and emotion; these were seen as the soul's diseases, which moral philosophical reflection alone could remedy.

In treating of the passion of sorrow in particular, seventeenth-century moral reflection emphasized the manifest physical complications and effects of grief. Comprised of historical examples of individuals dying from grief and of the descriptions of the physical suffering accompanying sorrow found in the Old Testament, the representation of sorrow as a fountain of disease and death was a well-established literary trope. In his *Treatise of the Passions* (1640), the English divine Edward Reynolds declared of grief:

> [I]n the body there is no other Passion that doth produce stronger, or more lasting inconveniences by pressure of heart, obstruction of spirit, wasting of strength, drynesse of bones, exhausting of Nature. Griefe in the heart ... stoppeth the voice, looseth the joints, withereth the flesh, shrivelleth the skinne, dimmeth the eyes, cloudeth the countenance, defloureth the beauty, troubleth the bowels, in one word, disordereth the whole frame.[14]

Reynolds gives no citations, but many of these phrases can be traced to the Psalms, Proverbs, and Jeremiah.[15] In *The Passions of the Minde in Generall* (1604), the Jesuit scholar Thomas Wright noted that "many have lost their lives with sadnesse and feare; but few, with love & hope, except they changed themselves into heavinesse and despaire." Wright acknowledged that the bodily disturbances caused by the passions deriving from pleasure could also prove fatal; it was more probable, however, that joy and love would harm the body through their natural lapse into grief and despair: "universally, after much pleasure and laughter, men feele themselves both to languish, and to be melancholy." Besides Proverbs 17:22 and Ecclesiasticus 30:23, Wright quoted Euripides in support of his point claim about the damaging effects of

---

13   See Nannerl O. Keohane, *Philosophy and the State in France: The Renaissance to the Enlightenment* (Princeton, NJ: Princeton University Press, 1980), 136–9, and J.H.M. Salmon, "Seneca and Tacitus in Jacobean England," in *The Mental World of the Jacobean Court*, ed. Linda Levy Peck (Cambridge: Cambridge University Press, 1991), 169–90. On the importance of Hellenistic moral philosophy in sixteenth and seventeenth-century works on the passions, see Anthony Levi, *French Moralists: The Theory of the Passions 1585 to 1649* (Oxford: Clarendon Press, 1964), 40–73.

14   Reynolds, *Treatise of the Passions*, 232.

15   Psalms 6:2, 6–7 and 31:10–12; Proverbs 17:22; Jeremiah 33:9.

sorrow: "Sorrowes to men diseases bring."[16] Later in the seventeenth century, grief appears as one of the categories of the causes of death in John Graunt's *Natural and Political Observations ... made upon the Bills of Mortality* (1662).[17]

Wright and Reynolds were here assimilating the indications medicine had used to mark out fear and sorrow as melancholic bodily distemper into a representation of sorrow intended to serve the philosophical aim of subduing emotional excess. According to the established wisdom of the medical art, the nature of melancholy as a bodily condition was evidenced by the variety of physical symptoms that accompanied excessive and irrational fear and sorrow. One of these symptoms was precisely the purported presence of black bile in the blood and the vomit, but the range of bodily complaints was much broader, and certainly included languishing and trouble of the bowels and of the heart, to name a few from Reynolds' list.[18] But in the context of these two treatises on the passions, the foregrounding of bodily complaints in no way indicated a distemper that was primarily physical in nature; rather, the debilitating physical effects of fear and sorrow to which biblical and classical sources attested offered a powerful rhetoric for representing the moral rather than the physical dangers of these passions.

Wright and Reynolds were engaged in the moral enterprise of anatomizing the passions. Such a dissection was intended to provide the intellectual resources necessary to interrupt the natural course of emotion by anticipating its manifestations and its errors. Their discourses were in this regard similar to the forms of spiritual exercise central Pierre Hadot has argued were central to ancient philosophy: they were modes of reflection designed to transform the self according to reason, and more specifically, to place the self beyond the influence of material interests acting through the emotions.[19] The language describing passion as mental disease was an outgrowth of such moral reflection, a way of re-describing common experience according to the insights of philosophical reflection, of straightening the untrained bent of apparently natural and all too human emotional reactions. The texts of Wright and Reynolds developed this language in important ways, elaborating what we might term moral pathologies of the emotions of fear and sorrow, with the hope that this knowledge would inoculate the soul against the excesses of emotion when absorbed into the soul through reflection.

Wright established empirically the connection between the painful emotions of the mind and physical disease, and turned to medical theory for a possible explanation: "The cause why sadnesse doth so moove the forces of the body, I take to be, the gathering together of much melancholy blood about the heart ... the which

---

16 Wright, *Passions of the Minde*, 61–4; cf. Coeffeteau, *Table*, 332–3; Senault, *Use of Passions*, 477–8.

17 The number of those killed by grief was small – 279 out of 229,250 – but it is the presence of the category that is significant. See Graunt, *Natural and Political Observations Mentioned in a following Index, and made upon the Bills of Mortality* (London: by Tho. Roycroft, for John Martin, James Allestry, and Tho. Dicas, 1662), 167.

18 See the discussion in Burton, *Anatomy*, I.iii.I.i: 439–42.

19 See Hadot, *Ancient Philosophy*, esp. Chapters 5–7 and 9.

humour being colde and drie, dryeth the whole body and make it wither away."[20] His primary aim, however, was not medical explanation, but moral representation; medical theory was enlisted to support the moral facts attested to by experience and by classical and biblical authority. Although Wright recognized a physiological component in some cases of fear and sorrow, he portrayed melancholic complication as an effect of emotional imbalance. He used physiological pathology to elaborate moral pathology, thereby subordinating medical theory to moral reflection.

Wright also recognized that melancholic humors could cause the emotions of fear and sadness. In this case, melancholy was more clearly a disease of the body, and Wright referred to the necessity of managing diet, exercise and rest in order to manage the passions:

> [S]ometimes wee feele ourselves, we know not why, moved to ... melancholy ... insomuch as any little occasion were insufficient to incense that Passion: for, as ... humors depend upon ... sleeping and waking, meate and drink, exercise and rest, according to the alterations of these externall causes, one or other Humour doth more or lesse over-rule the body, and causeth alterations of the Passions.[21]

But even this is not an exercise in medical theory: here knowledge of the human body is a form of rational self-knowledge leading to self-control. Diet and exercise were themselves forms of spiritual exercise in the classical moral philosophical tradition.[22] Deriving in early modern thought particularly from the Galenic medical-philosophical precept that the temperament of the mind follows the temperature of the body, regimen remained important in the effort to defuse and control passion in the seventeenth century. Medical language itself was an instrument through which to sift the dense matter of thought and feeling into the categories of body and soul, creating a critical disjunction between the self and the melancholic feelings by viewing them across the distance dividing soul from matter.[23]

Beyond its concomitant physical symptoms, the melancholic condition was by definition a pathological form of emotion; it was persistent, excessive, and unreasonable. In the medical tradition, an irrational tenacity of fear and sorrow indicated the force of the melancholic body acting on the mind, disabling the use of reason, which might otherwise rectify emotional excess. This linkage of irremediable fear and sadness with the melancholic humor had been instituted in the Hippocratic *Aphorisms*, which declared that "fear or depression that is prolonged means melancholia," a statement Galen later declared to be a commendably accurate

---

20   Wright, *The Passions*, 61–4.

21   Ibid., 65.

22   Hadot, *Ancient Philosophy*, 188–9; see also Galen, *De sanitate tuenda*, trans. Robert Montraville Green (Springfield, IL: Charles C. Thomas, 1951), 1.8: 26–7, and Michael Schoenfeldt, *Bodies and Selves in Early Modern England: Physiology and Inwardness in Spenser, Shakespeare, Herbert and Milton* (Cambridge: Cambridge University Press, 1999), 11–13.

23   See the comments in Bright, *Treatise of Melancholie*, 190–91.

characterization of the melancholic condition.[24] Yet moralists readily recognized such tendencies, as well as the presence of physical melancholic imbalance, in what could be considered the normal operation of the passion of sorrow, and to a certain extent that of fear. Reynolds added to his description of sorrow's physical effects the observation that "of all Passions, this of Griefe doth le[a]st admit of simple cure from the dictates of Reason, except it have a time given it too."[25] Nicolas Coeffeteau, whose *Tableau des passions humaines* (1620) was translated into English in 1621, declared that "there are many remedies against this *Passion*, but most commonly the *Griefe* is so obstinate, as all applications are unprofitable." Coeffeteau briefly raised the possibility that "the soule helpes to afflict herselfe" with sorrow through the effect of the melancholic humor, and like Wright, he drew on humoral theory to explain the bodily symptoms of sorrow. His analysis of the irrational persistence of sorrow was, however, psychological:

> If it be excessive, it quencheth the spirit, and takes from it all meanes to attend the search of truth. The reason is, for that all the powers of our soule, being tied unto their essence, as the branches unto the tree, it doth of necessity follow, that when shee is wholy busied in the functions of one of her powers, shee abandons the rest, and cannot assist them in their actions ... by consequence whereof, an exceeding heavines seazing upon her, it drawes her away; so as shee cannot thinke of any thing else, feeling her selfe opprest with *Griefe* as with a heavy burthen, which beares her downe and hinders the liberty of her functions.[26]

The cure of the condition was moral, according to Coeffeteau. Wine might be drunk to dispel the cold and dry humors, but "to cure [grief], we must first take away, or at the least diminish the opinion of the evil which afflicts us." As Coeffeteau acknowledged, this was difficult to do once the passion had settled in. The best cure was thus prevention, and Coeffeteau set out several classical moral philosophical exercises for strengthening the mind against sorrow, rehearsing many of the arguments found in Cicero's *Tusculan Disputations*. Like Cicero, Coeffeteau dismissed the therapy of simply allowing time to heal the pain of sorrow, and insisted that the excesses of sorrow could be prevented if we practice foreseeing "the accidents of this life," so that "if any crosse or misery shall fall upon us, we may bee the lesse amazed."[27]

The treatment of passions as diseases and the specifically moral reflection on the pathological effects of fear and sorrow by authors such as Wright, Reynolds, and Coeffeteau are an important intellectual context for the seventeenth-century use of moral philosophical therapy in cases of melancholy. Some of the most important

---

24 Hippocrates, *Aphorisms*, trans. W.H.S. Jones, in *Works*, vol. 4, *Loeb Classical Library* 150 (Cambridge, MA and London: Harvard University Press, 1992), 6.23: 185; on Galen, see Pigeaud, *La maladie*, 128.

25 Reynolds, *Treatise*, 228.

26 Coeffeteau, *Table*, 329–30. A similar description of the overwhelming and debilitating force of sorrow is given by Senault, *Use of Passions*, 476, 485.

27 Coeffeteau, *Table*, 334–6; Cicero, *Tusculan Disputations*, 3.x.23–xxxiv.84: 255–325, esp. xxii.52–xxiii.54: 287–91.

characteristics of the melancholic condition could be discussed as features of the emotions, understood as disorders of the mind to be remedied through philosophical reflection and practice. The language of emotion as irrational excess and mental disease and the specific pathologies of the emotions of grief and sorrow created the conceptual space for the philosophical treatment of melancholy; to put it slightly differently, melancholy neatly fit into the clinical categories developed in moral writing.

Burton recognized this in *The Anatomy of Melancholy*, where he devoted several sections to relaying philosophical therapies for the treatment of the melancholic mind. The treatment of the mind in *The Anatomy of Melancholy* was in part justified by the role Galenic medical theory ascribed to the management of the passions in the art of healing and hygiene. According to Galen, the emotions could interfere with the normal functioning of the body. The regulation of the mind's activities was thus a constituent of bodily health; and although he recognized that the mind was properly the province of the philosopher, Galen declared in *De sanitate tuenda* that the mind was not to be neglected by the physician. Writing in 1621, Burton pointed to a tradition of the medical care of the mind, finding in physicians as in philosophers the same recommendations for moderating the passions by reason, good counsel, persuasion, and diversion. He traced their advice back to "Galen, the common master of them all, from whose fountain they fetch water," and who "brags, *lib.* 1 *de san. tuend.*, that he, for his part, hath cured divers of this infirmity, *solum animis ad rectum institutis*, by right settling alone of their minds."[28]

But even if the subject of the passions in *The Anatomy of Melancholy* was justified by Galenic medical theory, Burton's treatment of the passions derived in large part from moral philosophical reflection on the passions, and in particular from the relatively compact and focused series of insights, techniques, and formulae for the consolation of grief found in the writings of Seneca, Cicero, and Plutarch.[29] These stood on their own authority as modes of therapy in cases of sorrow and discontent, without any reference to their physical effects or dispositions, and in defending himself against the possible accusation that his work was an illicit incursion into the territory of the medical art by a divine, Burton made a point of arguing that "it is a disease of the soul on which I am to treat, ... as much appertaining to a Divine as to a Physician." "Who knows not what an agreement there is betwixt these two professions?" he continued:

> They differ but in object, the one of the body, the other of the soul, and use divers medicines to cure: one amends *animam per corpus* [the soul through the body], the other *corpus per animam* [the body through the soul], as our Regius Professor of Physick well informed us in a learned lecture of his not long since. One helps the vices and passions of the soul ... by applying the spiritual physick; as the other uses proper remedies in bodily diseases.

---

28   Burton, *Anatomy*, II.ii.VI.i: 119, and II.ii.VI.ii: 129. See Galen, *De sanitate tuenda*, 1.8: 26–7.

29   George W. McClure, *Sorrow and Consolation in Italian Humanism* (Princeton, NJ: Princeton University Press, 1991), 1–27.

> Now this being a common infirmity of body and soul, and such a one that hath as much need of a spiritual as a corporeal cure … a Divine … can do little alone, a Physician in some kinds of melancholy much less, both make an absolute cure.[30]

Given the mutual influence of soul and body upon each other, the care of neither alone was primary. While the body acted upon the soul, and medical intervention was thus instrumental in correcting the melancholic passions of the soul, healing the vices and passions of the soul itself through "spiritual physick" was an essential ingredient in treating this compound disease. As Burton put it, the melancholic required "a whole Physician." Elizabethan medical texts had included the moral philosophical therapies of diversion and entertainment among their jumbled lists of medical recipes seen as effective for the cure of melancholy;[31] Burton saw that the treatment and prevention of melancholy through the mind in fact opened onto the full range of philosophical concerns about the rule of reason and the tranquility of mind and concluded from this that the cure of melancholy was as much under the authority of the physician of the mind as the physician of the body.

Moralists viewed the task of philosophy as one of disengaging the individual from patterns of thought, feeling, and behavior that seemed, as emotions often do, to be involuntary, spontaneous, natural reactions, outside of the effective jurisdiction of the will. Burton's insight was to argue that where melancholic feelings could not be cured through reason, by using reason the will could at least manage such feelings by putting them at a distance from a rational self that knew them to be irrational forces, produced in the mind by the body. He remained firmly attached throughout *The Anatomy of Melancholy* to the medical account of melancholy. "You may as well bid him that is diseased not to feel pain, as a melancholy man not to fear, not to be sad," he declared: "'Tis within his blood, his brains, his whole temperature." This statement is crucial to keep in mind when considering the early modern application of moral philosophy to melancholy. Such application did not result merely from the fact that the term "melancholy" included both "biochemical" and "psychological" forms of depression, to think anachronistically in terms of modern psychiatric terminology; rather, it followed from the insight that even if feelings of sorrow and fear originated in the body, there remained some level of psychic complicity in the final degree of melancholic suffering. *The Anatomy of Melancholy* was, in part, a moral philosophical anatomy of melancholy. The recognition that melancholy was a disease of the body itself gave to the sufferer a form of self-knowledge that created difference between the self and its melancholic passions. Burton's philosophic therapy for melancholy thus consisted partly of a rhetoric that emphasized and cultivated the domain of will in the melancholic individual, countering the passive posture of suffering a bodily disease by persuading the sufferer to see melancholic emotion as an object of choice.

---

30 Burton, *Anatomy*, "Democritus Junior to the Reader," 36. See also Rosalie L. Colie, *Paradoxia Epidemica: The Renaissance Tradition of Paradox* (Princeton, NJ: Princeton University Press, 1966), 437–9.

31 For example, Philip Barrough, *The Methode of Phisicke* (London: Thomas Vautroullier, 1583), 36.

If melancholic emotion is to a certain extent unavoidable, as Burton argued it was, the melancholic "may choose whether he will give way too far unto it, he may in some sort correct himself." Quoting Seneca, Burton exhorted the melancholic soul that "whatsoever the will desires, she may command: no such cruel affections, but by discipline they may be tamed."[32]

The discipline needed to tame melancholy consisted of a range of more specific philosophical therapies. Burton wrote that "though [the melancholic] be far gone, and habituated unto such phantastical imaginations, yet, as *Tully* [Cicero] and *Plutarch* advise, let him oppose, fortify, or prepare himself against them, by premeditation, reason, or as we do by a crooked staff, bend himself another way."[33] Burton here named three distinct philosophical strategies for managing the emotions. The work of bending, as Burton's homely analogy formulated it, referred to the philosophical remedy of driving out one particularly excessive emotion by cultivating its opposite. The spiritual exercise of premeditation, advocated most prominently by Cicero, was based on the notion that constant reflection on the possible vicissitudes of life accustomed the soul to the sight of ill fortune, which would otherwise disable the soul in shock and grief.[34] The melancholic soul, whose tranquility was already compromised by the body, could apply this therapy in order to deprive melancholy of matter through which to exacerbate itself. Finally, the melancholic could benefit also from the direct application of reasoning to its emotions. Burton prescribed "counsel, comfort, or persuasion" for the melancholic, which he himself delivered in his long "Consolatory Digression containing the Remedies of all manner of Discontent", a digest of the writings "of our best Orators, Philosophers, Divines, and Fathers of the Church."[35] The burden of such consolation was to suggest a series of perspectives through which the melancholic could limit the tendency of melancholic emotion to envelop the whole of thought and feeling, effectively blotting out non-melancholic perceptions of the world. They bent the thought of the reader from melancholy by focussing on the existing goods and comforts of life and by attempting to proportion sorrow and fear in reasonable relation to its objects.[36] Through such therapies, the melancholic individual could at least avoid becoming overwhelmed by melancholy. To put it differently, if melancholic feelings were at times inescapable, madness might still be avoided.

These kinds of philosophical therapies were available even in cases in which "the Patient of himself is not able to resist or overcome these heart-eating passions." Here Burton found timely and appropriate the advice of Seneca in cases of grief:

Lugentes custodire solemus, (saith *Seneca*), *ne solitudine male utantur*; we watch a sorrowful person, lest he abuse his solitariness, and so should we do a melancholy man. Set him about some business, exercise or recreation, which may divert his thoughts, and

---

32   Burton, *Anatomy*, II.ii.VI.i: 120–21.
33   Ibid.: 122.
34   Cicero, *Tusculan Disputations* 3.xxii.52–xxii.56: 287–91.
35   Burton, *Anatomy*, II.iii.I.i: 145.
36   Ibid., II.iii.I.i–viii: 145–238.

still keep him otherwise intent … if his weakness be such that he cannot discern what is amiss, correct, or satisfy, it behoves [the friend] by counsel, artificial invention, or some contrary persuasion, to remove all objects, causes, companies, occasions, as may any ways molest him, to humour him, please him, divert him, and if it be possible, by altering his course of life, to give him security and satisfaction.[37]

As I have indicated above, the moral therapy of diversion and company derived from Epicurus and from Seneca's *De tranquilitate animi*.[38] Counsel and persuasion are more straightforwardly philosophical. The aim of all of the efforts Burton here behoves the companions of the melancholic to undertake is to entice and command the thought of those who cannot otherwise help themselves away from melancholic patterns and preoccupations. A clearer example of the importance of moral philosophical therapy to the early modern treatment of melancholic madness would be harder to find.

We should not dismiss the incorporation of moral domains into the concept and treatment of melancholy as merely a feature of *The Anatomy of Melancholy*'s expansive tendencies, which one scholar has summed up in the statement that "all of human behavior as Burton sees it can be viewed and expressed in terms of melancholy."[39] Burton's was a detailed and learned elaboration of what was in fact a commonly accepted approach to the specific condition of melancholic emotion. We find the moral philosophical approach to melancholy illustrated also in a 1606 work by Bishop Joseph Hall, which was inspired by reflection on Seneca's *De tranquilitate animi*. Hall, who was known as the "English Seneca," warned those suffering in adversity to measure their discontentment with "wisdome, which shall teach us to esteeme of all eventes as they are, like a true glasse representing all thinges to our minds in their due proportion." "So as Crosses may not seeme that are not, nor little & gentle ones seeme great and intolerable," he continued, "give thy body Ellebore, thy mind good Counsell, thine eare to thy friend, and these fantastical evils shall vanish away like themselves."[40] The reference to hellebore, a traditional herbal remedy for melancholy, indicates that Hall did not rule out the possibility that melancholic humor might be at least partly responsible for exaggerated or groundless discontent. But wisdom, counsel, and consolation were sound physick for the soul, as Hall's reading of Seneca attested.

Hall's somewhat offhand remark reveals the extent to which the therapy of wisdom had become, like hellebore, common kitchen physick. Disseminated through a variety of works throughout the century, philosophical exercises were an established feature of the therapeutic repertoire for conducting oneself and others through cases

---

37 Ibid., II.ii.VI.ii: 126.

38 Pigeaud, *La maladie*, 533.

39 Lyons, *Voices of Melancholy*, 148; see also Colie, *Paradoxia Epidemica*, 455–6.

40 Joseph Hall, *Heaven upon Earth, or, Of True Peace and Tranquilitie of Minde* (London: John Windet, 1606), 73–4. On Hall, see Salmon, "Seneca and Tacitus."

of melancholy and discontent alike.[41] Appeals to moral philosophy in the treatment of melancholy were not comprised of the dogmatic assertion that overwhelming fear and sorrow were entirely in the control of the sufferer, that all was merely a matter of will. Both Burton and Hall clearly recognized that the melancholic condition was partly the result of a physical distemper beyond the immediate control of the individual's will. But melancholy displayed to both philosopher and physician the complex intersection of soul and body, and it was thus thought necessary to appeal to both sides of this dense system of mutual influence.

Melancholy and the moral physiology of Thomas Willis

The writings of Thomas Willis on melancholy are particularly important and suggestive texts in understanding the relation between moral philosophical language and the concept of melancholy in the seventeenth century. A physician who was also deeply interested in the moral nature of the passions of the soul, Willis' writing shows that where the physician dealt with sorrow and fear as melancholy, attempting to effect a change in the material basis of these emotions through both mental and physical means, the moralist could treat melancholic fear and sorrow as part of a moral problem calling for philosophical and spiritual self-government. Willis drew attention to melancholy as a form of emotion in his Sedleian lectures on natural philosophy and medicine given at Oxford, and this insight formed a central part of his later analysis of melancholy in the treatise on the organically based diseases of the mind in his major work on the soul, *De anima brutorum* (1672; the English translation, *Two Discourses concerning the Souls of Brutes ... and that which is the Sensitive in Man*, was published in 1683). And in relaying his fully formulated doctrine of the nature and faculties of the human soul in the first treatise of *De anima brutorum*, he described fear and sorrow in much the same terms as he had defined the melancholic condition itself in his lectures, and dealt with them explicitly and extensively as difficulties in the moral life.

Willis is known today primarily as a prominent Restoration natural philosopher, active in the several experimental circles in Oxford in which Robert Hooke, Robert

---

41   See Robert L'Estrange, *Seneca's Morals, by way of abstract* (London: Thomas Newcombe for Henry Broome, 1678); Antoine Le Grande, *Man without Passions, or, The Wise Stoic according to the Sentiments of Seneca*, trans. G.R. (London: for C. Harper and J. Amery, 1675), and Charleton, *Epicurus' Morals*. Certain seventeenth-century pastoral works drew extensively on classical moral philosophy as well: see John Downame, *Consolations of the Afflicted: or, The Third Part of the Christian Warfare* (London: John Beale for W. Welby, 1613), 1.v.3–10: 61–81, and Simon Patrick, *Hearts Ease, or, A Remedy against all Troubles, with A consolatory Discourse particularly directed to those who have lost their Friends and dear Relations* (London: Fr. Tyton, 1671). On Downame and Patrick, see pages 57–8, 92–8 and 112–13 below.

Boyle, Richard Lower, and others were also engaged.[42] His early interests related mainly to the study of chemical processes as a way of understanding physiological phenomena. Robert G. Frank has traced Willis' later philosophical interest in the nature of the soul, its faculties and its means of functioning, to his appointment in 1660 as Sedleian Professor of Natural Philosophy at Oxford.[43] The strictures of the professorship involved lecturing on substantial parts Aristotle's natural philosophical texts, including *De anima* and *Parva naturalia*, two of the founding texts for the study of the soul in the Western philosophical tradition. Willis took this broadly to mean that he "should Comment on the Offices of the Senses, both external and also internal, and of the Faculties and Affections of the Soul, as also of the Organs and various provisions of all these."[44] While his account of the soul was to be fully articulated in 1672 in *De anima brutorum*, his Sedleian lectures of the early 1660s contained several indications of his later psychological thought.

Willis initially expounded on the nature of the passions of the soul in a lecture to his Oxford audience on "Occasional Melancholy." He had in a previous lecture on melancholy explained what he called habitual melancholy as a distemper of the animal spirits, a theoretical entity thought to be the operative agent of the nerves and the brain in early modern medical thought. In the idiom characteristic of his natural philosophy, he explained the mental symptoms of melancholy as a function of a kind of imbalance in the chemical consistency of the animal spirits. Willis explained the symptomatic feeling of sadness by the failure of the animal spirits to activate properly the heart, causing the stagnation of the blood in the heart and circulatory system; fear, he argued, was the result of the dilation of the body's vessels, which then "impede the flow of blood from the heart."[45] Willis here assumed, without articulating any metaphysical argument, that certain mental functions depended upon the instrument of the body, and that changes in the body produced changes in mental habit and ability. But this was a common enough assumption in both Galenic medicine and in medieval and Renaissance Aristotelian science of the soul, and so there was hence no need to address at this point the nature of the soul, its powers and affections.[46]

---

42   See Robert G. Frank, Jr., *Harvey and the Oxford Physiologists: Scientific Ideas and Social Interaction* (Berkeley, CA: University of California Press, 1980).

43   See Robert G. Frank, Jr., "Thomas Willis and his Circle: Brain and Mind in Seventeenth-century Medicine," *The Languages of Psyche: Mind and Body in Enlightenment Thought*, ed. G.S. Rousseau (Berkeley, CA, Los Angeles, CA, and Oxford: University of California Press, 1990), 107–46.

44   Willis, "Preface," *Anatomy of the Brain*, in *Dr. Willis's Practice of Physick, Being the Whole Works of that Renowned and Famous Physician*, trans. S. Pordage (London: for T. Dring, C. Harper, and J. Leigh, 1684), 8.

45   Kenneth Dewhurst, ed. and trans., *Thomas Willis's Oxford Lectures* (Oxford: Sandford Publications, 1980), 122–4.

46   See Katherine Park, "The Organic Soul," in *The Cambridge Companion of Renaissance Philosophy* , ed. Charles B. Schmitt, Quentin Skinner, Eckhard Kessler, and Jill Kraye (Cambridge: Cambridge University Press, 1988), 464–84.

Occasional melancholy, however, raised an altogether different issue. Willis represented it as a disorder of the soul itself rather than of the soul's physical instrument – indeed, as a disorder relating to the soul as the locus of a self possessed of the typical features of conscious human life, including the passions:

> In the preceding lecture we discussed habitual melancholy: there is also an occasional [type]. For it is certain that nobody enjoys such a sanguine and gay constitution that he does not at some time become melancholy. But in order to delve deeper into this condition we must consider the nature and constitution of the *animus sensitivus*. This seems to consist of a contexture of animal spirits and is a sort of aetherial man made up of the most subtle atoms being coextensive with our body. Furthermore this genius of ours sometimes expands beyond our body, as in joy, eagerness and boldness; other times it contracts so as not to be coextensive with our body or is removed into a smaller sphere of activity.[47]

The *animus sensitivus* was to become Willis' answer in *De anima brutorum* to the Cartesian assertion that animals were, like machines, devoid of sense, feeling, and voluntary motion because they lacked an immaterial soul.[48] Not only could a certain kind of matter, in the form of the *animus sensitivus*, think; according to Willis, this material soul explained certain features of human thought as well. In particular, as Willis indicated in the lecture, it explained the physical and mental characteristics of the emotions. The topic of occasional melancholy thus opened up onto the matter of human emotion in a way that the etiology of diseased animal spirits and blood in the account of habitual melancholy did not. Occasional melancholy was not merely the condition of animal spirits making up the sensitive soul, but a condition effected by the powers and affections of the sensitive soul itself. It could indeed be caused for chemical reasons by "eating food which is salty or hardened in smoke." But, Willis continued, "sorrow and fear," "even worry and other efforts of the *animus* etc. constrict the systasis of the spirits, causing melancholy, with the consequence that other operations of the *animus* are neglected."[49] The distinguishing features of certain kinds of melancholy were therefore simply the features of its constituent emotions; occasional melancholy was an emotional constriction of the corporeal soul, caused in the normal way by the apprehension of an unpleasant object, or the perceived privation of some good.

In the chapter on melancholy in *De anima brutorum*, Willis drew out the implications of this insight, indicating that melancholy could and should be approached as a passion of the soul. He referred to precisely the same kinds of therapies as Burton had in his gloss on Seneca's advice to companions of the mournful.[50] Engagement in various activities draw the melancholic mind away from its habitual passions and thought into "chearfulness or joy: pleasant talk, or jesting, Singing, Musick, Pictures, Dancing, Hunting, Fishing, and other pleasant Exercises

---

47   Willis, in Dewhurst, *Oxford Lectures*, 125.
48   Willis, *Two Discourses concerning the Souls of Brutes*, in *Works*, 3–4.
49   Willis, in Dewhurst, *Oxford Lectures*, 126.
50   Burton, *Anatomy*, II.ii.VI.ii: 126.

are to be used." He framed this regimen by stating that "the intention of the *Physician* is so much to lift up, make volatile, and corroborate the more fixed or dejected Animal Spirits." This statement recognized that the proper sphere of the physician was the body, but in drawing upon the philosophical therapy of driving out one passion with its opposites, Willis recognized that fixing the animal spirits involved the "discipline and institution of the mind." Indeed, he argued that while in cases of long or inveterate melancholy the government of the mind was to supplement medical intervention, a fresh melancholy could be healed by the government of the mind alone.[51] Like Galen, Willis recognized that in treating a range of melancholic conditions, the physician must play the philosopher.

Michel Foucault has written that "the cure by passion is based on a constant metaphor of qualities and movements; it always implies that they are immediately transferable in their own modality from the body to the soul, and vice versa ... Between a cure by the passions and a cure by the prescriptions of the pharmacopoeia, there is no difference in nature; but only a diversity in the mode of access to those mechanisms which are common to both."[52] This analysis of passion and madness is the basis for his statement that there was no moral cure of madness in the early modern period. I understand this statement to mean that calling the cure by passion a moral cure is something of a category mistake: the conceptualization of the interaction and interpenetration of body and soul in the seventeenth century is incommensurable with our own understanding of the work of mental therapy.

Foucault is probably right to argue that in early modern thought the emotions were considered to be qualities of posture and bodily process as well as of thought, unified phenomena manifesting across the mind–body divide. Willis' account of the passions illustrates his point perfectly: passions are represented under a dual aspect as both physiological postures of the soul and patterns of thought. From this perspective, to act on one aspect of the mind–body substance was to act on the whole. But in the context of the moral therapy of melancholy, acting on the passions was not merely another means of acting on soul. When Willis introduces sadness and fear as symptoms of melancholy in *De anima brutorum*, he briefly discusses the physical posture of the corporeal soul, but ends the discussion by saying that "[t]he formal reasons of these Distempers, and their causes, we have before exposed."[53] It is clear from the context of the passage that Willis is referring to his discussion in the first part of *De anima brutorum* on the operation of the passions in the imagination, judgment, and appetite. There he takes them as complex mental phenomena proceeding the soul's judgment of an object as either good or bad and resulting in a particular form of pleasure or grief depending on the context of the perception. Sadness is the opinion of evil which has occurred; fear the estimation that an evil is about to occur. In commenting on the formal causes of fear and sadness in the chapter on melancholy, he thus seems to have had in mind something of the

---

51   Willis, *Souls of Brutes*, in *Works*, 194.

52   Foucault, *Madness and Civilization*, 181.

53   Willis, *Souls of Brutes*, in *Works*, 191.

distinction made by Aristotle in the *De anima* between the formal cause of anger, defined as "a craving for retaliation," and the material cause, "a surging of blood and heat around the heart."[54]

Foucault's point about the unity of body and soul in mad phenomena, including melancholy, thus ignores the important distinction between the physical force of melancholic emotions and their logic or sense – in Aristotelian language, between their material and formal causes.[55] Furthermore, this distinction was important to how melancholy was treated *vis-à-vis* other forms of madness. The therapy of the passions in the case of melancholy was not simply an alternative means of acting the mechanisms common to body and mind as it was in mania, but was peculiarly psychological. Mania, like melancholy, had an emotional aspect – boldness and audacity. But there was an altogether different relation between emotion and disease in each case. The emotional symptoms of mania were considered secondary: their cause was located entirely in the violent force of the confused animal spirits that were the evident cause of the primary symptoms of delirium and fury, whereas the fear and sadness of melancholy were introduced as primary symptoms themselves, resembling the emotions caused through the apparatus of perception and opinion rather than being related immediately to the diseased animal spirits.[56] Melancholy could be substantially defined by its emotions – its emotions made it the kind of thing it was – and indeed its causes were often precisely these emotions. If mania could be produced by violent or excessive passion driving the animal spirits into confusion, this cause bore a relation to its secondary, emotional symptoms only through the force of the animal spirits. Melancholy, too, could be caused by "violent passions ... which, when they remain long, they bend the whole Soul, yea and the Body, from their due temper and constitution"; but Willis singled out "vehement sadness, panick fears" and care in particular. It was especially clear that in cases of what Willis terms "particular melancholy," where unrequited love, a suspicious jealousy of the beloved, or a "despair of *Eternal Salvation*" was the precipitating cause, and where delusion and diseased emotion tended to limit themselves to the locus of the cause, there was a continuity and similarity between emotion and melancholy, involving both mental and physical aspects of the soul.[57]

It therefore made sense for Willis to recommend for the cure that the "Evident Cause of this Disease, if any noted thing went before, should be enquired into; and if it may be, either presently removed, or else its removal to be in some sort feigned."[58] Here were formal causes of fear and grief. Nothing of this sort could be recommended for mania. Mania took from the passions only the violent force of confused physical

54   Aristotle, *On the Soul*, trans. W.S. Hett, *Loeb Classical Library* 288 (Cambridge, MA: Harvard University Press/London: William Heinemann, 1986), 1.1: 17.

55   The distinction between *force* and *sens* in the pathology of emotion is suggested by Jackie Pigeaud in "La théorie des passions de Pinel à Mireau de Tours," *History and Philosophy of the Life Sciences* 2 (1980): 123–40.

56   Willis, *Souls of Brutes*, in *Works*, 205.

57   Ibid., 199–200; see also *Oxford Lectures*, 128–9.

58   Willis, *Souls of Brutes*, in *Works*, 193.

movement, whereas melancholy was also structured by their sense or logic. Thus, the use of "punishments and hard usage" in mania to produce reverence and awe "of such as they think their Tormenters," if it was intended to compel "the Corporeal Soul ... to remit its pride and fierceness," had as its object "the furies and exorbitances of the Animal Spirits" rather than any formal cause.[59] Melancholic passions, too, acted by the chemical force of the animal spirits, and therapies of the passions in which "Sadness is ... opposed with the flatteries of Pleasure, Musick, a desire of vain glory, or also a *panick* terror" were the physical cancellation of melancholic emotion. But at the same time, melancholy could be sustained in the way that passions in general were, by an object acting in the imagination. Therapy, then, must involve forcing the mind's attention away from the objects of melancholic passion, "for the mind being busied with necessary cares or duties put aside, and at last deserts more easily, vain and mad cogitations." Thus, "pleasant talk, or jesting, Musick, Pictures, Dancing, Hunting, Fishing ... sometimes *Mathematical* or *Chymical* Studies, also travelling, do very much help," partly because they encourage emotional movements contrary to fear and sadness, but also simply because the mind becomes otherwise engaged than by its melancholy. *Pace* Foucault, this was not merely the opposition of a set of qualities, but a therapeutic strategy aimed specifically at the mechanism of the mind.

In advocating the government of the mind for melancholy, Willis was working well within the strictures of the medical profession. Diversion and conversation were an established feature of the early modern physician's therapeutic battery for cases of melancholy.[60] In an important sense, the physician played the role of Burton's (and Seneca's) wise and careful friend in taking over the management of the patient's mind. In terms of the aims and intention of the medical art, the object of the physician was, as Willis recognized, the material cause of melancholic emotion in the movement of the animal spirits. Willis thus framed the prescription of the institution of the mind as a means of acting on the body through the mind. This in itself is important, since it shows the extent to which the care of the mind was a central feature of the early modern care of melancholy, even within medical practice. But medical practice was not Willis' only intellectual horizon. While his early understanding of melancholy as emotion informed his published account of melancholy in important ways, he expanded considerably the moral elements of melancholy indicated in his Sedleian lecture when he turned to deal with the emotions more generally, drawing attention to the pathological nature of melancholic-like states in a largely moral vocabulary.

We may point out in this regard that Willis' description in his Sedleian lecture of the constriction of the soul in melancholy is of a piece with the representation of sorrow as a force which allowed for no other concern or thought found Coeffeteau

---

59   Ibid., 206, 191.

60   See note 27 above. See also Felix Plater, Abdiah Cole, and Nicholas Culpeper, *A Golden Practice of Physick* (London: Peter Cole, 1662), 36–7.

and also in Senault.[61] It is significant as well that Willis' description of melancholy as a constriction of the soul is strikingly similar to Cicero's description of *aegritudo* as a condition to which "fools are subject ... in the face of expected evil," in which "their souls are downcast and shrunken together in disobedience to reason."[62] The seventeenth-century English translator of the *Tusculan Disputations* rendered the passage as: "a Fool hath that wherewith men are affected in conceited Evils, and let their Spirits sink, and are Melancholly, not obeying Reason."[63] By all accounts, the melancholy did not obey reason, and were possessed with merely imagined evils. But the point made by Burton, and which seemed implicit as well in Willis' analysis, was that it was not the body alone which was the source of the melancholic condition.

Early modern thought marked a point at which the medical concept of melancholy had, in spite of Cicero's criticisms, gained an undisputed foothold in understanding the emotions. Yet, unlike Cicero, early modern moralists did not worry that the medical diagnosis of melancholy would reduce cases of excessive, irrational, even mad emotion to a bodily disorder. Melancholy could be analyzed with reference to its physiology; but it could also, and in the very same breath, be analyzed with reference to the moral representations of its passions. Indeed, at this point in the history of the concept of melancholy, its physiology was precisely a representation of its moral nature. Thus, the description of melancholy as a condition of the soul's constriction and paralysis through grief, fear, or anxiety was developed at length in *De anima brutorum* not in the chapter on melancholy, but in the several chapters relating to the passions of the soul and the need for their rational conduct. Willis there gives an expanded description of the contractive posture of the melancholic soul portrayed in the lectures:

> [I]n Grief, whil'st the Soul sinks down, contracted into a more narrow space, the Spirits inhabiting the Brain, as it were struck down by flight, and troubled, put on only sad and fearful Imaginations, from whence the Countenance is cast down, the Limbs grow feeble, and the *Præcordia* being contracted or bound together by reason of the Nerves carrying the same affection from the Brain, restrain the Blood from its due Excursion, which being therefore heaped up in the same place, with a weight, brings in a troublesome oppression of the Heart, and in the mean time, the Exterior Parts being deprived of its wonted afflux, languish and Contract a paleness.[64]

---

61   Coeffeteau, *Table*, 329–30; Senault, *Use of Passions*, 476. Senault states that the notion that sorrow is the most "complete" of the passions derives from Aristotle. I have not been able to trace this reference. But see Cicero, *Tusculan Disputations*, 3.xii.27: 259.

62   Cicero, *Tusculan Disputations* 4.vi.14: "Stultorum aegritudo est, eaque adficiuntur in malis opinatis animosque demittunt et contrahunt rationi non obtemperantes. Itaque haec prima definitio est, ut aegritudo sit animi adversante ratione contractio."

63   Cicero, *The Five Days Debate at Cicero's House in Tusculum* (London: for Abel Swalle, 1683), 219.

64   Willis, *Souls of Brutes*, in *Works*, 48. Willis' description of grief, it should be noted, was a general description for all grievous, as opposed to pleasurable, passions, and hence included sadness, fear, and worry.

This is not merely a clinical description: Willis was engaged in precisely the same mode of moral rhetoric as Wright and Reynolds, and like them, was constructing a pathology of sadness and fear in which ethical considerations were depicted and reinforced through physiological language. Fear and sorrow were a kind of moral bondage, on Willis' account, for they dominated almost entirely the thoughts and concerns of the soul. Against this bondage to passion, reason is called to govern and moderate "all Concupiscences, and Floods of Passions, that are wont to be moved … within the Phantasie."[65] Willis echoed the classical precept that the passions be moderated according to the correct estimation of an object's importance, calling attention to the moral virtues of temperance and self-control:

> A Wise and Strong man easily moderates the passions of pleasure or Grief, lest these… should affect the Phantasie and the *Præcordia*, by too great a waving; For the Brain and Heart, which are the supports of the soul, ought not to be moved much, by the more light Objects of the Senses; nor are these principal Powers, at leisure to be present at every small thing.[66]

The passions, Willis argued, besides being particularly concerned with material objects to the neglect of rational goods, tended to exaggerate the value and importance of material concerns.[67] Like both ancient and early modern moralists, Willis was advocating the philosophic therapy of correcting opinion in order to alleviate suffering and promote well-being.

Willis was drawing attention to the spiritual and rational aspect of human nature, which set it apart from the animal nature and which had its own criteria of well-being, one less concerned with material enjoyment than with virtue and piety, both of which thus became acts of self-control. Health was, on his account, a state of harmony and tranquility governed by reason and altogether free from vehement emotion. Having described the "floods" and "too great a waving" of passion, Willis depicted the ideal state of the soul: "The whole Corporeal Soul, so long as she is quiet and undisturbed, she is fitted to her proper Body equally, as to a certain Chest or Cabbinet, and waters all its Parts gently, both with little Rivulets of Blood Circulating, and actuates and inspires them every where with a gentle falling down of the Animal Spirits."[68] This condition of tranquility was the norm of both moral and physical health that reason was to maintain through the exercise of moral meditation. Importantly as well, Willis, himself a devout churchman, portrayed prayer as a particularly salubrious activity.[69]

---

65   Willis, *Souls of Brutes*, in *Works*, 43.

66   Ibid., 48.

67   Ibid., 50.

68   Ibid., 45.

69   Ibid., 48–9. On the religious dimension of Willis' work and thought, see Robert L. Martensen, "'Habit of Reason': Anatomy and Anglicanism in Restoration England," *Bulletin for the History of Medicine* 66 (1992): 511–35. The extent to which Willis' moral psychology

I have argued throughout this chapter that moral philosophy provided one particularly important approach to melancholy in the seventeenth century, that the moral philosophical analysis and representation of sorrow and fear as emotional "diseases of the soul" contributed to recognizing and treating philosophically the psychological aspects of melancholic suffering. Moralists such as Wright, Reynolds, and Coeffeteau embroidered their emphasis on the dangerous nature of sorrow with some of the central features that defined melancholic pathology – namely, the overpowering and irrational force of its emotions and the presence of bodily symptoms. Wright's text in particular suggested that melancholic pathology itself could be understood as a physical complication arising ultimately from intemperate fear or sorrow, a suggestion which Burton fully articulated in arguing that melancholy was as much a disease of the soul as of the body, and thus that philosophy was of central importance in treating melancholic affliction. Writing as both a philosopher and a physician, Willis clearly regarded melancholy as a condition of the mind in a way that other forms of madness were not. Moreover, while Willis treated melancholy as a medical category, in the moral philosophical part of his work he recognized melancholic symptoms as a moral condition, to be treated through rational self-government.

Early modern physicians and philosophers interested in melancholy did not feel that they first had to pin down the nature of the melancholic condition as either bodily or mental before deciding on the appropriate therapy. Operating in the context of a moral psychology that took the emotions themselves as dangerous mental diseases which affected the mind powerfully in part through the body, the early modern concept of melancholy encompassed both the perspective of the moralist and that of the physician. It was thus the standard wisdom that the successful treatment of melancholy required both the treatment of the body and the correction of the mind.

---

and his very brief mentions of religious despair and of prayer can be attributed to Willis' High Church affiliations and sympathies is more difficult to determine than Martensen suggests.

CHAPTER THREE

The Pastoral Care of Melancholy in Calvinist England

In the second act of *Hamlet*, Hamlet wonders if the ghost he has seen is in fact a delusion produced by the devil acting on his "weakness and [his] melancholy" to incite him to murder and so to damn him.[1] The association between the devil and melancholy was a common way of accounting for the apparently deluded, and sometimes sinful, beliefs which melancholic persons tended to have; here, Hamlet conveniently uses it to bypass once more his obligation to act courageously to avenge his father's death and punish Claudius. Similarly, individuals suffering from specifically religious fear and sorrow in the late sixteenth and early seventeenth centuries had their suffering dismissed *en toto* as melancholic by Renaissance wits familiar with the popularized Galenic dictum that the mind's temperament followed the body's temperature. The poet Ben Jonson wrote in *To Heaven*: "Good, and great God, can I not thinke of thee / But it must, straight, my melancholy bee? / Is it interpreted in me disease / That, laden with my sinnes, I seeke for ease?"[2] According to the frequently published narrative of the case of Francis Spira, a sixteenth-century Venetian lawyer and a Protestant, the mental agitation and emotional turmoil produced by his public renunciation of the Protestant religion against his conscience was attributed by some to "his Melancholicke constitution; that overshadowing his judgment, wrought in him a kinde of madnesse."[3]

The trajectory of Spira's case is similar to Hamlet's. Both are burdened by conscience – one for sin, the other for morally weak inaction – and the result in both cases is intense despair, self-laceration, and a longing to die. In both cases, melancholy seems to be a possible cause of their suffering. But just as it is clear in *Hamlet* that Claudius is right in his diagnosis of Hamlet's apparent madness and that Hamlet's own suspicion of his melancholic temperament is wrong-headed, the Spira narrative emphasizes that the attempt to reduce cases of religious despair entirely to

---

1   *Hamlet*, II, ii, 554.

2   *Poems of Ben Jonson*, ed. Bernard H. Newdigate (Oxford: Clarendon Press, 1936), 82, as cited in Noel L. Brann, "The Problem of Distinguishing Religious Guilt from Religious Melancholy in the English Renaissance," *Journal of the Rocky Mountain Medieval and Renaissance Association* 1 (1980): 63–72.

3   *A Relation of the Fearefull Estate of Francis Spira, in the Yeare 1548* (London: I.L. for Phil Stephens, 1638), 32. On this narrative, see Michael MacDonald, "*The Fearefull Estate of Francis Spira*: Narrative, Identity and Emotion in Early Modern England," *Journal of British Studies* 31 (1992): 32–61.

bodily dysfunction is both impious and medically unsound. Spira himself, perhaps more courageously than Hamlet, eschewed such a diagnosis, affirming that the problem lay in his soul:

> Alas poore men, how farre wide are you; doe you thinke that this disease is to be cured by potions; believe mee there must bee another manner of medicine, it is neither potions, plaisters, nor drugs, that can helpe a fainting soule cast downe with sense of sinne, and the wrath of God; it is onely Christ that must bee the Physician, and the Gospel the sole Antidote.[4]

Even the three physicians consulted in the Spira case differ significantly from those who, "not looking so high as the Judgement of God," suggest that Spira's suffering was merely melancholic, and are indeed much closer to Spira's own judgment (although they appear not to know the case history). Spira's body was not "afflicted with any danger or distemper originally from it selfe," they asserted; rather, his malady "did arise from some griefe, or passion of his minde, which being overburthened, did so oppresse the spirits, as the wanting free passage, stirred up many ill humours, whereof the body of man is full; & these ascending up into the braine, troubled the fancie; shadowed the seat of judgment and so corrupted it." Thus Spira's physicians, although they attempted to heal his melancholy "by purgation," agreed in the end with Spira's own self-diagnosis "after they had understood the whol truth of the matter, and therefore they wished him to seeke some spirituall comfort."[5] Indeed, the narrator states that "for remedy all agreed in this, to use both the wholesome helpe of Physicians, and the pious advise of Divines."[6]

From a medical point of view, then, the minister was thus expected to provide comfort by assuring the patient that he was not damned, that the Gospel declared God's promise of salvation for the repentant. (The Spira narrative is chock-full of such arguments of consolation.) But at this point the specific concerns of the spiritual physician supervened on the concern for bodily health. If the spiritual comfort which was to calm the passions and heal the body was to be true and effective, repentance had to be deep and profound, yet such repentance was not a comfortable procedure. Honestly facing one's sins and humbling oneself often entailed terror at the thought of God's just damnation of such sin, and it was easy to lose sight of God's grace and to despair in practicing the Christian virtue of humility. Thus, evangelically minded divines in the Elizabethan and Jacobean Church concerned with the health of the soul often complained that persons suffering from the terrors of their conscience themselves used the notion of melancholy as Hamlet does – to avoid facing certain uncomfortable moral and spiritual demands. From a modern perspective, such spiritual purgation is likely to be seen in the same light as the physical purges and bleedings early modern physicians prescribed for melancholics. For their part, however, early modern spiritual physicians insisted that if the health of the soul and

---

4   Ibid., 36.
5   Ibid.
6   Ibid., 32.

the body were interdependent, as Galenic medicine maintained, then the healing of religious melancholy, and indeed of melancholy in general, demanded that the soul find its rest and its health in God.

Yet within the context of evangelical spiritual therapy itself, there were often pressing reasons for de-emphasizing the need to practice thorough repentance and humility and encouraging the suffering individual to meditate on the more comfortable aspects of the Christian faith. As *Hamlet* indicates, it was commonly thought that the devil used melancholy and religious despair as the instruments in driving people to self-murder, to blaspheme against God's power or willingness to save, or to despair sinfully of salvation.[7] Burton cited a list of medieval and Renaissance medical and religious authorities who supported the idea that melancholy was the "*Balneum Diaboli*, the Devil's Bath":

> [T]he Devil, spying his opportunity of such humours, drives them many times to despair, fury, rage, &c., mingling himself amongst these humours … this humour invites the Devil to it, wheresoever it is in extremity, and, of all others, melancholy persons are most subject to diabolical temptations and illusions, and most apt to entertain them, and the Devil best able to work upon them.[8]

The notion of melancholy as the *balneum diaboli* entailed that medicine itself was an important part of the battery of dispossession and the cure of the demonic affliction of conscience in some English Protestant circles. But it also underscored the importance of combating the lies and temptations of the devil in cases of religious melancholy through spiritual comfort and theological argument. These were the same means through which ministers consoled non-demonic forms of religious melancholy and despair. As in all cases of religious melancholy, if the body was ill, it was very clearly the soul that was at stake.

Religious despair and religious melancholy

In the last quarter of the sixteenth century, and well into the seventeenth century, many of England's most respected divines and theologians addressed themselves in print and in practice to the consolation and cure of religious despair, or what was known more commonly in contemporary religious language as the "affliction of conscience." The consolatory literature on religious despair, written by an expanding body of university-trained Reformed clergy concerned with the evangelization of their nation, appeared to be immensely popular, most works going through several editions up to the 1640s; and divines who had a reputation in resolving "cases of conscience" were tremendously esteemed among English Protestants who took seriously the demands and beliefs of Reformed Christianity. The numerous literary works, treatises, popular autobiographical and biographical accounts of spiritual

---

7   See also Kiblansky, Panofsky, and Saxl, *Saturn and Melancholy*, 77.
8   Burton, *Anatomy*, I.ii.I.ii: 228–9.

crises, and anecdotes of contemporary observers all indicate that the penetration of the discourse on religious despair into English culture was deep and profound.[9]

Spira's worldly friends had pointed to the possibility that what was properly to be regarded as mere melancholy could express itself, deceptively, in the vocabulary of religious despair. Cases such as Spira's, which involved both melancholic disease and the terrors of conscience for sin, were termed "religious melancholy" by Burton in *The Anatomy of Melancholy*. Burton discusses a huge variety of cases in this category, at times using the notion of melancholy to critique and dismiss various religious groups, especially Catholics and radical heterodox Protestants such as the Anabaptists. Some scholars have taken the term "religious melancholy" to be equally dismissive of cases of affliction of conscience more generally, aligning Burton's position with that of Spira's medically minded friends.[10] On this reading, Burton was joining those who criticized the more evangelical, "Puritan" ministers among the established English Church, who insisted that terror for sin and despair over salvation could in fact be spiritually salubrious, and sought to promote such feelings through their preaching. In his widely cited study of the medical practices of the seventeenth-century clergyman Richard Napier, Michael MacDonald notes that such spiritual physicians were criticized by Napier for exacerbating rather than consoling fear and sorrow by stressing the need to intensify the terrors of conscience.[11] In contrast to the "Puritans," MacDonald argues, Napier believed that "the antidotes to religious worry were relatively simple." "It is unlikely," he writes, "that [Napier] explored their doubts in depth or engaged in theological dispute with" his melancholic and troubled patients.[12] MacDonald goes on to enlist Robert Burton's discussion of religious melancholy and despair in *The Anatomy of Melancholy* in order to construct the notion of an "Anglican" style of "spiritual physic," distinguished from the "Puritan" methods in its "simplicity" and its emphasis on formal and liturgical prayer and comfort rather than emotional introspection. Burton, who, according to MacDonald, "abhorred" the "Puritans," asserted that "faith, hope, repentance, are the sovereign cures and remedies, the sole comforts in [despair]; confess, humble thyself, repent, it is sufficient."[13]

Quoted out of context, such a prescription for melancholic feelings of despair may sound simple. Yet it is embedded in a detailed theological and consolatory discussion which was, like "Puritan" works on the affliction of conscience, informed by a long theological and spiritual tradition going back to the letters of Paul that stressed the need for sorrow for sin, even desperation over salvation, as crucial in the turn away from reliance on the self towards the acceptance of God's grace.

---

9   See John Stachniewski, *The Persecutory Imagination: English Puritanism and the Literature of Religious Despair* (Oxford: Clarendon Press, 1991), esp. 27–60. On the pastoral concerns of the English Reformation, see William Haller, *The Rise of Puritanism* (New York: Columbia University Press, 1937).

10   Stachniewski, *Persecutory Imagination*, 227–8.

11   MacDonald, *Mystical Bedlam*, esp. 217–31.

12   Ibid., 220–21.

13   Ibid., 221.

Furthermore, among Burton's authorities in his concluding section on the cure of religious despair are several "Puritan" ministers well known for their work in healing spiritual affliction. Burton thus uses and cites with approval the work of the well-known late sixteenth and early seventeenth-century English evangelical preachers and thinkers Richard Greenham, William Perkins and Robert Bolton as among the many "excellent Exhortations" that are appropriate "for such as are in any way troubled in mind."[14] And where Burton acknowledged that religious despair could be mixed with melancholy and that "melancholy alone again may be sometimes a sufficient cause of this terror of conscience," he was merely following his evangelical sources.[15] Ministers of all stripes concurred with the advice given Spira, that both spiritual and bodily physick were required for healing. Burton agreed, warning of the cure of religious despair that although the physician Felix Platter claimed to cure "many by Physick alone … they take a wrong course, that think to overcome this feral passion by sole Physick."[16]

Noel L. Brann argues that both "Anglican" and "Puritan" Elizabethan and early Stuart divines "failed to come to satisfactory terms, at least on a practical level," with the distinction between spiritual affliction and melancholic disease.[17] But here we reach what is perhaps the most important idea governing one of the major modes of perceiving melancholy in late sixteenth and early seventeenth-century England, for it was precisely on the practical level that they did not think it important to attempt to discriminate between the two. Many ministers recognized that certain genuine cases of conscience were mixed with melancholic disease, and some went so far as to argue that the influence of melancholy in cases of the affliction of conscience was common. William Perkins included a discussion of melancholy as a special form of spiritual "temptation, or trouble of minde" in his *Cases of Conscience* (1602). Concluding his discussion of the various forms of temptations, he wrote:

> [I]f we make examination of the state of such persons as are troubled with any of these five temptations, we shall not usually finde them single, but mixed together, especially

---

14 Burton, *Anatomy*, III.iv.II.vi: 468.

15 Ibid., III.iv.II.iii: 453.

16 Ibid., III.iv.II.vi: 469. Any analysis of Burton's treatment of religious melancholy and despair must now take into account Angus Gowland's intelligent and exhaustive study of Burton in *The Worlds of Renaissance Melancholy* (Cambridge: Cambridge University Press, 2006). Gowland makes a compelling case that Burton regarded the Calvinist inability to secure assurity of salvation as making impossible the comfort of despair, and that he recommended and rehearsed Calvinist practical divines largely parodically. Gowland argues as well that Burton may well have been a crypto-Catholic who regarded the efficacy of the sacraments as providing a sound basis of comfort. Regrettably, this work came too late to my attention to consider at length here. However, I think there is still a case to be made for the fact that Burton did not regard all religious despair as proceeding from and reinforced by Calvinist worries about salvation, and that Burton and the "Puritans" did share a common ground in emphasizing the importance of humility and repentance for comfort, which, even in Catholic theology, was a condition of the efficacy of the sacraments: see page 54 below.

17 Brann, "Religious Guilt," 64.

Melancholy, with terror of Conscience ... For the distraction of the mind will often breede a distemper in the body, and the distemper of the body likewise will sometimes cause distractions of mind.[18]

Perkins' formulation of the interaction of body and soul drew on a commonplace of Galenic medical theory and was entirely uncontroversial. Spiritual physicians argued, like Spira's doctors, that it was necessary to consult both a physician in cases of the affliction of conscience.[19] Yet the possible presence of melancholy in the body did not make the care of the afflicted soul any less important, or provide cause to interpret feelings of damnation and abject humility themselves as merely melancholic. From a practical point of view, the fact that many cases of conscience were, like Spira's, "mixed" cases entailed that both spiritual and bodily physick were necessary. Nor did it matter if a "mixed" case arose when terror of conscience was caused initially by melancholic disease alone, as we might expect. Even as a "medical" condition, cases of mere melancholy were to be subjected to the proper spiritual cure of the soul. "Thou must repent and renew thy repentance," John Abernethy counseled the melancholic in his *A Christian and Heavenly Treatise, containing Physicke for the Soule* (1622).[20]

But repentance was precisely the kind of spiritual exercise which tended to generate despair in the soul, as it reminded the sinner of the enormous and properly unforgivable burden of his sins. Abernethy thus added that "thou must bee also comforted with the promises of mercy," which was the standard course of spiritual physick for cases of extreme religious despair. To the modern mind, this sounds like a much more appropriate treatment. The task of the historian is to make sense of the perceived need to push the melancholic through a course of spiritual meditation which would take him even closer to the despair to which his melancholy already dangerously exposed him. And to perform this task, we must understand the nature of the late sixteenth and early seventeenth-century discourse on despair which provided both a form of expression for melancholy and a mode of healing.

What needs to be appreciated above all else is the extent to which early modern English Protestants (and Catholics) thought of moments of despair as both common occurring features of the Christian life and as spiritually healthy, or at least health-bringing. This has been generally obscured by the view that the literature on the consolation of despair in late sixteenth and early seventeenth century was part of an effort to remedy the terrifying consequences of Calvinist predestinarian theology.

---

18   Perkins, *The Whole Treatise of Cases of Conscience* (Cambridge: John Legatt, 1642), 116.

19   See Richard Greenham, *A Most Sweete and Assured Comfort for All Those that Are Afflicted in Conscience, or Troubled in Minde* (London: John Danter, for William Jones, 1595), sig. F. See also Perkins, *Cases of Conscience*, 196–7; Burton, *Anatomy*, III.iv.II.vi: 490; Bright, *Treatise of Melancholie*, 198, and John Abernethy, *A Christian and Heavenly Treatise, Containing Physicke for the Soule* (London: Felix Kingston for John Budge, 1622), 135–6.

20   Ibid., 135.

On this view, which has been argued since at least the early seventeenth century, high levels of anxiety and despair regarding salvation are a phenomena particular to the Calvinist stress on the doctrine of double predestination, according to which God has decreed the eternal fates, whether damned or saved, of all persons irrespective of their own beliefs and choices. Indeed, while Burton commended the writings of certain "Puritan" divines as therapeutic for cases of melancholic religious despair, he also criticized "our indiscreet Pastors," who, "whilst they speak so much of election, predestination, reprobation *ab æterno*, subtraction of grace, præterition, voluntary permission, &c. by what signs and tokens they shall discern and try themselves, whether they be God's true children elect, they … thunder out God's judgement without respect … they so rent, tear, and wound men's consciences, that they are almost mad, and at their wits' ends."[21] More recently, the German sociologist and historian Max Weber argued in his influential *The Protestant Ethic and the Spirit of Capitalism* that Calvin's assertion that the reprobate could evidence the same signs of grace as the elect confounded the believer's attempt to ascertain what was thought to be the most important element of their existence: whether or not they were saved. The result of Calvin's irresolvable paradox was potentially a great deal of anxiety, for which no comfort could be had.[22]

For most English Reformers of the late sixteenth century, the Calvinist assertion that absolute assurance of salvation was given to the elect through divine predestination remained a central orthodoxy. One of the reasons it was insisted upon was that it countered what English Protestants saw as the unsettling implication of the idea that salvation was contingent on human moral performance. This is what English Protestants took to be the Catholic view, and as Peter Lake argues, the related positions of absolute assurance and anti-Catholicism were two of the defining features of late sixteenth-century Protestantism in England.[23] Yet Calvin's writing on the signs of election had rendered the effort to attain assurance highly problematic, and the anxiety caused by this double bind should not be minimized or ignored, as modern-day apologists for Calvin and for Calvinism have attempted to do.[24] Godly Protestants who accepted the established Church's basically Calvinist theology scrutinized their lives for the signs of grace and strained to conduct their lives free from sin in the effort to improve upon the graces which they had been granted; yet they were agonizingly forced to draw back from claims to certainty for

---

21   Burton, *Anatomy* III.iv.II.iii: 457; see also Susan Snyder, "Left Hand of God," 29–30.

22   See Max Weber, *The Protestant Ethic and the Spirit of Capitalism*, trans. Talcott Parsons (London and New York: Routledge, 1992), 98–128.

23   Peter Lake, *Moderate Puritans and the Elizabethan Church* (Cambridge: Cambridge University Press, 1982), 99, 219.

24   See Basil Hall, "Calvin against the Calvinists," in G.E. Duffield, ed., *John Calvin* (Appleford: Sutton Courtney Press, 1966); Richard A. Muller, "Perkins' *A Golden Chaine*: Predestinarian Scheme or Schematized *Ordo Salutis*?", in *Sixteenth-Century Journal* 9 (1978): 69–81; cf. Ian Breward, "The Significance of William Perkins," *The Journal of Religious History* 4 (1966–67): 113–28, esp. 113, and Lake, *Moderate Puritans*, 116–68.

fear of unraveling the evidence of their election by presumptuously claiming grace through their righteous acts.[25]

However, the "culture of despair" that the literary historian John Stachniewski and others point to in describing the milieu of late Tudor and Stuart England is not best understood as a phenomenon produced simply by Calvinist predestinarian theology acting through what Stachniewski terms a "persecutory imagination" on passively fearful individuals who could not help but try to guess their status. It is plausible that Burton had some worries about the implications of Calvinist theology in creating religious melancholy and despair, as Stachniewski has argued. But we should note as well that Burton broke off his discussion of the doctrine of predestination and assurance in his discussion of religious despair by declaring that "the last main torture and trouble of a distressed mind, is, not so much this doubt of Election, and that the promises of grace are smothered and extinct in them … but withal God's heavy wrath, a most intolerable pain and grief of heart seizeth on them."[26] If Burton is correct, late sixteenth and early seventeenth-century religious despair was not primarily the result of being trapped in the inescapable logic of Calvin's horrible doctrine, but of a simple feeling of wrath and damnation. And Burton likely is correct: this at least would make sense of the fact that complaints of feelings of condemnation and divine abandonment continued well after the Calvinist theological framework had been abandoned in the last half of the seventeenth century.[27]

Furthermore, to point to Calvinist predestinarian belief as a direct source of experiences of religious anxiety ignores the extent to which despair was actively cultured as a token of God's favor and as something of a spiritual exercise. The godly Protestant could not claim grace through the performance of works. This, according to English clergy, was papism. Forced continually to the recognition of their moral insufficiency and corruption, the spiritually minded believer cultivated a fear and sorrow appropriate to the acknowledgement of human moral worthlessness as both the substance of godliness and the means to certainty of salvation. Pastoral consolations of religious trouble of mind were not simply an attempt by "Puritans" to remedy the psychological damage done by the logic of their predestinarian theology; they were prescriptive and normative accounts of the godly temperament. As Peter Iver Kaufman has rightly pointed out in accounting for the plentiful evangelical Protestant urgings to "rippe up all the inwarde and secrete corners of conscience" through prayer, late sixteenth and early seventeenth-century religious despair can be regarded in large part as a performative effect of prayer and meditation, a posture actively cultivated through a close inward scrutiny and meditation which intensified religious feeling precisely to the end of assurance.[28] Kaufman quotes Edward

---

25   Ibid., 151, 161–3; Kenneth L. Parker and Eric J. Carlson, eds., *'Practical Divinity': The Works and Life of Revd Richard Greenham* (Aldershot: Ashgate, 1998), 87.

26   Burton, *Anatomy*, III.iv.II.vi: 485.

27   See pages 95–8 and 101–2 below.

28   Laurence Chaderton, *An Excellent and Godly Sermon most needeful for the time wherein we live in all Securitie and Sinne* (London, 1610), 32–3, as cited in Kaufman, *Prayer,*

Dering's pithy paradox several times: "Care not for hell, for the nearer we feele it, the further we are from it."[29] In the Reformation tradition of Calvin and Luther, hell was understood by the English Protestants as a state of divine abandonment, the condition of being forsaken by God to which despair was the appropriate response.[30] Dering was thus explicitly encouraging the cultivation of despair while at the same time circumscribing its impact by fashioning it into a sign of grace. A similar approach was replicated in many other pastoral works.[31]

William Perkins, in speaking of the various causes of desperation in Christian life, commented on the case of Spira that "[t]hey are much overseene [*sic*] that write of him as a damned creature. For ... in the very middest of his desperation, he complained of the hardnesse of his heart, which made him that he could not pray: no doubt then he felt his hardnesse of heart: and the feeling of corruption in the heart, is by some contrary grace."[32] Perkins' analysis of the Spira case is representative of a typical therapeutic strategy in cases of despair and affliction of conscience. It can be found in many works of consolation, Burton's included.[33] The feeling of hardness of heart might induce and contribute to despair. It indicated that an individual was not sorry enough for the enormous burden of sin that Reformation theology asserted was theirs; that the Holy Spirit's gift of repentance had been withdrawn; in short, that God had indeed abandoned the soul. But that an individual was concerned enough with the matter of salvation to sense and lament hardness of heart betrayed to the minister and to the godly community a secret, profound and difficult movement of the Spirit in penetrating the soul, paradoxically linking hope to the substance and feeling of despair itself.

More broadly, then, Perkins' reading of the Spira case is indicative of the extent to which English Protestants were willing to see despair not simply as a spiritual danger and, except in a few cases, not at all as a sin, but as an act of grace and a sign of saintliness. This is further reinforced in the hagiography of John Glover in John Foxe's massively popular *Actes and Monuments* (1563). Foxe included John alongside his martyred brother Robert because John's acute pains of conscience, no less than the burning of Robert's body, accounted him a saint and a martyr. Glover became inconsolably tormented by the idea that he had sinned the unpardonable sin against the Holy Ghost. It was obvious to Foxe, as it was obvious to most others when one of the godly feared this, that John had done no such thing; but Foxe

---

Despair and Drama: Elizabethan Introspection (Urbana, IL: University of Chicago Press, 1996), 19.

29   Dering, *Certaine Godly and verie Comfortable Letters full of Christian Consolation* (London, 1590), B3r, quoted in Kaufman, *Prayer*, 20.

30   Snyder, "The Left Hand of God," 27.

31   See, for example, Parker and Carlson, *'Practical Divinity'*, 90–91, 162, 168, 175–6, 188–9.

32   Perkins, *A treatise tending unto a declaration, whether a man be in the estate of damnation, or in the estate of grace*, in *The Workes of ... William Perkins. The First Volume* (London: John Legatt, 1612), 378.

33   Burton, *Anatomy*, III.iv.II.vi: 475, 481.

skipped over completely the delusional aspect of John's experience to hallow the sufferings themselves: "For as the said Robert was speedily dispatched with the sharp and extreme torments of the fire in a short time; so this no lesse blessed Saint of God [John] what and how much more grievous pangs, what sorrowfull torments, what boiling heats of the fire of hell in his spirit inwardly he felt and sustained, no speech outwardly is able to express." John, like Robert ushered into heaven through a martyr's death, had left behind worldly concerns while he was still alive, the flesh almost completely mortified through the terrors of conscience.[34] If the martyr took up the cross of death, imitating the ultimate act of Christ's crucifixion, the afflicted of conscience took up the cross of God's abandonment, also in imitation of Christ. "My God, my God, why hast thou forsaken me?": there was hardly a pastoral treatise addressed to the afflicted of conscience which did not exploit Christ's quotation of the psalmist to show the sufferer that what he bore was in imitation of Christ.

In an important sense, then, ministers encouraged and cultivated despair, and this formed part of their consolation for the despairing. Those who were disturbed by such feelings could be shown that they were participating in the work of salvation. Furthermore, although ministers were concerned in their pastoral work with providing hope for the afflicted conscience, they warned against the desire for easy comfort, against the pragmatic use of the comforts of the work of atonement. Richard Greenham, who was highly respected in the late Tudor and early Stuart Church for his pastoral skill in ministering to the afflicted conscience, wrote in *A Most Sweete and assured Comfort* (1595):

> [I]t is good to mark that there be many who are more troubled for vexation and disquietness of the mind being distempered, than for the vileness and horribleness of their sin committed; who are wounded more with the fear of shame, with the fear of being mad, or with the fear of running out of their wits, than with the conscience of sin. Which thing if we find them in, it is our part to travail with them that they make a less matter of the outward shame, and more conscience of the inward sin.[35]

For some, trouble of conscience was perceived as one of many forms of mental agitation, worryingly near to distraction and madness. "They are wont to have recourse to Ministers for ease and helpe," declared the casuist and divine Robert Bolton, exasperated. The spiritual physician most appreciated in such cases was one who was most ready to apply the comfortable portions of the scripture. From the perspective of those like Greenham and Bolton, however, although the Gospel provided inestimable comfort, it did so only for those truly humbled by the magnitude and import of their sins. This was the essential point from whence the soul might begin to mend, to proceed towards the wholeness for which it was intended, through justification to the work of sanctification. They therefore cautioned against

---

34   Foxe, *Actes and Monuments of Matters Most Speciall and Memorable, Happening In the Church* (London: for the Company of Stationers, 1610), 1: 1551.

35   Greenham, *A Most Sweete ... Comfort*, sig. Giiij; cf. Robert Bolton, *Right Comforting*, 203.

the inappropriate application of the comforts of the Gospel. The message of God's free grace was misapplied if applied too soon.[36] The intention might be good, but more often, many of these writers criticized the "daubers," who covered over the ugliness of sin and gave men and women the appearance of righteousness in their own eyes.[37]

It appears that Richard Napier's concerns about the "Puritan" ministers were thus correct. The immediate concern of medicine was to alleviate dis-ease; the likes of Greenham and Bolton seemed intent on exacerbating it. The evangelical approach was equally perverse from the perspective of moral philosophical ideals as well. But on this point the evangelicals, as well as many other early modern intellectuals, followed the Augustinian critique of heathen moral philosophy. Writers such as Francis Bacon and James I criticized Stoic teaching as prideful, asserting that unaided philosophical exercise alone was viewed by many as inadequate to the cultivation of mental tranquility.[38] Joseph Hall admired the philosophy of the Stoics, but argued in his *Heaven upon Earth* that although the heathen ancient philosophers correctly perceived tranquility of mind as a worthy good, they "knew not the way to it."[39] This was because one of the main sources of distress was conscience of sin, and humans had become helplessly sinful through Adam's original sin. The human condition of wretched emotional suffering could thus not be remedied through philosophical exercise, but only through the Christian life aided by divine grace. In his *Consolations of the Afflicted: or, The Third Part of the Christian Warfare* (1613), the "Puritan" minister John Downame drew extensively on the writings of Seneca, Cicero and Plutarch in order to urge Christians to mortify their earthly sorrows "with spirituall joy, and meeke submission of our will to the pleasure of God" so as to keep "from bursting out into murmuring [complaining] and repining, or from sinking into desperate sorrow and deepe despaire" in times of outward affliction.[40] But Downame insisted against his philosophical sources that such moderation of sorrow within its natural limit was impossible except through the help of divine grace. Furthermore, he argued that Stoic "insensibility" to emotion was not wisdom, but hard-heartedness; at the same time that sorrow was to be moderated, Downame argued that "sorrow and greefe is appointed by God to be a medicine proper and peculiar for the curing of sinne; and being rightly applied unto it, and in fit proportion, it doth cure and heale it."[41] Worldly sorrow was never to be eradicated, so long as it was not out of "our judgement, choyce, and will, but onely so much as nature and necessity compelleth us unto."[42] But the sufferer was to sanctify his painful suffering; the pain of sorrow

---

36 Ibid., 211, 268.
37 Ibid., 151–64, 257–310; Perkins, *Cases of Conscience*, 55–7.
38 See Salmon, "Seneca and Tacitus," 170–71, 174, 185–6.
39 Hall, *Heaven upon Earth*, 13.
40 See Downame, *Consolations of the Afflicted*, 1.v.3–10: 61–81.
41 Ibid., 2.i.5: 101.
42 Ibid.

was to be experienced as the sting of chastisement for having loved an earthly finite object such that one could be pained by its absence.[43]

Augustine had understood his spiritual suffering during conversion to be God's discipline for sin, and the idea of sorrow and anguish as a crucial preparatory experience for the healing of the soul through divine grace remained as an important feature of Christian thought and experience in the early modern period. Augustine's *Confessions* were translated into English and published several times throughout the seventeenth century, and similar descriptions of moments of deep despair and sudden infusion of light and grace could be found in the many evangelical spiritual autobiographies circulating in Tudor and Stuart England. William Perkins, one of England's foremost Reformed theologians and pastoral writers, discussed the idea under the denomination of "holy desperation: which is, when a man is wholly out of all hope ever to attaine salvation by any strentgh [*sic*] or goodnes of his owne, speaking and thinking more vily of himselfe then any other can doe, and heartily acknowledging himselfe to have deserved not one onely, but even ten thousand damnations in hell fire with the devill and his angels." Through this desperation, he asserted, God "maketh the heart fitte to receive faith."[44] This is Augustine's experience, transposed into an early modern Protestant idiom (with its characteristic and perhaps regrettable emphasis on hell and damnation). And, glossing his assertion that "faith, hope, repentance are the sovereign cures and remedies, the sole comforts" for feelings of God's wrath and judgment, Burton cited a similar Augustinian sentiment from the exposition of Psalm 52: "*Parcam huic homini*, saith *Austin* (*ex persona Dei*) *quia sibi ipsi non pepercit*; *ignoscam, quia peccatum agnovit*. I will spare him because he hath not spared himself; I will pardon him, because he doth acknowledge his offence."[45]

English evangelical descriptions of "holy desperation" and "godly sorrow" contain often violent images of self-excoriation and self-condemnation. It is crucial to understand that early modern English evangelical Protestants were not fostering a peculiarly abject and tormented "Puritan" psychology when describing such spiritual experiences; they were rather explicating commonly held theological ideas which had been emphasized recently by Reformation thinkers such as John Calvin and Martin Luther and which had roots in the early Church Fathers. Many medieval writers had similarly stressed the importance of despairing at human sinfulness and sorrowing for sin as both a stage in the soul's turn towards Christ and as a recurring trial of the saint to build faith and hope. In his magisterial study of guilt in the Christian West, Jean Delumeau has uncovered a deep-rooted and persistent notion of the absolute sinfulness and worthlessness of the human and a tendency

---

43   Ibid., 2.i.5–6: 101–3.

44   Perkins, *A treatise tending unto a declaration*, 365.

45   Burton, *Anatomy* III.iv.II.vi: 488. See also the commentary by J.B. Bamborough and Martin Dodsworth in *The Clarendon Edition of Robert Burton's "The Anatomy of Melancholy,"* ed. Thomas C. Faulkner, Nicholas K. Kiessling, and Rhonda L. Blair (Oxford: Clarendon Press, 1989–2000), 6: 293.

to cultivate fear, sorrow and anxiety in spiritual reflection throughout the history of Christianity.[46] Delumeau laments the early turn to such patterns of thought. More sympathetically, however, we should remind ourselves that as human pride and self-love was seen in the Augustinian interpretation of Christianity to be the root of vice, humility was one of key virtues, without which no other virtue could be obtained.[47] In moral philosophical terms, the humble soul was a healthy soul; but the cultivation of humility was itself painful, and the moral philosophical goal of happiness and tranquility of mind was deferred to the next life, while this one was given to the application of uncomfortable spiritual medicine.

In the context of this *longue durée* of Christian thought, writers like Bolton, Perkins, Greenham, and Burton were, like Chrysostom and Augustine, arguing for a dialectic of sorrow and joy in the Christian life, a fruitful tension curbing presumption through despair and despair through grace, ultimately centering the soul in a posture of humble hope in the efficacy of he work of Christ.[48] Bolton showed this idea clearly in his cautions to the would-be physician of the soul in his *Instructions*:

> A man may presse, and apply Gods justice, and the terrours of the Law *too much*; therefore also mercy and the comforts of the Gospell, too much. The consequent if cleare. For as the former may plunge into the Gulph of despaire; so the other may cast upon the Rocke of presumption.[49]

Bolton thought that the danger of presumption was far greater, "because wee are farre readier to apprehend, and apply unto our selves mercy, then judgement. And thousands are endlessly overthrown thorow presumption, for one by despaire."[50] This perception of human nature is the reason why Bolton published a book like *Helpes to Humiliation* (1631), and the reason he pressed home the need for the continual cultivation of godly sorrow throughout one's life:

> When the anguish of thy guilty Conscience, is upon sure ground something allayed, and supplied with the oyle of comfort; and thy wounded heart warrantably revived with the sweetnesse of the Promises, as with *marrow and fatnesse*: Thou must not then, either shut up thine eyes from further search into thy sins, or dry them up from any more mourning. But comfort of remission must serve as a pretious *Eye-salve*, both to cleare their sight, that they may see more, and with more detestation; and to enlarge their Sluces, as it were, to poure out repentant tears more plentifully. Thou must continue ripping up, and ransacking that hellish Heape of thy former rebellions, and polutions of youth: still dive and digge

---

46   Delumeau, *Sin and Fear: The Emergence of a Western Guilt Culture, 13th to 18th centuries*, trans. Eric Nicholson (New York: St. Martin's Press, 1990).

47   See Alasdair MacIntyre, *Whose Justice? Which Rationality?* (Notre Dame, IN: University of Notre Dame Press, 1988), 157, 160, 163.

48   Snyder, "The Left Hand of God," 35; Augustine, *Tractates on the Gospel of John, 28-54*, trans. John W. Rettig, *The Fathers of the Church*, vol. 3 (Washington, DC: The Catholic University of America Press, 1993), 41.8: 142–3.

49   Bolton, *Right Comforting*, 282.

50   Ibid.

into that body of death thou bearest about thee, for the finding out, and furnishing thy selfe with as much matter of sound humiliation as may be; that thou maist still grow viler and viler in thine owne eyes, and bee more and more humble untill thy dying Day.[51]

Early modern evangelicals were here again following Augustine and other patristic writers. "Hee that thinkes, He hath sorrowed enough for His sinnes, never sorrowed savingly," Bolton wrote, glossing Augustine's "Si dixisti, sufficit, perusti."[52]

Bolton also echoed Augustine's point that such sorrow was done not out of fear alone, but out of a love of God. The repentant soul, Bolton wrote, having seen the extent of its sin and its offence to its savior, "canst not chuse, but mourne more heartily, Evangelically ... and sweetly perpetuate the spring of godly sorrow, more pleasingly unto God."[53] Yet for the apparently few people poised dangerously on the abyss of terminal despair, the moment of holy desperation and godly sorrow had to be persistently countered with hope, otherwise an individual might become sinfully despairing, rejecting such instruments of grace as prayer and scripture, blasphemously asserting a divine inability or unwillingness to save, or committing the sin of self-murder. Thus Bolton, whose descriptions of legal terror were particularly vivid, sought to convey a more balanced representation of the Christian temper. Bolton warned the individual "truly and heartily humbled for all his sins, and weary of their weight" against continuing in mere mourning in the experience of conversion, "tho' the degree of his sorrow be not answerable to his own desire": "Thou maist, by the unsettledness of thy heavie heart, unnecessarily unfit and disable thy self for the duties and discharge of ... thy callings" and gratify the Devil, who, through his "lying suggestions, will "detain thee in perpetual horror."[54] Echoing Chrysostom, he asserted that evangelical sorrow, far from being terrifying, "is mingled with abundance of spiritual joy which doth infinitely surpass in sweetness and worth, all worldly pleasures and delights of sense."[55]

The two moments of grief and joy which made up the substance of the Christian life were both of central concern in ministering to the religious melancholic. In the context of his emphasis on the necessity of godly sorrow and legal terror, Bolton asserted that melancholy was a potentially positive constituent of spirituality. The melancholy, he said:

> have a passive advantage ... by reason of their sad dispositions, and fearefull spirits, to be sooner affrighted, and dejected by comminations of judgments against sinne; more feelingly to take to heart the miseries, and dangers of their naturall state; more easily to tremble and stoope under the mighty hand of God, and hammer of his Law, Guiltinesse, and horrour, damnation and hell beget in their timerous natures stronger impressions of

---

51 Ibid., 298–9.
52 Ibid., 288–9; 296. The marginal citation is of Augustine, but no work is given.
53 Ibid., 297; see also 171.
54 Ibid., 297.
55 Ibid., 293.

feare: whereupon they are wont to taste deeplier of legall contrition, and remorse; and so proportionably to feele and acknowledge a greater necessity of *Jesus Christ*.[56]

After conversion, the melancholic has "more watchfulnesse over their wayes, tendernesse of conscience, impatiency of loving spirituall peace, sensiblenesse of infermities, and failings, awfulnes to Gods Word, &c." And they are readier to cultivate godly sorrow, "improving naturall sadnesse to mourne more heartily for sinne," while holding fast, of course, to all the Gospel promises to the repentant.[57]

This last requirement seemed to have proved rather difficult for many pious individuals, and this helps to explain the enormous literature of consolation for religious despair. Evangelical protestant ministers themselves recognized that some Christians were unable to sustain the difficult dialectic of holy desperation and salvific joy, and found themselves slipping into terminal despair. Even after they had received the comforts of the Gospel, and had heard arguments for the evidence of grace in their lives, many earnest Christians could not shake the feeling that they were nevertheless damned. But where historians such as Stachniewski have blamed the confluence of Calvinist theology, social frustration and authoritarian child-rearing practices for what he regards as widespread despair in the sixteenth and seventeenth centuries, English divines themselves looked to melancholy for an explanation of the spiral into inconsolable doubt.[58] Even Bolton's estimation of the spiritual value of the melancholic humor was prefaced by the prescription of "the art, and aide of physicke" to "abate and take off the excesse and phantasticalnesse of this horrible humor."[59] And against the criticism of those like Richard Napier, evangelical ministers urged would-be spiritual physicians to be sensitive to the temperaments of their patients in their efforts to heal their souls. In his popular consolatory work *The Bruised Reed and Smoaking Flax*, Richard Sibbes advised against "austerity" and "dark speeches" in ministering to those who, weak in their grace, were prone to doubt and fear.[60] Likewise, Greenham cautioned that legal terror might be used to harmful effect in individuals given to fear and sadness and urged specifically that pastors "find out whether by nature" an afflicted individual is "more fearful or melancholy or no."[61]

More controversial was the application of the Gospel's purgative medicine to those suffering from cases of melancholy apparently unmixed with religious despair or affliction of conscience. In defending against the criticism that Puritan religiosity drove men mad, Bolton claimed that far from making individuals mad, the Gospel was something of a universal panacea. Quoting Chrysostom, Bolton set forth that

---

56 Ibid., 211.

57 Ibid., 212; cf. Thomas Cooper, *The Sacred mysterie of the government of the thoughts* (London: B. Alsop, 1619), 189–90, 196–7.

58 Stachniewski, *Persecutory Imagination*, 60–61.

59 Bolton, *Right Comforting*, 203.

60 Sibbes, *The Bruised Reed and Smoaking Flax* (London: J.G. for R. Dawlman, 1658), 55.

61 Greenham, *A Most Sweete ... Comfort*, sig. Gv.

"there is no malady, either of body, or soule, but may receive a medicine out of Gods Booke."[62] He touted the same line when it came to melancholy:

> A melancholicke man, let him turne ... which way hee will, is like without the light of grace, to live, a very miserable life upon earth, and as it were in some part of hellish darknesse: to which also at length, shall be added the torment, if he dye impenitently. But now let them addresse themselves to the *Booke of Life*, and thence onely they may *sucke, and be satisfied with the brests of consolation.*[63]

Greenham, too, encouraged the cure of melancholic trouble of mind through the Gospel. In ministering to the those suffering from trouble of mind, Greenham declared, one must first bring "them to the sight of sin, as to some cause of their trouble."[64] Here he dealt with the classic mental expression of melancholy – unspecific emotional upset – and moved quickly to fix the object of fear and sorrow on sin. Whereas physician Timothy Bright had emphasized that the feature distinguishing melancholy from affliction of conscience was the presence of a clear and reasonable cause in the case of the latter, Greenham sought to create the presence of this cause in the conditions of general sorrow.[65] Or, if we ignore the curious hypothetical conjunctive phrasing, and the indefinite adjective describing the cause – "as to some cause of their trouble" – Greenham sought to uncover the conditions he believed lay unrecognized at the root such trouble. Perkins recognized that it was melancholy he was treating, but he was no less explicit in his prescription of spiritual treatment than was Greenham. In the case of melancholics, Perkins wrote, "search and triall must be made, whether he hath in him any beginnings of grace, as of faith and repentance, or no. If he be a carnall man, and wanteth knowledge of his estate, then meanes must be used to bring him to some sight and sorrow for his sinnes, that his melancholy sorrow may be turned into a godly sorrow."[66] Later in the century, the minister Richard Baxter would qualify his therapeutic work to exclude those melancholic souls who merely aped the affliction of conscience; late sixteenth and early seventeenth-century practical divines in fact encouraged the expression of melancholy in the language of spiritual affliction.[67]

This may seem a rather duplicitous practice, and an exceptionally unhelpful one from a therapeutic point of view. Richard Napier certainly thought so.[68] Yet even works which intended specifically to console melancholy followed this line of thought. Burton prefaced his consolation of melancholic despair by presupposing "that which *Beza, Greenham, Perkins, Bolton,* give in charge, the parties to whom

---

62 Bolton, *Right Comforting*, 204–10.
63 Ibid., 212.
64 Greenham, *A Most Sweete ... Comfort*, sig. Fij.
65 Bright, *Treatise of Melancholie*, 188.
66 Perkins, *Cases of Conscience*, 114.
67 On Baxter, see below, pages 105–114.
68 See MacDonald, *Mystical Bedlam*, 217–31.

counsel is given be sufficiently prepared, humbled for their sins."[69] Furthermore, from a broader perspective than the discourse on melancholy or religious despair, the call to repentance can be seen as an expression of a common conceptual and symbolic structuring of sin and disease shared by most early modern Christians. Illness in general was viewed as an important occasion for evaluating the state of the soul and the individual's relation to God. This is most obviously because illness was a threshold experience, in which the soul began to loosen from the body, its concerns turned towards the after-life. On a level no less profound, the relation between the disease of sin and natural diseases was in fact basic to the Christian perception of both. In was generally held that the Fall of humankind had introduced natural diseases, which were still the means of God's providential punishment for sin. In the preface to *The Anatomy of Melancholy*, Burton framed the phenomenon of melancholic affliction as a whole in relation to the fallenness of humankind.[70] The pious who suffered from physical pain and disease turned to examine their life for sin, with the understanding that disease was a part of the process of purification of the soul. Disease was one of the many trials and temptations which nudged the believer towards acknowledgement of their dependence on God, fostering patience, hope and faith, and administering the bitter vinegar which revealed sin to the humbled Christian.[71]

These sensibilities concerning disease and sin were merely applied to cases of those troubled in mind by those like Abernethy, Burton and Puritan ministers. In his *Short rules sent to a gentlewoman troubled in mind* (1621), Greenham suggested the ends of Providence as a way of understanding mental affliction: "Believe always your estate to be the work of God, and vary not therein: for your humiliation, your consolation, the glory of God, and the good of many others."[72] It was to be understood that melancholy was itself a means of Providence:

> Beware that you do not often alter your judgement of your estate; as saying, sometimes it is Gods work, sometimes melancholy, sometimes your weakness and simplicity, sometimes witchery, sometimes Satan: you may think melancholy to be an occasion, but no cause, and so of the rest. Therefore look steadfastly to the hand of God, surely trusting on this, that he

---

69   Burton, *Anatomy*, III.iv.II.vi: 468–9.

70   Burton, *Anatomy*, "Democritus Junior to the Reader."

71   See Keith Thomas, *Religion and the Decline of Magic* (New York: Charles Scribner & Sons, 1971), 90–132; Lucinda M. Beier, *Sufferers and Healers: The Experience of Illness in Seventeenth-century England* (London: Routledge & Kegan Paul, 1987); Andrew Wear, "Puritan Perceptions of Illness in Seventeenth-century England," in Roy Porter, ed., *Patients and Practitioners: Lay Perceptions of Medicine in Pre-industrial Society* (Cambridge: Cambridge University Press, 1985), 71–6.

72   Greenham, *Short rules sent to a gentlewoman troubled in mind, for her direction and consolation* (London: T. Suodham for T. Pavier, 1621), rule 15. It is significant that Greenham is addressing a gentle*woman*: the gendered dimension of spiritual therapy and melancholy is dealt with below, on pages 77–81.

not only knoweth thereof, but that whatsoever is done directly, or indirectly, by means or immediately; all is done and governed (by his divine providence) for your good.[73]

That melancholy was to be thought an occasion, but no cause, was a caution against dismissing the work of conscience. The temptation to dismiss the affliction of conscience as mere melancholy was, as I have suggested, the reason why writers attempted to show that the two disorders could be distinguished by their symptoms and that a given case could be clearly identified as either a spiritual malady or a physical disease. But the providential understanding of disease itself directed the mentally troubled to explore a spiritual dimension to their condition. Bright drew a sharper distinction than most of the evangelical ministers between the case of God actively withholding "the comfort of his spirite from you for a season" and the melancholic "frailtie wherein you stand [diminishing] the sense thereof," yet in the case of the body's weakness he gave a providential gloss and emphasized the practice of the passive spiritual virtues. In the case of melancholy, he wrote, "knowe that nothing befalleth you straunge herein more then to other of Gods children before you, and that to wade through these violent streames, patience and constancie is most needfull, with a resulute mind to abide the Lords wil, who in the end wil come, and will not tarie."[74] Melancholy was simply one of the many trials allowed by God to exercise the faith, patience and hope of the elect.

The devil's bath

Burton pointed out in *The Anatomy of Melancholy* how melancholy grossly exaggerated sources of fear and worry.[75] The religious melancholic was thus often thoroughly and incorrigibly convinced not only that they were a sinner and justly condemned by the law, but that the were damned for ever, that God could not or would not save them. As the author of *The Wonderfull History, Case and Cure of Mrs. Drake* (1647, 1654) wrote in his account of the melancholic suffering of Joan Drake: she everywhere "read her own damnation," and "hearde judgments and arraignements herself."[76] For most early modern English Calvinists, these fearful and condemnatory perceptions recalled the biblical figure of the devil as

---

73 Greenham, *Short rules*, rule 16.

74 Bright, *Treatise of Melancholie*, 234.

75 Burton, *Anatomy*, I.iii.I.ii: 447.

76 [John Oh-ni, pseud.], *The Firebrand taken out of the Fire, or, The Wonderfull History, Case and Cure of Mrs. Drake* (London: for Thomas Mathewes, 1654), 56–65. This account was first published as [John Oh-ni, pseud.], *Trodden downe strengthe, or, Mrs. Drake Revived* (London: R. Bishop for Stephen Pilkington, 1647). All references will be made to the 1654 edition, unless otherwise noted. There is an important difference in the prefaces to the two editions, which I deal with below (see page 116). On the authorship of this narrative, see George Hunston Williams, "Called by Thy Name, Leave Us Not: The Case of Mrs. Joan Drake, A Formative Episode in the Pastoral Career of Thomas Hooker in England, Part II," *Harvard Library Bulletin* 16 (1968): 278–300.

"the accuser of the brethren," who "deceiveth the whole world," working hard to convince God's children that they were not forgiven.[77] It was the devil who, in the words of Greenham, made sin the size of "the smallest prick of a pin" into "a globe of the whole earth" in the perception of the tempted believer, in order to discourage the convicted soul of applying to the grace of God for salvation.[78] If the proximate cause of melancholic spiritual affliction was a disorder of the body, often the content of the religious melancholic's thoughts was regarded as demonic. The devil himself was "mixed with our melancholy humours," as Burton put it.[79]

The account of the case of Joan Drake is a particularly illuminating illustration of the demonological approach to religious melancholy. Recounting the case of a religiously melancholic gentlewoman which took place in Esher (Surrey) in the 1620s and involved the counsel of a series of well-known Puritan divines, the narrative draws simultaneously on melancholy and the devil to explain Drake's spiritual suffering and temptation, illustrating perfectly the interpenetration of the demonic and the physical which the concept of melancholy enabled.[80] It illustrates as well the specific therapies used by evangelical ministers in treating the religious melancholic, the aim of which was not as much to cure melancholy as to place the demonic utterances and beliefs of the melancholic in a theological context that disarmed their despairing effect. Like moral philosophical therapies, religious therapies limited and contained melancholy, which otherwise all too often ended in madness.

Mrs. Drake Revived conforms in part to what scholars have termed the "Puritan conversion narrative," the general structure of which provided for the godly community a pattern of experience and expression to be copied and cultivated.[81] Like Augustine's *Confessions*, the "Puritan" conversion narrative moved from emphasizing a profligate life of sin through a moment of conviction and legal terror to eventual comfort in the hope of the Gospel. *Mrs. Drake Revived* begins by noting that although Joan Drake was a "Good Gentlewoman," full of love, courtesie, mercy and meekness, affable in conversation...tender-hearted, free and bountifull, in nothing covetous but of grace; the freest alive from hypocrisy, unless it were to belie herself," she was not "acquainted with the powers of godliness" before her episode of spiritual affliction.[82] Indeed, she would, "sometimes in a little mirth," "vex and jest with the supposed worser sort [the godly]." But her teasing of the godly belied a

---

77 Revelation 12:9–10; 2 Corinthians 2:11; see also 1 Peter 5:8 (KJV).

78 Greenham, *A Most Sweete ... Comfort*, sig. E.

79 *Anatomy*, I.ii.I.ii, 229. See also Michael MacDonald and Terence R. Murphy, *Sleepless Souls: Suicide in Early Modern England* (Oxford: Clarendon Press, 1990), 59.

80 Biographical details of Mrs. Drake, her family and the ministers involved in her case can be found in George Hunston Williams, "Called by Thy Name, Leave Us Not: The Case of Mrs. Joan Drake, A Formative Episode in the Pastoral Career of Thomas Hooker in England, Part I," *Harvard Library Bulletin* 16 (1968): 111–28.

81 Patricia Caldwell, *The Puritan Conversion Experience: The Beginnings of American Expression* (Cambridge: Cambridge University Press, 1983); Owen C. Watkins, *The Puritan Experience: Studies in Spiritual Autobiography* (New York: Schocken Books, 1972).

82 *Mrs. Drake*, 6–7.

secret admiration, as a "strange presaging" comment to one of her ladies-in-waiting evidences: "Doest thou see these people, some of whom I doe so jeare at and vex; of my conscience, I shall one day 'ere I die bee one of them; for those of them who are right, are the only happy souls." Thus, as the narrator presents the case in a summary at the end of the account, the story of Mrs. Drake was a case of a convicted conscience leading eventually through despair to salvation:

> A Good creature, in her natural estate … accidentally encountering with some grand difficulties, which a little overcame her natural parts. By the way, being surprized with admiration and wonder at the power of godliness in some eminent Professors her Neighbours (the reflex whereof struck her with a strong conviction, not to be yet the same, as to be saved she must needs be) with her other concurring crosses, wrought so upon her, as she became very melancholy, yet with an enforced mirth to cloke the same; which advantage Satan espying (who still loves to work out his ends by that doleful temper) he assaults her with fearful night-dreams, seconded with divers wild-fire temptations to have driven her unto final despair.[83]

As we have seen, it was not unusual to recognize the contribution of melancholy to the conversion moment. Robert Bolton argued that "there is a kind of natural power, besides God's special hand, in sickness, sorrow, darkness, melancholy, the night, extraordinary crosses, the Bed of Death, to represent the true number, and heinousness of sins with greater horror, and more unto the life."[84] The devil was also regarded by many early moderns as an instrument of God's spiritual affliction, and the temptation of the Devil in the affliction of conscience was a common way of accounting for the sustained severity of some spiritual afflictions. "Satan is Gods Beadle, or Master of his correction-houses," noted the preface to the 1654 edition of *Mrs. Drake*; "but his discipline is sore and severe."[85]

In the case of the Mrs. Drake narrative, however, the presence of the devil shifts the emphasis almost entirely from her melancholic case of conscience as a moment of the legal terror in the process of conversion to a moment of dangerous diabolical temptation to despair. To put it differently, the "normal" sense of just condemnation is magnified into the sense that she is *irredeemably* damned. This, among other features of her behavior such as attempts to kill herself, betrays to the godly community presence of the devil. The story thus is structured somewhat along the lines of a Christian morality play as a struggle between the devil and the godly for the soul of Mrs. Drake. The precipitating event is Mrs. Drake's afflicted conscience; but the substance of the action is generated in the battle between the godly community, who seek to heal Drake's afflicted conscience, and the devil, who seeks to create out of her legal terror the entrenched belief that she is necessarily damned. As the preface put it, echoing Greenham: "this wound is such that the Devils claw is awaies in, to prick and gall it, and to give scarce any respite of torment or time to close and heal."

---

83 Ibid., 165–6.
84 Bolton, *Right Comfort*, 480; see also 488, 490.
85 *Mrs. Drake*, "To the Christian Reader."

The natural course of conversion through legal terror is interrupted by melancholy and the devil, and the full weight of spiritual consolation, the application of the Gospel against the terrors of the Law, is necessary.

This explains why, in the course of the effort to comfort Drake, her natural goodness is emphasized throughout the narrative. It was highly unusual for a conversion narrative to emphasize the natural goodness of an individual in their pre-conversion state, as did the author's summary of the case.[86] Calvinist theology represented the soul without grace as entirely depraved; in the Augustinian framework which so profoundly informed Reformed theology, natural virtue was taken to be ultimately motivated by self-interest and pride.[87] But in the context of Joan Drake's life, her sudden affliction of great horror revealed to the godly community not a moment of truth, the revelation and acceptance of her worthlessness as a human creature, but of diabolical deception. It was a *"strange hypocrisie,"* writes the narrator, that "shee was pitifull and mercifull unto others, but in secret so hid and clokt with words and shewes of the contrary, that it was treason against her for any she entrusted, to bewray any part of parcell of her goodnesse; because shee would gladly have beene thought past hope."[88] Her natural goodness functioned in spiritual therapy as a sign of grace with which others countered her claims to know her damnation. Calvinist orthodoxy emphasized the depravity of the unregenerate, but the godly could be quite flexible in their theology when it came to comforting those oppressed by the devil and in danger of despair, the outcome of which was to turn away from the means of grace and ultimately to kill oneself.[89] To emphasize further the point developed above: from the perspective of most pastoral writers, melancholy was often seen as the root of the inability to hold legal terror and evangelical hope in productive tension, and it was urged that those intending to win souls had need to be sensitive to the psychophysiological intolerance of certain individuals to the more condemnatory and difficult passages of Scripture.

Mrs. Drake Revived thus moved between a conversion narrative and what might be termed the affliction narrative, the purpose of which was to provide both hope against despair and a warning against presumption. In his posthumously published *Narration of the grievous visitation, and dreadfull desertion of Mr. Peacock in his last sickness* (1641), Bolton asserted that the story of Thomas Peacock's deathbed religious despair was a "Mirror of Gods justice and Mercy, being as well an antidote against despair … on the left hand; and also … a curb of restraint unto, a warning piece, and counterpoison against Presumption, on the right hand." Peacock was a respected and eminently pious sixteenth-century Oxford fellow and one of Bolton's

---

86 See Watkins, *Puritan Experience*, 231–2.

87 See John Calvin, *Institutes of the Christian Religion*, ed. John T. McNeill, trans. Ford Lewis Battles (Philadelphia, PA: The Westminster Press, 1960), 2.iii.4, 3.xiv.3; on Augustine, see E.J. Hundert, "Augustine and the Sources of the Divided Self," *Political Theory* 20 (1992): 86–104, esp. 96–7.

88 *Mrs. Drake*, 25.

89 See Williams, "Called by Thy Name … Part I," 125–6.

own spiritual mentors, and the counterpoison here was thus the fact that even a man as godly as Peacock could be afflicted with such "temptations, griefes of conscience, and restless terrors" that "none can understand, much less express, but *he* which felt them." Righteousness was not itself any protection against despair, and however godly Christians were in life and conduct, they were forced to rely on God's mercy for ultimate comfort.[90] *Mrs. Drake Revived* similarly urged the need for God's mercy: "if smaller sins discovered thus set on and torment, yea, some only, as in this Good Gentlewoman; oh! what may the greater doe, if [God] should aggravate them, discovering the wrath due unto them, without a suitable sight of mercy."[91] The intended hope in both narratives came from the eventual triumph over despair. The 1647 edition of *Mrs. Drake Revived* bore a notice of permission to print written by John Downame, famous for his work in practical divinity, who declared there that the book was "well worthy to be Printed and published, as a singular antidote to preserve others in her condition, from being plunged into and quite swallowed up with deep despaire."[92] Although Joan Drake was plagued with "dangerous tentations and fearefull desertions," "her blessed recovery, and joyfull issue out of all her troubles" upheld the point of comfort urged in many pastoral works that spiritual affliction was to be seen as a matter of God's "correcting Justice" rather than his lasting withdrawal, part of the work of bringing his children back onto the path of righteousness and faith rather than an effect of his condemnation. As Foxe argued in the case of John Glover, Glover's final triumph showed that God did not allow his saints to be tempted above their capacity.[93]

John Glover, Thomas Peacock, and Joan Drake were thus represented as being patterns and parables for the *via media* between presumption and despair. They demonstrated the great humility and self-excoriation of the saint; and in emphasizing the sudden moment of divine comfort after long periods of despair, they gave afflicted readers hope in their own struggles with despair. In the case of Drake, the author acknowledged at the same time that her experience of spiritual affliction was caused by her melancholy. But her melancholic body does not put into question the legitimacy of her spiritual experience. Melancholy was simply considered by the narrator and the ministers treating her as the natural cause through which the devil worked, which exacerbated her affliction of conscience, but did not cause it.

Joan Drake's was a classic case of disappointment and emotional distress transformed into a melancholic temperament, irrupting into a more acute melancholic madness through complications at childbirth. She was married to "such a one … whom at first she could not affect," and so against her own desire. This, the narrator

90   Bolton, *A narration of the grievous visitation, and dreadfull desertion of Mr. Peacock in his last sicknesse* (London: for Robert Milbourn, 1641), 11–12; *Mrs. Drake*, "To the Christian Reader."

91   *Mrs. Drake*, 174.

92   *Mrs. Drake* (1647).

93   Foxe, *Actes and Monuments*, 2: 1552.

declares, "first bred in her the foundation of those stormes and tempests, which in time were in danger to have overthrown her":

> [T]hough she were obedient and dutiful to her Parents; yet it stuck close unto her, though her strength of spirit and jovial temper endeavoured with all her strength to have shaken it off, out-worn it, and by all meanes out-faced it, without of discontent, by merry company and divers journeys (which usually divert melancholy thoughts) as though there had been no such matter. But griefe being like unto fire, which though for a time smothered, yet could not be concealed, her discontent did secretly work upon her a habit of sadness in the midst of her mirth with her friends.[94]

The heading in the margin reads "Cause of her melancholy," and we can see here the conventional wisdom concerning melancholy. It is generated from strength of passion, which, if it is not subdued, breeds changes in the body towards a settled emotional disposition of sadness. Mrs. Drake, of a "natural jovial constitution", became "accidentally melancholy."[95] Later, in delivering a daughter, she was, as the result of "being wronged by her Midwife":

> ever after troubled with fumes and vapours mounting up unto her head, which bred in her for the most part a continual head-ach, like unto a megrum, together with somewhat like unto a fire continually burning in her stomach, which no physick could remove, or was not God's pleasure it should; the which drew her towards a more constant constitution of sadness and distemper, though yet with her usuall strength of spirit and chearfull disposition, shee out-faced, as though she had been well. But a fire of discontent being kindled full of sad thoughts in her; which bred and encreased all the time she lay in of her daughter.[96]

Medical authorities often listed headaches and gastro-intestinal discomfort among the physical symptoms of the melancholic condition, while the etiology, since it involves the female reproductive system, suggests what Burton termed "Maids', Nuns' and Widows' Melancholy."[97] The story, however, moves immediately on to her spiritual affliction: "Thus it fell out, That … in the fore-part of the night she fell asleep, but not long after fell into terrible shrieks and out-cryes to this purpose, that *she was damned, and a cast-away, and so of necessity must needs go to Hell,' and therewith shook, dropt down with sweat, and wept exceedingly.*"[98] These were immediately recognized by those caring for her as the lies of the devil. Her mother (whom the narrator does not identify as one of the godly) comforts her during this first fit by telling her "not to believe illusions, that the Devil was a liar."[99] Mr. Dod, the famous and respected practical divine who had ministered to Thomas Peacock and whom the

---

94 *Mrs. Drake*, 9.
95 Ibid., 6–7.
96 Ibid., 11–12.
97 See Burton, *Anatomy*, I.iii.I.i: 439–42; I.iii.II.ii: 472–5; and I.iii.II.iv: 476–8.
98 *Mrs. Drake*, 11.
99 Ibid., 12.

narrator persuades to help Mrs. Drake, was to urge the same against her fears using the logic of predestinarian theology: it was impossible *"for the Devil ... to know the decree of God, either for salvation or reprobation*; but that this revelation came in the use of meanes God blessing the same; for which cause all must use the meanes who would be saved."[100]

Mr. Dod makes considerable progress in refuting the lies of the devil, but her melancholic disease continues to provide a basis of demonic resistance. Mr. Dod addresses many of the possible grounds of her fears that she is damned, convincing her that she had not sinned against the Holy Ghost; that her alleged indisposition to godliness was no sign of damnation; that only the use of the means – prayer, preaching, communion – revealed one's estate; and that "all experiences since the beginning of the world have shewed, that it never yet was in vaine, or unsuccessefull, but alwayes advantageous and prosperous to use the meanes, waite and depend upon God."[101] The narrative records that she became convinced of these points, and that "she were contented to do what she could in using the meanes, if she might bee assured to reape benefit thereby." However, against Mr. Dod's assertion that her indisposition to godliness was entirely in her will, she pleaded her disease, "that the accidental indisposition both of her body and mind were such as in this case could do nothing to help herself, no more than a stark dead creature could; and therefore, that God must do all; in which case, if hee were so pleased to give her strength and grace to work, then she would; otherwise she could do nothing." Although convinced by Mr. Dod's arguments that she could not know God's will as to her estate and that God saved through the human use of the appointed means, she was apparently still gripped by fear and anxiety: "she could not pray; and for reading of the Word, to what purpose were that, so to read her own damnation, or to heare judgements and arraignements against herself." The narrator draws attention to her refusal of the means as an indication of the devil: it was "a sore temptation, which even until her last she could hardly shake off." For his part, Mr. Dod noted the influence of her physical distemper. Hopeful because of the ground gained, Dod declared that her recovery still "seemed a tough task to effect: because the indisposition and melancholy temper of her body was such as hindered much the work, she therewith being adverse to Physick."[102]

Some improvement in her spiritual state did appear over time, although interrupted by lapses. For a time, she joins in the singing of Psalms, and goes to hear sermons. Indeed, "willingly shee would have lived under some powerfull Ministry, hoping, that thereby some such work might be wrought upon her, as might enable her to performe duties," although plans to live with Mr. Rogers of Dedham, renowned for his powerful, indeed thunderous preaching, did not materialize. Secretly she began to be comforted with the words of the book of Micah: "He wil turne againe, *and* have compassion upon us: he wil subdue our iniquities, & cast all their sinnes into

---

100 Ibid., 50–51.
101 Ibid., 58.
102 Ibid., 56–65.

the bottome of the sea" (Micah 7:10). However, afraid that if she claimed comfort it would vanish as an illusion in the self-accusations of pretension, she did not voice her comfort. The narrator sums up the slow course of recovery under the hindrance of illness as "now up, now down, the better she grew in her mind, having still therewithall the greater weakness and indisposition of body."

It is tempting for the historian of psychiatry and madness to assess the efficacy of spiritual therapy in subduing melancholic distemper. H.C. Eric Midelfort has thus speculated favorably on the parallel between modern modes of therapy and early modern religious understandings and treatments that invoked the devil, and MacDonald implies in his indictment of the late seventeenth-century medicalization of the treatment of madness that the psychological healing of those like the "Puritans" was therapeutically sounder than the techniques of the medical art.[103] Yet the question of efficacy is impossible to answer; even in the contemporary world of mental illness; where some clients see spiritual transformation towards recovery, others see the work of medications, and efforts to transform the process of recovery into the observable lose the crucial ingredient of the patient's perception in statistical generalization. More importantly for our historical understanding, however, we should note that the narrative of Mrs. Drake is concerned with different issues than therapeutic efficacy in curing melancholic disease. Even though the story ends with Mrs. Drake gaining a triumphant sense of assurance about her salvation, the point of the story is not to show recovery from melancholy – that is clearly seen as the job of physick – but to encourage perseverance against melancholy and its demonic dangers within and supported by the community of the godly.

In one sense, it is apparent that she does not recover from the weakness of her body. Even in what the author terms the "Comical Conclusion" of the "tragick-comedy" of *Mrs. Drake*, there is a recurring question about her mental stability. Her moods continue to swing erratically, and her thought seems at times fevered. First, she takes on a "posture of discontent" for some "strong distaste [that] was given her from a near friend."[104] Then she becomes convinced that she is about to die and insists on returning to her father's house, where, "being in a surpassing extraordinary strange humour of talking of the best things perpetually night and day without intrusion, not having any jot of sleep almost day or night ... her spirits were both much spent and tyred out." Mention of her concern with "the best things" is buried here amid bafflement at her mental agitation and concern about her health.[105]

Then at last comes the moment of beatific vision, the moment of absolute assurance for which she has waited all along. At eight o'clock in the morning, the household is aroused by a "strange and uncouthe cry" by one "in shew of rapture of another world":

---

103 Midelfort, *History of Madness*, 106; MacDonald, *Mystical Bedlam*, 217–31.
104 *Mrs. Drake* (1647), 132.
105 Ibid., 134–5.

> She heaved and heaved up still all the time with fixed eyes towards the house-top, as though she had seen some vision, and would have flown away from them all, making a hole through the chamber roof ... This fit of a sudden, extreame, ravishing unsupportable joy, (beyond the strength of mortality to retaine or be long capable or) being over, and shee layd again; who formerly had striven to have got away from them all.

Apparently, this righteous frenzy was physically restrained. And the godly around her do not at first know what to make of it. When she asks them, "[W]hat did you think of me lately in this strange posture I have been in? did you not imagine me to have been mad all the time?", Mr. Dod replies: "that it was very strange unto them all, having never heard or seen the like." She relates that after a prayer for God to "open the brazen gates of this hard heart of mine, that the King of Glory might enter in ... this sudden out-crying fit of unsupportable joy and feeling surprized me with such violence rushing upon me, as I could not containe myself." The godly did indeed rejoice with her as "she lay in her former joyful posture, rejoycing to speak of the best things unto everyone near unto her." They also order a "weakening cooler to keep her down low," lest "she should be lifted through her former revelation, joyes and rapture, so short which endured not, surpassing her strength."[106]

Her joyfulness of temper does not last unabated. She "is surprized with an extreame fainting and weakness of spirits, being for ten days and nights over wearied, watched and toiled out, so as now she bewrayed some weakness in her expressions, not being as formerly so lively and substantial." And it is not just a matter of physical weariness, as the euphemisms would lead us to believe. After she at last falls asleep and wakes up "in a very milde gentle temper", she asks her cousin if she had "not lately in some speeches forgot [herself]?" The cousin's answer suggests some culpability in her manner: "Truly Cousin, so you did, but we imputed the same to your many days and night-watchings, and over-wearying your spirits, unable so to hold out."[107] It seems likely that she continued to struggle with the "harsh and untowards" temper which was the result of her indisposition, and the suggestion in the summary that she *regained* her comfort after this episode of weakness more damagingly suggests that she continued to struggle with fear and doubt.[108] As evidenced in the reaction of the godly community to her behavior, melancholic distemper remains a concern until her death.[109]

The sudden outpouring of feeling which marks the happy ending, although clearly establishing absolute assurance in a struggling soul, is ultimately downplayed through the concern with the physical dangers of such raptures, encapsulated in a bit of moralizing at the end of the story: "Seeing too eager desire of feeling cost this Gentlewoman so deare though she had her desire, therefore not to dote too much upon it ... Let them be contented of what measure thereof God of his infinite wisdom

---

106 *Mrs. Drake*, 132–58.
107 Ibid., 159–61.
108 Ibid., 122–3, 168.
109 Ibid., 159–60.

thinks best for them."[110] The triumph is not in the vision which so weakens her spirits, and perpetuates her bodily distemper, but in the peace that can be built up in the slow process of spiritual therapy, by addressing gross misconceptions and lies, and by turning the patient towards the practice of godliness without regard to the feeling of absolute certainty.

If she still suffers from physical distemper, however, it is clear that the devil has been defeated; she has been gradually dispossessed, even before the vision of assurance. This is evidenced in her gradual willingness to use the means and to find comfort in scripture; but it can also be seen in the withdrawal of the Devil from the bodily distemper in the telling of the story. Mrs. Drake's relapse into spiritual weakness after her vision, as well as her frenetic and at times unruly behavior, is referred only to the weakness of her body, an understanding which she apparently shares in. She concurs with her cousin's explanation of her spiritual lapse after her vision of assurance: "So it was, said she, My spirits were spent and gone, which caused that weakness."[111] Her struggle shifts from a struggle with the devil to a too eager desire for a strong measure of feeling in her faith and the disorder of body that follows. Essentially, she is transformed from one possessed to a typical "Puritan," filled with vexing questions, troubled by the doldrums of religious feeling, desirous of assurance, but using the means of grace and holding fast to the modicum of comfort she has found.

Anthropologists have analyzed the rituals surrounding dispossession according to culturally defined roles which the possessed can adopt and the set of prescribed actions and text through which the possessed and the community perform the dispossession.[112] The affliction of Mrs. Drake can be thought of in similar terms. It is clear that the godly community sees in her erratic behavior and fearful thoughts the possession of the devil. The preface of the 1654 edition makes clear that the case was one of possession, rather than demonic suggestion or temptation alone: "While this Intruder was Master and Governer of this Gentlewoman, her tongue uttered his Oracles, and was taught to speak nothing but what favoured the spirit that ruled her."[113] Her text is the self-accusation of damnation. She complains that "God had forsaken her, and given her over unto a reprobate sense, her hard heart could not repent, and that in all her actions shee but heaps up wrath against the day of wrath to her further condemnation; and that in that whee could not grieve, nor be sorrowful, for that woefull estate she was now in, this shew the desperateness thereof."[114] Michel de Certeau has shown that Catholic exorcists were keen on identifying the demon possessing the individual in order that the possession could

---

110 Ibid., 174–5.

111 Ibid., 161.

112 See Clark, *Thinking with Demons*, 396–400.

113 *Mrs. Drake*, "To the Christian Reader." The element of demonic possession and temptation was strongly present in the 1647 edition of *Mrs. Drake* despite the difference in preface.

114 *Mrs. Drake*, 23.

be located within the discourse of demonology, which then provided the necessary techniques for dispossession according to the nature of the demon in question.[115] Evangelical Reformed ministers, who had rejected the Catholic rituals of exorcism, sought to render the language of self-accusation and spiritual complaint in terms of the discourse of theology; they sought to uncover the specific diabolical lies that were at the root of the individual's determined self-accusation, which they could then address with theological and scriptural argument.

The devil, the narrator of *Mrs. Drake* related, uses secrecy to create private delusions which then feed fear and despair:

> to make mountaines of molehils, and of mole-hils mighty mountaines; never suffering them to come unto the knowledge of the quality and nature of their disease, whilst the thing oppressing and seeming great unto them, is usually little, and nothing at all in respect of that he makes it; sometimes but a lie, a delusion, such as parties themselves upon such discoveries in relating become ashamed of.[116]

Mr. Dod's first triumph is thus to have her disclose to him "the cause and ground of all her distempers and trouble, and what just cause she thus had to have complained, as hopeless."[117] She confesses privately to Dod that she believes herself to have sinned the unpardonable sin against the Holy Ghost. Dod then walks her through the reasons why this was not true, pointing out that she had not wilfully turned away from God's calling to faith. In the end:

> all she could alleadge against herself, consisting only in a matter of thoughts … which were only things wrept up in that we call *tentatio Foeda*, strange injected thoughts of God, as *Rom.* 1:23, representing him to the fancy in abominable similtudes, likening him to the vilest and basest things; which were only Satans wild fire tentations; for which seeing she even then, and since, abominated them, being sorry for them, Satan must answer for, *they being hers no further than as she entertained and allowed of them.*[118]

When she insists none the less that she simply knows that she is damned, Dod counters with the predestinarian assertion that this knowledge is God's alone and is revealed only through the use and pursuit of his appointed means for salvation – hearing the word, prayer, meditation, repentance. When she claims that her heart is hard, that she had no inclination to repent, pray, and listen to the Scripture, and that therefore she is damned, it is countered that there are degrees of faith, and that even second-order desire, the desire to desire to repent, pray, and feel godly sorrow, were indications of faith; and furthermore, the willingness to perform outwardly the duties of the godly manifested an obedience to God, even where an inward inclination

---

115 De Certeau, *The Writing of History*, trans. Tom Conley (New York: Columbia University Press, 1988), 244–68.
116 *Mrs. Drake*, 34–5.
117 Ibid., 32–3.
118 Ibid., 46–7.

was absent.[119] Dod sought throughout to hold her responsible to reason, encouraging her to provide a defense of the legitimacy of her feelings, then using theological discourse to show the weakness of these reasons. Recognizing that the weakness of her body influenced her mind, he insisted that she concentrate on theological argument instead of melancholic feeling.

Attempts by ministers to exorcize demons, such as the apparently unsuccessful vigils and fasts that were held on several occasions for Joan Drake, were a focal point of tension between the more evangelical Protestants of the Church and the Church authorities and part of the impetus behind the move of some intellectuals to replace demonological perceptions with diagnoses based solely on medical theory and natural philosophy.[120] Writing in response to claims that the demoniac Mary Glover had been dispossessed through prayer and fasting, Dr. Edward Jorden argued in *A briefe discourse of a disease called the suffocation of the mother* (1603) that although it was not to be denied that there were real cases of possession and witchcraft, men and women were far too ready to describe as demoniacs persons who could be more accurately diagnosed with a natural disease.[121] The activity of one of the most notorious of the "Puritan" exorcists, the minister John Darell, had earlier provoked John Walker and John Deacon's *Dialogicall Discourses of Spirits and Divels* (1601), an attempt to block systematically any possibility of invoking demons as a category of explanation in the examination of physical or behavioral phenomena. The age of possession and exorcism was past, the authors argued, and cases of alleged possession were either fraudulent or the result of diseases which could appear strikingly similar to possession, like epilepsy and melancholy.[122]

The motivation for both Darrell's widely publicized exorcisms and the official reaction was largely polemical. After the Elizabethan Puritan movement had failed to reform the English Church along Presbyterian lines, some took up the practice of exorcism as a test of ecclesiastical legitimacy. The true Church, they argued, was distinguished by the power to cast out demons. Like all Protestants, the "Puritans" eschewed the allegedly "magical" forms of exorcism practiced by the Catholics in favor of prayer and fasting which, according to Protestant sensibilities, was considered the only correct way of dealing with demons, sanctioned as it was by Christ's instruction to his disciples that "this kind [of demon] only comes out by prayer and fasting."[123] But because of the obvious threat to the Church hierarchy's authority and credibility, the very popular exorcisms of Darrell in the opening years of the seventeenth century were a source of concern and embarrassment to the

---

119 Ibid., 50–51, 74–6, 85–6.

120 See Clark, *Thinking with Demons*, 417.

121 On Jorden, see Michael MacDonald, ed., *Witchcraft and Hysteria in Elizabethan London: Edward Jorden and the Mary Glover Case* (London: Routledge, 1991), and Keith Thomas, *Religion*, for example 490, 571–2; Clark, *Thinking with Demons*, 182.

122 On the Darrell controversy and its background, see Keith Thomas, *Religion*, 479–86.

123 See Burton's censure of the "unlawful" and "magical" elements of Catholic exorcisms: *Anatomy*, II.i.i: 5–9.

officials of the Church. In a Church canon of 1604, praying and fasting for the sake of exorcism was prohibited except with the permission of the bishop of the diocese.

Dod and his associates clearly contravened this canon in their vigils and fasts for Joan Drake, and "Puritans" as well as others continued to perceive the activity of the devil in cases of melancholy.[124] Burton, for instance, clearly thought that the devil worked through melancholy. Moreover, in the chapter on lawful cures, coming immediately after his discussion of Catholic exorcism as unlawful and "magical," Burton condoned treatment by prayer and fasting, quoting Christ's words to his disciples in Mark 9:29:

> Some kind of Devils are not cast out but by fasting & prayer, & both necessarily required, not one without the other. For all the physick we can use, art, excellent industry, is to no purpose without calling upon God.[125]

Thus, while the godly community caring for Joan Drake may have contravened the 1604 canon, they were operating well within a broad consensus regarding the presence of the Devil in melancholic affliction. In spite of anti-supernatural arguments like those of Walker and Deacon and ecclesiastical injunction, the time-honored idea of melancholy as the devil's bath continued to provide an important and powerful medium of experiencing and treating the melancholic condition.

The position of Walker and Deacon was, as Stuart Clark has argued of Reginald Scot's anti-supernaturalist view in *The Discoverie of Witchcraft* (1586), an extreme position in early modern demonological discourse.[126] Furthermore, the kinds of arguments which Walker and Deacon put into circulation failed to deal satisfactorily with the notion of the devil's bath. Walker and Deacon asserted that the devil no longer possessed the human mind, but they did admit that he was still present in the world through his power of obsession. Obsession involved things like the devil's physical afflictions, but also his temptations and vexing thoughts. The models for this idea were Job and his physical afflictions, and Christ in the desert tempted by the devil, rather than Saul being overtaken by an evil spirit, and the demoniacs of the Gospels. But when it came to melancholy, the obsession/possession distinction was simply unserviceable, and against the defined and substantial relation between the devil's lies and the delusions of melancholy, the distinction tended to vanish into theoretical thin air. When Burton approached the issue of the extent of the power of demons and the nature of their operation some twenty years later, in 1621, he asserted that the devil worked through melancholy, perhaps even causing melancholy for the purpose of bending its fear and delusion to the soul's destruction, but equivocated on how this well-documented feature of melancholy related to the obsession/possession distinction: "this humour invites the Devil to it, wheresoever it is in extremity, and, of all the other [humors], melancholy persons are most subject to diabolical

---

124 For instances of prayers and fasts for Joan Drake, see *Mrs. Drake* (1647), 20, 22, 26, 27.

125 Burton, *Anatomy*, II.i.II: 10.

126 Clark, *Thinking with Demons*, 417.

temptations and illusions, and most apt to entertain them, and the Devil best able to work upon them; but whether by obsession, or possession, or otherwise, I will not determine; 'tis a difficult question."[127]

H.C. Erik Midelfort suggests that, in the context of Protestant Germany at least, the abandonment and repression of Catholic rituals of exorcism left those expressing forms of possession to languish under medical care as mad rather than being treated according to the language through which they themselves articulated their affliction.[128] I have argued here that there was a language of dispossession in the English Reformed tradition: it was that of the afflicted conscience. Furthermore, medical care was not at all alien to the pastoral concern with the afflicted conscience. The understanding that the devil worked through natural means, and in particular through melancholy, ensured that the treatment of the body was central to the treatment of the soul. Medical and spiritual care were combined as mutually reinforcing approaches in the evangelical ritual of dispossession. Mrs. Drake was regarded, by herself and others, as both sick with melancholy and afflicted of the devil. If she never totally recovered from the various manifestations of a melancholic distemper, supported by other believers she was gradually able to withstand the devil as one of the many weak but hopeful souls whom the enormous pastoral literature consoling the afflicted conscience was intended to encourage.

Ministers, madmen, and women

Katharine Hodgkin points out in her study of Dionys Fitzgerald's autobiographical account of religious despair, written in the seventeenth century, that "the language of the soul in spiritual torment comes dangerously close to that of insanity, and is frequently identified by the unsympathetic as a consequence or a symptom of excessive (unreasonable) emotion."[129] Thus, Richard Greenham noted that many suffering from the affliction of conscience feared the shame of the imputation of madness more than they did the consequences of the sinful condition of their afflicted soul.[130] The stigma of insanity in the early modern period consisted of both the image of madness as bereft of reason, and therefore of humanity, and the suspicion that what had caused the loss of reason was in fact a moral weakness of the soul. Fitzgerald was therefore insistent on proving wrong those who attributed her suffering to "melancholy, or I know not what turning of the braine," framing her suffering, as Spira had his, in terms of "a religious calling and a subsequent fall

---

127 Burton, *Anatomy*, I.ii.I.ii: 229.

128 Midelfort, "Catholic and Lutheran Reactions to Demon Possession in the Late 17th Century," *Daphnis* 15 (1986): 623–48.

129 Hodgkin, "Dionys Fitzherbert and the Anatomy of Madness," in Kate Chedgzoy, Melanie Hansen, and Suzanne Trill, eds., *Voicing Women: Gender and Sexuality in Early Modern Writing* (Keele: Keele University Press, 1996), 76.

130 See page 56 above.

from grace, duly punished by God."[131] As Hogdkin argues, Fitzgerald was claiming the dignity of reason and personhood and attempting to put madness at a distance by casting her state of mental agitation as affliction of conscience.

Timothy Bright had written his *Treatise of Melancholie* motivated in part to counter "the prophanes of othersome, who ... accompt the cause [of the affliction of conscience] naturall, melancholy, or madness, but many physicians of the soul expected a certain amount of distraction of mind and "madness" to accompany conscience of sin.[132] Bolton wrote of the affliction of conscience:

> this extreamist of miseries, *a wounded spirit*, is tempered with such strong, and strange ingredients of extraordinary fears, that it makes a man *a terrour to himself and to all his friends: To flee when none pursues, at the sound of a shaken leafe:* To tremble at his owne shadow: *To bee in great feare, where no feare is*: Besides the insupportable burthen of too many true and causefull terrours, it fills his darke and dreadfull fancy with a world of fained horrors, gastly apparitions, and imaginary hells, which notwithstanding, have reall stings, and impresse true tortures upon his trembling and wofull heart.[133]

The italicized phrases were quotations of Jeremiah 20:4, Leviticus 26:37, and Psalm 53:5 respectively. Yet it appears that this language had been absorbed into the experience itself, for others painted a similar scene with no biblical allusions.[134] Furthermore, such mad terrors and fears were thought to be rather persistent. Perkins wrote that "he that is the comforter, must not be discouraged, though after long labour and paines taking, there follow small comfort and ease to the partie distressed ... for ... usually it is long before comfort can be received."[135] It was thus in spite of such apparent madness that evangelical ministers insisted that the afflicted of conscience were indeed persons who required and deserved pastoral consolation and comfort rather than medical treatment alone. In the case of the melancholic, spiritual therapy may have been a vehicle through which some transfigured a self held passively to sorrow and fear by their bodies into saints exercising patience, forbearance, and hope in the face of affliction, and a reliance on the promises of the gospel in the face of doubt and despair. The suffering of melancholy was thus given meaning, a moral horizon, and the melancholic's life was structured by Christian responsibilities and duties appropriate to their condition of spiritual affliction.

This is not to suggest that evangelical spiritual therapy was efficacious in curing or managing melancholic disease. For one thing, the kind of therapeutic encounter Greenham, Perkins and the *Mrs. Drake* narrative describe and the kinds of virtues it required no doubt approach an ideal. For another, we have to keep in mind the

---

131 Hodgkin, "Dionys Fitzherbert," 70.

132 Bright, *Treatise of Melancholie*, 187–8.

133 Bolton, *Right Comforting*, 80–82.

134 Perkins, *Cases of Conscience*, 62; Robert Yarrow, *Soveraigne Comforts for a Troubled Conscience* (London: for Ralph Rounthwaite, 1619), 2–3, and Burton, *Anatomy*, III.iv.II.iv: 464.

135 Perkins, *Cases of Conscience*, 62.

perspective of ministers like Napier, who argued that evangelical therapy did more harm than good. But it is important to recognize as well that evangelical therapy must have been immensely attractive for many emotionally troubled individuals. The evidence suggests that the experience of religious despair and affliction of conscience was fairly common in the late sixteenth and early seventeenth century, for reasons we have explored above. On the strength of the Renaissance popularization of the medical theories of melancholy, those who suffered acute fear and sorrow in a religious form were often thought to be merely melancholy, or even mad. The refusal to accept a naturalistic interpretation merely confirmed the presence of a stubborn delusion. The religious melancholic was caught between the world of his experience of religious despair and the medical diagnosis used by others to explain the "truth" of their feelings. The evangelical pastoral care of religious melancholy, while it clearly recognized that its patients' complaints were likely compounded by the melancholic humor, viewed the patients' ideas and feelings as instances of the pattern of religious thought and feeling which formed a central part of the evangelical religious experience, and the intensity of melancholic feeling was matched by the prescribed intensity of "normal" religious emotion in evangelical writing.

Katharine Hodgkin has argued that it would have been particularly attractive for women to express melancholic affliction as the affliction of conscience. Since female melancholy in particular pointed to the weakness of female reason and the subsequent inaptitude of women in the work of the disciplining the passions that virtue required, finding religious meaning in episodes of melancholic madness would have transformed female weakness into Christian piety.

There is much to recommend this view. Certainly, it was commonplace in early modern thought that women were morally weak, prone to emotional excess, and fit only for the "virtue" of obedience to male authority. Various Scriptural passages were taken as evidence of this; and from a physiological point of view, the female constitution was understood as wet and spongy, and therefore inhospitable to the rule of the rational soul, which was thought to require the drier and hotter embodiment provided by the male body.[136] The evidence also suggests that it was by and large women who sought out help concerning their spiritual doubts and anxieties, which oftentimes grew out of grief over the deaths of family members, and sometimes out of what was described as melancholy. Greenham's *Short rules* are thus "sent to a *gentlewoman* troubled in mind," and, of course, the *Mrs. Drake* narrative is about a woman. Seventy-two out of the 91 spiritually afflicted individuals who consulted with the Reverend Richard Napier were women.[137] Surviving letters written by godly

---

136 See the important work by Ian McLean, *The Renaissance Notion of Woman: A Study in the Fortunes of Scholasticism and Medical Science in European Intellectual Life* (Cambridge: Cambridge University Press, 1980); see also Phyllis Mack, *Visionary Women: Ecstatic Prophecy in Seventeenth-century England* (Berkeley, CA: University of California Press, 1992), 25–6; Sara Mendelson and Patricia Crawford, *Women in Early Modern England 1550–1720* (Oxford: Clarendon Press, 1998), 19–20; Schoenfeldt, *Bodies and Selves*, 35–7; Hodgkin, "Anatomy of Madness," 73.

137 Macdonald, *Mystical Bedlam*, Appendix D, Table D.1, 244; see also 220.

women give a picture of the substantial and intimate therapeutic relationships often formed between practical divines and godly women, which were a source of comfort and consolation for women and sometimes of patronage, livelihood and support for ministers.[138] (In the case of Joan Drake, 12 ministers were involved at one point or other in her comfort, including Dr. Ussher, then Archbishop of Ireland; and the young Thomas Hooker, recently graduated from Cambridge, was provided with his first clerical appointment in a local parish precisely because Mr. Drake and the godly community wished to have an attentive minister for Mrs. Drake close by.)

Perkins urged sufferers to entrust their judgment to the skilled physician of the soul, and this certainly had additional meaning when it is *her* judgment which is to be entrusted: they are features of an entirely conventional understanding of early modern gender relations.[139] Women, understood as less rational and more passionate, were also thought to rely more on their senses and feelings in the life of faith and less on their understandings. Thus, while Joan Drake's melancholy is not moralized as the weakness of emotional control in *Mrs. Drake Revived*, her desire for *sensible* consolation and comfort is. It was thought that women needed male reason to guide them to ensure that they did not become overwhelmed by feeling or mislead in their pursuit of feeling into erroneous doctrine.

But this is not the whole story. For women were encouraged not simply to rely on male authority and "reason," but to cultivate strength of mind for themselves. Greenham urges his gentlewoman interlocutor not to rely on the excuses of "melancholy," "weakness or simplicity" to put off grappling with her spiritual doubts and anxieties, but to cultivate a posture of steadfast courage in facing what he argued were Providential trials.[140] John Dod encouraged the same of Joan Drake. Courage was one of the virtues which women were thought not to be able to possess, precisely because of their "softness" and passivity, their weakness.[141] In some early modern academic discussions, women were seen as less responsible for their conduct because less capable of controlling their action and cultivating their temperament.[142] But in some Reformed evangelical writing, godly women were often held up as models of "male" virtue which put men themselves to shame. Moreover, as Christine Peters points out, "in emphasizing the naturally weak and sinful nature of all christians in relation to God," English Reformation piety "rendered the difference in male and female capacities largely irrelevant." Stories celebrating the godly lives of devout women thus emphasized the powers of grace over natural human weakness, as did stories of godly men. The recognition of such weakness was itself a Christian virtue:

---

138 See Diane Willen, "Godly Women in Early Modern England: Puritanism and Gender," *Journal of Ecclesiastical History* 43 (1992): 561–80; Crawford, *Women and Religion*, 77, 83; Patrick Collinson, "The Role of Women in the English Reformation Illustrated by the Life and Friendship of Anne Locke," in *Godly People: Essays on English Protestantism and Puritanism* (London: The Hambledon Press, 1983), 274–5.

139 Perkins, *Cases of Conscience*, 61.

140 See above, pages 63–4.

141 See McLean, *Notion of Women*, 47–67.

142 McLean, *Notion of Women*.

both men and women were to adopt "feminine" humility and submissiveness in relation to God.[143]

Even women's propensity to cultivate faith through experience and feeling rather than through the correct understanding of Scripture and doctrine was seen by men as valuable. Spiritual experiences were, after all, immensely valued elements of faith in godly circles.[144] They imparted both wisdom and fervency which could be a comfort and lesson to others. Godly women were sought out by men and women for comfort and spiritual wisdom in times of affliction.[145] Thus, Joan Drake's spiritual vision towards the end of her life was transcribed in full by the author of *Mrs. Drake Revived*. And, as George Williams points out, Thomas Hooker later universalized the experiences of Mrs. Drake into general descriptions of conversion and religious doubt without even bothering to change the feminine pronouns.[146] The story of Joan Drake was intended as one example among others, of both men and women, of saintly humility and perseverance, and as a powerful lesson of God's gracious revelation of himself to those who suffer under his wrath.

Evangelical Protestant views on the relationship between gender and piety are thus quite complex. In some ways, they accept the notion of female weakness and so reinforce the perceived need for male rationality and power. On the other hand, female weakness undergoes a transvaluation, becoming Christian virtue. Godly women, even melancholics such as Joan Drake, are held up as examples of righteousness and devotion and as emblems of God's grace. Evangelical religious discourse on the affliction and comfort of conscience thus situated female "madness," which in other discourse appears as the terminus of female moral and physical weakness, as a moment in a spiritual pilgrimage towards God enabled by grace, and ruled by Providence. In the case of Joan Drake, it was acknowledged that her condition was to some extent "madness" – but it was at the same time much more.

Christine Peters writes of gender and piety in Reformed circles that "[i]deally ... the process of spiritual edification was best pursued by a partnership of man and wife, or minister and godly lay-woman, in which both the complementarity [*sic*] and the essential nature of the two contributions was recognized."[147] This ideal of complementarity describes the practice of piety that late sixteenth and early seventeenth-century practical divinity attempted to formulate and foster more generally; it is what allows for the spiritual consolation, even valuation, of melancholy. Spiritual experiences and feelings were to be held in a productive tension with the

---

143 See Christine Peters, *Women in Early Modern Britain 1450–1640* (Basingstoke: Palgrave Macmillan, 2004), 149–52, 154, 161; Willen, "Godly Women," 565–6, and Jacqueline Eales, "Samuel Clarke and the 'Lives' of Godly Women in Seventeenth-century England," in W.J. Sheils and Diana Wood, eds., *Women in the Church* (Oxford: Basil Blackwell for the Ecclesiastical History Society, 1990), 365–87.

144 Peters, *Women*, 151–2.

145 Willen, "Godly Women," 572–3.

146 Williams, "Called by Thy Name ... Part II," 278–300.

147 Peters, *Women*, 152.

understanding provided by doctrine and Scripture. For some Christians, feeling could provide hope and assurance. Evangelical ministers' understanding cautioned that unless this was built on repentance and humility, it was false hope and unfounded assurance. For many, it seems, and for those prone to melancholy especially, feeling declared nothing but damnation. Here, ministers insisted that there were manifold reasons for hope, taking the feeling of despair itself as a sign of God's favor.

Like the art of medicine, practical divinity consisted of universal concepts applied to particular cases, and this required wisdom and prudence in its application. This is why the spiritual therapies of the late sixteenth and early seventeenth centuries are not easily characterized as either wholly despair-inducing or entirely comforting, as either "Puritan" or "Anglican." Practical treatises on the Christian life constantly exhibit a kind of double movement between despair and presumption. To take one example out of many, Bolton, like others, stressed that one could not sorrow enough for one's sins; but he warned as well that too much sorrow would invite the devil to "detain" the soul in "perpetual horror."[148]

While they recognized that some pastoral clumsiness could throw pious individuals into unnecessary and dangerous despair, evangelical ministers were committed to the belief that the true saint would, by the grace of God, persevere in the faith through even the darkest despair. This is why Perkins displayed some resistance in taking even the story of Francis Spira's despairing death as hopeless, in spite of the fact that it was often cast as a story of God's retribution against backsliders and apostates. Such moves reinforced the idea that the spiritual postures of godly sorrow and holy despair English ministers helped to popularize were seen as ultimately spiritual beneficial and could be taken as signs of grace. But in the context of the anti-Calvinism which began to develop in the 1630s and became institutionalized in the established Church after the demise of the Commonwealth and the Restoration of Charles II to the throne, both the practical divinity of late sixteenth and early seventeenth century and its theological assumptions were seriously challenged. And one of the issues on which anti-Calvinist criticism turned was precisely the pastoral care of melancholy. The consolation and care of religious melancholy was by no means abandoned by the Restoration Church, but the language through which care and consolation was performed was significantly altered.

---

148 See above, page 60.

CHAPTER FOUR

Anglicanism, Melancholy, and the Restoration Critique of "Enthusiasm"

During the 1620s and 1630s, English Protestantism became increasingly divided between those who insisted on the Calvinist interpretation of the doctrine of predestination and those who, following the views of the Dutch theologian James Arminius, saw a greater role for the human will in the work of salvation. Opinion was also virulently divided between those who argued that the Church should be a body of the godly alone and others who argued that the Church was a national body, whose spiritual service was to be made available not only for the edification of those "Puritans" who alone seemed to consider themselves godly but, more broadly, for the salvation of all English subjects. These were certainly not the only issues which led to the English Civil War, but they were important sources of tension and conflict within the Church and in English society more broadly. And it proved somewhat difficult after the Restoration of the monarchy to settle on a form of Church government and a unifying theological vision. The final Act of Settlement (1662) resulted in a nation divided into two groups, legally very sharply defined, but in fact rather heterogeneous. There were those who conformed to the new requirements of the Church of England and those who did not – conformists and nonconformists, or "Anglicans" and "Dissenters."[1]

The lines dividing the two groups were somewhat artificial. There were anti-Calvinists on both sides, and nonconformists comprised a range of theological positions, from the more moderate Presbyterians through the more separatist Congregationalist and Independent Christians to the heterodox (and, in the eyes of their detractors, somewhat politically subversive) Quakers.[2] Moderate Dissenters resented being lumped together with more radical religious groups, and they, along with many Anglicans, sharply condemned the religious sects that had arisen in the 1640s and 1650s, whose forms of religious expression often involved spontaneous outbursts of politically radical, theologically heterodox, and emotionally heightened

---

1   See John Spurr, *The Restoration Church of England, 1646–1689* (New Haven, CT and London: Yale University Press, 1991).

2   On the differences between these religious groups, see Isabel Rivers, *Reason, Grace and Sentiment: A Study of the Language of Religion and Ethics in England, 1660–1780*, Volume 1: *Whichcote to Wesley* (Cambridge: Cambridge University Press, 1991), 91–109; John Spurr, *English Puritanism, 1603–1689* (New York: St. Martin's Press, 1998), and Michael Watts, *The Dissenters*, Volume 1: *From the Reformation to the French Revolution* (Oxford: Clarendon Press, 1978), 89–179.

utterances. Where groups like the Quakers perceived such "prophesyings" as manifestations of the Holy Spirit, many Restoration divines and philosophers viewed these experiences as proceeding from an imagination ungoverned by what they argued was the proper and sovereign principle of the human mind, the faculty of reason.[3] Some writers went wider in their critique of forms of religious life, implicating the practices of more mainstream evangelical English Protestants in fostering the extremities of religious emotion and the theology which supported it. This group of critics, most of them Anglican churchmen but also some important Dissenting ministers, used the idea of melancholy disease to dismiss a range of religious experiences as delusion and madness.[4] The feelings of divine withdrawal and despondency, which had been considered by many English Calvinists earlier in the century to be expressions of the state of the soul, were thus traced by Restoration critics to a humoral imbalance of the body instead.

This reaction to more emotive forms of religion has become known to historians as the critique of "enthusiasm," which was a contemporary term for the possession or indwelling of the human psyche by a spirit. The Restoration critique of enthusiasm was an incisive and critical moment in the discourse on melancholy, as in the history of English thought more generally. The rhetoric that represented the nonconformist as dangerously under the sway of sense and feeling cemented an approach to religious thought and experience that rejected many of the central elements which had informed the approach to melancholy and to spiritual affliction of late sixteenth and early seventeenth-century pastors. Where previously the melancholic element of religious melancholy had often been overshadowed by a language that described the affliction of conscience in terms of a harrowing and distracted dark night of the soul, the medical concept of melancholy as a disorder of the body was now foregrounded as the central and perhaps the sole cause of religious despair and disconsolation. Henceforth this would remain a central feature of the pastoral writing on melancholy among the Anglican clergy; and, as we will see in the next chapter, it figures in some of the most important Dissenting pastoral work as well.

---

3   On the religious and political radicals of the English Revolution period, see Christopher Hill, *The World Turned Upside Down: Radical Ideas during the English Revolution* (New York: The Viking Press, 1972); on the Quakers in particular, see Mack, *Visionary Women*.

4   See Daniel Fouke, *The Enthusiastical Concerns of Dr. Henry More: Religious Meaning and the Psychology of Delusion* (Leiden: E.J. Brill, 1997), 130–80; George Rosen, "Enthusiasm: A Dark Lanthorn of the Spirit," *Bulletin of the History of Medicine* 42 (1968): 393–421; Michael Heyd, "Robert Burton's Sources on Enthusiasm and Melancholy: From a Medical Tradition to a Religious Controversy," *History of European Ideas* 5 (1984): 17–44; Heyd, "Medical Discourse in Religious Controversy: The Case of the Critique of enthusiasm on the Eve of Enlightenment," *Science in Context* 8 (1995): 137–57; *'Be Sober and Reasonable': The Critique of Enthusiasm in the Seventeenth and Early Eighteenth Centuries* (New York: E.J. Brill, 1995); John F. Sena, "Melancholic Madness and the Puritans," *Harvard Theological Review* 66 (1973): 293–309; Hillel Schwartz, *The French Prophets* (Berkeley, CA and Los Angeles, CA: University of California Press, 1980).

Michael MacDonald has argued that the critique of enthusiasm was responsible for making mental illness into much less of a pastoral problem and much more of a strictly medical problem. But while the trenchant criticisms of Restoration divines may seem merely dismissive of the religious melancholic, their critique of English Calvinism was driven by strongly therapeutic concerns. Religious melancholy, they argued, was comprised of both the melancholic humor and a religious vocabulary which misidentified melancholic feelings as spiritual. The roots of this misidentification were seen to be in Calvinist theology. Restoration anti-Calvinists argued that by insisting that the soul is totally passive in the matter of salvation, English Calvinism threw the Christian onto the introspective scrutiny of their sensations and feelings for evidence of the state of their soul. Every mental event was thus read as a possible sign of damnation or salvation. And, pointing to a certain perverse fashionability of both despondent and ecstatic spiritual experiences in Calvinist circles, anti-Calvinists argued that the language of spiritual complaint was naturally but mistakenly adopted by those suffering from cases of mere melancholy. Helping the religious melancholic thus meant providing them with what critics of Calvinism took to be the correct theological understanding of salvation, on which the cultivation of feeling was seen as much less important in securing salvation than the performance of moral and religious duties.

The critique of enthusiasm had ensured that the discourse on religious despair that shaped late sixteenth and early seventeenth-century religious culture largely disappeared in eighteenth-century Anglican culture, and the emotionally charged rhetoric associated with that discourse was, until the religious revivals of the Methodists and others in the 1720s and 1730s, excised from the Anglican spiritual vocabulary. But to concede this point does not mean that we need to buy into a representation of the Anglican clergy as dismissive of the spiritual and mental trouble of their parishioners. For at least some critics of enthusiasm, theological polemic against the dissenters was motivated by pastoral rather than strictly theological concerns. Furthermore, the pastoral advice embedded in the more polemical texts of Restoration continued to be expounded in the context of what became something of a standard *topoi* in Anglican sermons and tracts into the 1740s: the consolation of religious melancholy. The complaints which Anglican clergy continued to treat echoed those of Elizabethan and early Stuart Calvinist melancholics: they were possessed of blasphemous thoughts; they could not go about their Christian duty with any amount of enthusiasm, or were motivated only by fear; they felt abandoned by God, even damned. They were told by Anglican ministers that they suffered from diseased bodies; but they were also provided with specifically theological and spiritual modes of comfort.

Anti-Calvinist antidotes: Simon Patrick and the Latitudinarians

The Restoration critique of English Calvinist religious experience addressed the tendency of Calvinists to invest all that passed in the sphere of the mind and heart with a great deal of spiritual significance. The spiritual lives of many "Puritans" were occupied with the thoughts and pictures which suddenly appeared to them, with the feelings which suddenly came upon them and were often perceived as direct communications and revelations from God. Language to this effect litters the Baptist itinerant preacher John Bunyan's prose, for example.[5] For the anti-enthusiast critics, this preoccupation with feeling and sensation in spiritual life was of a piece with pretensions of groups like the Quakers to prophetic utterance. Without the control and discrimination of reason in the interior life, thought and emotion were left to be effected entirely by the forces of the body. What the devout nonconformist thought was grace or abandonment, or the prophet thought was the voice of God, could not, the anti-enthusiast argued, be distinguished from the wanderings of the human imagination and movement of fluids in the brain.

Thus, the critique of enthusiasm was not simply the dismissal of the heterodox or politically seditious as in need of medical treatment; it was the assertion that all human thought stood in need of the governance of reason. The anti-enthusiast critics went further than just casting suspicion on the experiences of the prophet and the Calvinist puritan. Elaborating a moral psychology which stressed the supremacy of reason in human life, they argued that for those who denigrated or ignored reason, the only other source of conduct and thought was the body, its sensations, its passions, and its diseases.

In his influential polemic against the enthusiasts, *Enthusiasmus Triumphatus* (1656), Henry More gave the standard account of the human psyche on which this was based. The brain receives the impressions of the external senses, through the vehicle of the subtle, quasi-spirituous substance known as the animal spirits flowing in the nerves. The vigor with which impressions are received as "figures" in the brain affects the "inmost seat of sense" so as to create the "opinion of truth." But the same inmost seat of sense can in a like manner be effected purely through the imagination. Where normally the force of external sensation keeps the soul within the sphere of reality, if the movement of the imagination in the brain is strong enough, "the enormous strength of the imagination ... thus peremptorily engages a man to believe a lie," as with "mad or melancholy men, who have confidently affirmed that they have met with the devil or conversed with angels, when it has been nothing but an encounter with their own fancie."[6]

Importantly, however, although the enthusiast was often dismissed as mad, madness was here figured as the terminal condition of a much less visible fault. In his discussion on the preventatives of enthusiasm, More argued that the imaginations of the brain were to be weighed against the claims of reason. The movement of the Holy Spirit should not, More argued, be understood as contrary to, or even "above," the principle of reason. Rather, "that Spirit of illumination which resides in souls of the faithful, is a principle of the purest Reason that is communicable to the human

5   See, for example, Bunyan, *Grace Abounding*, ed. John Stachniewski, Oxford World's Classics (Oxford and New York: Oxford University Press, 1998), 1–94.

6   More, *Enthusiasmus Triumphatus* (London: J. Flesher, 1656), Sections 5 and 6.

nature. And what this Spirit has, he has from Christ (as Christ himself witnesseth) who is the eternal [logos], the all-comprehending wisdom and reason of God." On More's analysis of the sources of religious experience, one who does not make the exercise of reason a part of their spiritual life is of necessity under the dominion of the imagination, the strength of which More called the soul's weakness and unwieldiness: it was a weight under which the soul sinks, eventually preventing entirely the "use of her more free faculties of Reason and Understanding."[7]

Others made much the same point without adopting More's neo-Platonic Christology. Speaking more directly to the "Puritan" religious experience, the influential Restoration divine Edward Fowler glossed the idea of the inward testimony of the Spirit to the truth of the Gospel. Previously, the inward testimony of the Spirit was understood as an important moment of divine illumination confirming the calling of the elect, overcoming the doubt and prevarication of human sense and reason with the power of immediate certainty and so providing the bedrock of faith. It was often referred to as the spirit of adoption of Romans 8:15. As Perkins put it, it consisted of the "full perswasion … that they are the children of God," for which "the holy Ghost draweth not reasons from the workes, or worthinesse of man, but from Gods favour and love." When such persuasion is true, Perkins added, it "is most lively and stirring."[8] Fowler made the spirit of illumination all but indistinguishable from the normal operation of reason in determining truth:

> I say that the external and rational Motives of Credibility are sufficient to give unprejudiced persons an undoubted belief of the truth of our Religion; as any rational Arguments are to perswade a man of the truth of any thing, he desireth satisfaction concerning: But yet because our Grand Adversary useth all Arts to make it as much suspected as may be, and to shake our faith therin; and we are moreover in regard of the Contrariety of our Religion to our carnal and fleshly interests very apt to be strongly prejudiced against it, (and we are not easily brought fully to believe what we would not have true) God is ready without all question, to assist our weakness by his grace and Spirit, in this as well as other particulars, when humbly sought to: but we have no reason to think that he doth this *ordinarily* in an immediate manner, but by blessing the use of means, *i.e.* the consideration of the motives he hath given us to believe: and that he confirms our Faith, by giving us to see such strongly-convincing demonstration in those Arguments, and by so *closely* applying the evidence of them to our understandings, as that they come to be even *perfectly* over-powerer'd, and against all opposition to have full assent, and such as hath a powerful influence upon our practice, as it were, even *forced* from them.[9]

---

7   Ibid., Sections 6 and 54. On More's psychology of religious experience and the importance of his moral psychology in dismissing the experiences of the Quakers, see Fouke, *Dr. Henry More*, esp. 151–80.

8   Perkins, *A Golden Chaine, or, The Order of Causes of Salvation and Damnation* (London: John Legatt, 1621), Ch. 57. See also Calvin, *Institutes*, 3.ii.11.

9   Fowler, *The Principles and Practices of Certain Moderate Divines of the Church of England, abusively called Latitudinarians*, 2nd edn. (London: for Lodowick Lloyd, 1671), 56–8.

The experience of faith Fowler was describing was very different from what the "Puritans" had described. For the English Calvinist schooled under those like Perkins, it was a question of some uncertainty whether one had true saving faith or fleeting, hypocritical faith. The believer sought assurance of election, and searched for the signs of true faith listed by the minister. Alternately, if the searching after signs did not convince, doubters were urged to rely on the promise of the Gospel that God would not abandon those who sincerely desired to be saved. Thus, particularly in the Baptist and Congregationalist forms of English Calvinism that emerged in the middle of the seventeenth century, the contrite soul was encouraged to "rest in the promises of Christ" for the assurance of her salvation.[10] For Fowler, who rejected the Calvinist doctrine of predestination and its corollary of irresistible grace for the Arminian position affirming the possibility of universal redemption and the exercise of human freewill, the question of whether one had faith was much less tortuous. There were only two conditions, easily recognized. The first was that the truth of revelation was apprehended; the second, that the will embrace the conditions under which grace was offered in that revelation. As John W. Marshall sums up the difference, this description of faith "inclined towards *fides*, the intellectual assent to theological propositions, rather than *fiducia*, the loving, trusting relationship with Christ that brought its own sense of conviction."[11]

Fowler was identified with a group of Restoration divines known as latitudinarians. The label indicated that many of this group had served in the Church during the years of the English Commonwealth, while others who stood more firmly on royalist or episcopalian principles had been ejected from their positions. They insisted in Restoration times that "matters indifferent," about which the scriptures did not comment one way or another, did not give believers or clerics cause to dissent or withdraw from the established church, whether Presbyterian or Episcopalian. Thus, they conformed to Restoration episcopacy as they had to the theological creed of the Westminster Assembly (1647), and thus they argued against the Restoration Dissenters that the possibly exceptionable portions of the official Book of Prayer and Westminster Confession regarded indifferent matters and did not justify the Dissenters resistance to join the established Church. While Dissenters objected on the grounds that to support and participate in certain ceremonies and institutions went against their consciences, the latitudinarians insisted that the established Church alone had the authority to decide such matters.[12]

---

10   See Spurr, *English Puritanism*, 95–6.

11   Marshall, *John Locke: Resistance, Religion and Responsibility* (Cambridge: Cambridge University Press, 1994), 124.

12   See Richard Ashcraft, "Latitudinarianism and Toleration: Historical Myth versus Political History," in Richard Ashcraft, Richard Kroll, and Perez Zagorin, eds., *Philosophy, Science and Religion in England, 1640–1700* (Cambridge: Cambridge University Press, 1992), 151–77. See also Spurr, *Restoration Church*, 29–104; N.H. Keeble, *The Literary Culture of Nonconformity in Later Seventeenth-century England* (Leicester: Leicester University Press, 1987), 25–67.

The theology articulated by the latitudinarians thus aimed at limiting appeals to individual conscience and inner experience as authoritative sources of religious belief and action.[13] In light of the kinds of claims asserted by the radical Protestant sects throughout the Interregnum, the latitudinarians and other churchmen tended to regard all forms of religious authority grounded on individual experience as suspect, given to fostering political and religious sedition and anarchy. Concerned as well to defend the truth of revealed Christianity against deists who advocated a philosophy of natural religion, latitudinarians drew away from speaking of grace and faith in terms of incommunicable experiences of assurance and instead identified the apprehension of the Gospel's truth with the light of reason correctly exercised, emphasizing the congruity of theology and philosophy, of faith and reason.[14] One of their particular contentions was that revealed religion could be regarded primarily as a powerful and necessary improvement on the "Motives and Arguments" regarding moral behavior available to the heathen philosophers.[15]

By defining the essence of religion to consist in the notions of natural law available to all through reason, and limiting the import of Christianity to the effective reinforcement of these moral duties, latitudinarians hoped to advance beyond the bitter sectarian strife over doctrine and to cut off theological and ecclesiastical dissension. This was the intellectual attitude which informed their accusations that the Dissenters devalued both the practice of virtue and the exercise of reason in favor of supposed spiritual experiences. The very active anti-enthusiast writer and divine Joseph Glanvill argued that the religious vocabulary which had grown around assertions such as William Perkins' that the witness of the Spirit "be most lively and stirring" gave free play to the human imagination, and so perverted the correct order of the human faculties. Talk of "*Incomes, Illuminations, Communions, Lights, Discoveries, Sealings, Manifestations* and *Impressions*, as the Heights of Religion," along with a denigration of reason as "merely carnal" and opposed to the spiritual, created a mentality in which people could not "easily avoid looking upon the *glarings* of their own *Imaginations*, and the *wants* and impulses of their *Melancholy*, as *Divine Revelations* and *Illapses*."[16]

As Richard Ashcraft points out, Dissenters defended against the imputation that they denigrated reason, and many recognized the importance of rational inquiry in the life of faith. Indeed, many Dissenters gave as great a reign to the exercise of reason as the latitudinarians in arguing that the individual was to be entrusted with

---

13   See Ashcraft, "Latitudinarians and Toleration," 163–4.

14   See Margaret C. Jacobs, *The Newtonians and the English Revolution, 1689–1720* (Brighton: The Harvester Press, 1976), 52–3; H.R. McAdoo, *The Spirit of Anglicanism: A Survey of Anglican Theological Method in the Seventeenth Century* (New York: Charles Scribner's Sons, 1965), Chs 5 and 6, esp. 157–62; John Spurr, "'Rational Religion' in Restoration England," *Journal of the History of Ideas* 49 (1988): 563–85.

15   Fowler, *Principles*, 89.

16   Joseph Glanvill, "Antifanatickal Religion and Free Philosophy," Essay 7 in *Essays on Several Important Subjects in Philosophy and Religion* (London: J.D. for John Baker, 1676), 19; see also Glanvill, *Philosophia Pia* (London: J. Macock for James Collins, 1671), 224.

the task of discerning for himself the true nature of religion and of the Church, where the latitudinarians espoused submission to what they argued was the more informed and rational opinion of the instituted clergy.[17] Furthermore, for the Elizabethan and early Stuart English Calvinists, the devaluation of reason often took place in a context where faith in the promises of the Gospel stood opposed to reliance on a sensible assurance of election. Carnal reason followed the evidence of the senses rather than the insights revealed to the faithful. A person could have faith in spite of a weakness of feeling or an illegibility of the other signs of grace. Carnal reason was also the voice of the devil insisting that according to the standards of the natural moral law, one stood condemned before God without hope of redemption. The place those like Fowler assigned to reason in the act of faith was simply irrelevant to the Calvinist experience. In the Reformed predestinarian context, assent to the truth of the Gospel, even if it provided the will with ample reason for obedience to Gospel precepts, mattered little; in straining towards blessed assurance, the search for the signs of election demanded the suspension of what Calvinist divines took to be the normal mechanisms of belief, or more radically, the rupture into consciousness of divine assurance, as in the case of Joan Drake, John Peacock, and others.

But the Arminian perspective of the latitudinarians entailed that faith be defined by the acts and faculties under substantial human control, and on their religious and moral psychology, feelings and sensations were thereby excluded as the grounds of faith. This endeavor to secure religious experience and vocabulary in the common, recognizable, and transparent acts of understanding and will was in part the motive of the latitudinarian critique of the popular language of faith as a "resting in Christ" and the doctrine of imputed righteousness undergirding this language. On the doctrine of imputed righteousness, which defined English Protestant orthodoxy until the middle of the seventeenth century, faith was a matter of believing that Christ's righteous obedience unto death had fulfilled the conditions of the New Covenant established between God and his people; upon believing, itself an act of grace, the righteousness of Christ was imputed to us as our own, and in this way we were justified before God. In the context of predestinarian theology, "resting in Christ" and other cognate terms indicated a withdrawal from both a human effort at righteousness and from the need to feel sensible assurance, which, however valued, was not always available. Assurance was provided by the promises of God; faith was the act of believing those promises applied to oneself. The latitudinarians and other Restoration churchmen were deeply critical of this doctrine on at least two counts. First, they asserted that it relied on feeling for verification. As Fowler commented on the doctrine of imputed righteousness: "Christs righteousness or inherent holiness is as *completely* made *theirs*, as if they themselves were *completely* and *perfectly* righteous: and that upon no other condition or qualification wrought in them, but onely *believing*; whereby too many of them mean strongly *fancying* this righteousness to be *theirs*."[18] The phrases used to describe the act of saving faith were thus so much cant, according to

---

17   Ashcraft, "Latitudinarianism and Toleration," 160–67.
18   Fowler, *Principles*, 128.

these churchmen. Glanvill wrote that all the talk of "*closing with Christ, getting in to Christ, falling upon Christ, relying upon Christ,* and *having an interest in Christ,*" though it made "silly people believe that there was something of Divine Mystery, or extraordinary spirituality under the sound of these words," was entirely vacuous; if it had substance at all, it was only in the realm of feeling and imagination.[19]

Second, whether or not these words described grace or imagination, dissenters and their opponents agreed that it described an experience in which the individual was entirely passive. The individual's effort at righteousness or belief did not contribute to the inward turn to belief and assurance. But since grace was not in the exercise of will or understanding, critics of the doctrine argued that the doctrine of imputed righteousness meant that salvation was possible without conversion or repentance, for a person could believe wholeheartedly that Christ's righteousness was his while still living in willful sin.[20] This, Fowler and his colleagues argued, was basically antinomian, raising the Interregnum specter of the alleged Ranter belief that all was morally permitted under the terms of the new covenant. Fowler and his colleagues were persuaded that belief as a condition of justification was belief in Christ as Lord, one to whom repentance and obedience was due. They still adhered to a version of the doctrine of imputed righteousness; the condition, however, was not mere believing but repentance and sincere striving after moral perfection. Fowler put the matter clearly: "This ... is [the latitudinarian] notion of Christs Imputed righteousness: That those which are *sincerely* righteous, and from an *inward living* principle allow themselves in no *known sin,* nor in the neglect of any *known duty,* which is to be truly *Evangelically* righteous, in and through Christ, as if they were perfectly, and in a strict *Legal* sense so."[21]

Thus, the latitudinarians, along with other Restoration churchmen and even some Dissenters, made moral performance the condition of justification. The massively popular *The Whole Duty of Man* was without a doubt the primer in this school of religious sensibility. They understood righteousness not as a mysterious infusion of grace nor as a mere change in legal standing before God, but as actual moral righteousness, and the latitudinarians in particular argued that the very end of religion was to inculcate true moral righteousness. In response to the argument that biblical righteousness was somehow different than mere moral righteousness, Fowler stated "I know no Righteousness, but what is ... truly *moral.* And a righteousness in no sense so, seems to my understanding a most perfect Contradiction."[22] Their opponents, they knew, cried up the great difference between mere virtue and grace. A person could be perfectly virtuous yet without grace, it was said, if they did not possess that

---

19 Glanvill, "Antifanatickal Religion," in *Essays*, 19.

20 Fowler, *Principles*, 149–50, 181; on the doctrine of imputed righteousness, see C.F. Allison, *The Rise of Moralism: The Proclamation of the Gospel from Hooker to Baxter* (London: SPCK, 1966), esp. 186–8, and Spurr, *Restoration Church*, 296–311.

21 Fowler, *Principles*, 166; see also Glanvill, "Antifanatickal Religion," in *Essays*, 37–8.

22 Fowler, *Principles*, 124.

righteousness which alone could justify them, the imputed righteousness of Christ. But, the latitudinarians countered, they could not find in the act and manifestation of grace anything but virtue. As Samuel Parker put it:

> 'Tis not enough (say they) to be completely Vertuous, unless we have Grace too: But when we have set aside all manner of Vertue, let them tell me what remains to be call'd Grace, and give me any Notion of it distinct from all Morality , that consists in the right order and government of our Actions in all our Relations, and so comprehends all our Duty; and therefore if Grace be not included in it, 'tis but a Phantasm, and an Imaginary thing. So that if we strip those Definitions that some Men of late have bestowed upon it, of Metaphors and Allegories, it will plainly signifie nothing but a vertuous temper of Mind; and all that the Scripture intends by the Graces of the Spirit are only Vertuous Qualities of the Soul.[23]

It was misleading to claim that the idea of grace apart from virtue was inconceivable. If, as Perkins said, the grace of redemption was given not out of "reasons from the workes, or worthinesse of man," then virtue was irrelevant to saving grace. But grace and virtue came to be coextensive once it was argued that the condition of salvation is our obedience to the precepts of the Gospel. In this theological context, it was only logical that grace manifest itself as virtue, since this was all that mattered.

The notion of resting in Christ for salvation was, from this perspective, tantamount to resting in moral weakness.[24] Simon Patrick, who identified himself as a latitudinarian and helped to articulate it as a theological and political position, asserted that where the substance of faith was defined as laying hold of or resting in Christ, it amounted to *"Believing, without Doing."*[25] The dissenting ministers taught their listeners "to despise sober and plain Doctrine, which teaches them their Duty towards God and their Neighbour, entertaining them with finer Speculations of Pretended Gospel-Mysteries and Manifestations; with which we heard almost every Sermon stuffed." Likewise, the much vaunted "Stories of God's *Withdrawings* and *Desertings*; and again of his *Shinings in* and *Sealings*" were most often no less fanciful, according to Patrick.[26]

God's withdrawal could indeed be occasioned by "some provoking Sin," Patrick acknowledged. But, he continued, "I see that they who cannot charge themselves with any voluntary act of Sin, nor with any such Omission neither, fall into these Fancies ... of being forsaken by God." The fact was, he argued, the believer merely felt something of an abatement of zeal in the performance of duty, a perfectly natural occurrence having nothing to do with the presence or absence of grace. Addressing the dissenter in *A Friendly Debate*, Patrick declared that "all the occasion that ever I could find for such black thoughts is but some such thing as this, that they have not

---

23   Samuel Parker, *Discourse of Ecclesiastical Politie*, 3rd edn. (London: for John Martyn, 1671), 74.

24   See Spurr, *Restoration Church*, 279–330; McAdoo, *Anglicanism*, 172–3.

25   Patrick, *A Friendly Debate*, 33–5.

26   Ibid., 48.

such enlargements as they were wont; or cannot go to duty, as they speak, with the delight which formerly they took in it: which your ministers ought to teach them are no reasons, but only melancholic conceits."[27]

English Calvinist ministers recognized that there was often a melancholic complication in cases of spiritual affliction. Patrick, however, seemed to insist that they were only melancholic feelings, compounded, exacerbated, and perhaps dramatized by the language of affliction of conscience. He countered the dissenting experience of being abandoned by God by declaring that "if these be the things you call experiences, there are none of us but understand them as well as you, finding the same dullness and heaviness in ourselves. Only we are taught not to talk or complain of it, but to do our duty notwithstanding as well as we are able, and we shall find it will not last always."[28] Recognized as the work of fancy and silently born by the believer whose reason was not encumbered by the evangelical language of feeling, such melancholic conceits would disappear in time, under the pressure of the exertion of the will in duty. But to "lay too great weight upon" these troubles of mind as "Marks of a Gracious Soul," as Patrick argued the non-conformist did, "helps to put good (but weak) people into these Humours; and, I doubt, makes them lay hold on all occasions to fansy themselves deserted."[29] The set phrases describing the experiences of belief and doubt, grace and withdrawal, had become tokens of social esteem: "he was thought no-body that had not good store of them."[30]

The Dissenter, according to Patrick, was in characteristic fashion replacing the moral and pious duty of which the Christian life consisted with empty speeches by fostering the expression of melancholic complaints as an important Christian duty. The religious melancholic, while they had not committed any sin to deserve the perceived withdrawal of grace, was led by the Dissenter into the sinful and inexcusable neglect of moral performance. Patrick suggested elsewhere that to complain of a dullness and heaviness might even betray a spiritual pride. To those who are troubled when they "abate of the height of their zeal" where once "they did pray with some fervour," Patrick cautioned in his consolatory discourse *Hearts Ease, or, A Remedy against all Troubles* (1671): "Truly, we must not expect while we are here below in this cave or dungeon, to be quite free from all such damps. And it may be some degree of pride, not to be able to endure some dulness and coldness of spirit."[31]

To endure the "damps" of the earthly human condition was, however, as difficult for the pious latitudinarian as it was for the Calvinist, and Patrick, who was deeply committed to his clerical role as pastor and spiritual physician, recognized this in his

---

27 Ibid., 48–9.
28 Ibid.
29 Ibid., 49.
30 Ibid., 38.
31 Patrick, *Hearts Ease*, Epistle Dedicatory.

practical writing on the Christian life.[32] For the Calvinist, melancholic feelings led to despair by being interpreted in terms of the signs of grace as, in Abernethy's words, "sensible tokens of Gods displeasure."[33] The latitudinarian was not as concerned with possible signs of grace as he was with becoming a virtuous person.[34] Patrick included under the rubric of Christian righteousness "Passions more subdued to Reason," and in his highly regarded *Advice to a friend* (1673), Patrick oriented the whole of Christian life and discipline around the problem of the government of irrational appetites and desires, using a mixture of Stoic and Platonic moral philosophical language.[35] But although Christ was revealed to humankind both to inspire us with courage by "his glorious Example" and to comfort us "with the hopes of mighty power from above to aid and assist us in our Christian conflict with all unreasonable desires," Patrick acknowledged that the rational control of the appetites was immensely difficult to achieve. He encouraged his cures to reflect on their souls, "those Divine Inhabitants" which have knowledge of the greatest human good, "God and the Life to come." "Represent to yourself, as often and as sensibly as you can," he continued, "*the incomparable greatness of that invisible happiness in the World to come.*"[36] These were Christianized Stoic spiritual exercises intended to transform the individual's relation to the world and himself, raising his consciousness out of the particularity of his worldly "lusts and pleasures" into the realm of the "substantiall Good ... in heaven."[37] Such spiritual exercises were easy when the body is "more ready and forward to accompany [the mind] in the contemplation of Diviner objects. Then the mind is in fact able "to impress its perceptions upon the [animal] spirits," producing by their movement a "sensible delectation in the Borders of our Soul." At other times, however, "the body becomes like a lump of Clay, and cannot endure to be drawn any longer to these Holy Duties."[38] Faced by the body's unwieldiness, "the Soul it self (unless it duly consider) will begin hereat to be greatly dejected."[39]

The first stage of Patrick's therapeutic regime in such cases consisted of a course of mental hygiene similar to the cures recommended to the melancholic by Burton. Patrick relayed to the reader many of the received cures and preventatives of melancholy. Paraphrasing Seneca's *De tranquilitate animi*, he pointed to the diversions of Socrates and Cato to argue for the wisdom of recreation.[40] Good

---

32   On Patrick's pastoral activities, see *The Oxford Dictionary of National Biography*, s.v. "Patrick, Simon."

33   Abernethy, *Treatise*, 114–15.

34   Patrick, *A Friendly Debate*, 148–9.

35   Patrick, *Advice to a Friend* (London: for R. Royston, 1673), 5; see also the moral philosophical exercises derived from Marcus Aurelius' Meditations in Patrick's Hearts Ease, 26–7, 54, 132, 173–218.

36   Patrick, *Advice to a Friend*, 33.

37   Ibid., 27, and *Hearts Ease*, 132.

38   Patrick, *Advice to a Friend*, 5, 12–13.

39   Ibid., 101–4.

40   Ibid., 88–96; 155. See Seneca, *On Tranquility of Mind*, in *Moral Essays*, vol. 2, 17.4: 278–81.

company and friends in whom to confide also lighten the mind and relieve the oppressed movements of the spirits.[41] Patrick also argued that clearly recognizing that certain perceptions and feelings are influenced by the body provided a measure of consolation:

> [I]f in this state, the Mind recollect it self and consider, that, for its part, it doth what it did before (although it doth not feel it self and perceive its power in the same manner) and that it is not bound to produce these pleasurable motions in the lower man, and that they are more pleasing to us, than to God; it might presently have rational satisfaction & tranquility in its own breast (which is the best of all other joys) and be perswaded to hold on in its course, notwithstanding this seeming discouragement.

Patrick added that where the body provides no reward in the practice of piety and virtue, the merit accruing is all the greater.[42]

This was a point transposed from earlier Calvinist consolations of religious melancholy, where it was argued that a course of faith in the use of the means and in holding onto the promises of Christ in spite of the lack of sensible signs showed all the more powerfully the evidence of grace and faith. Importantly for Patrick, the consolation derived from the constancy of the human powers of reason and will. But just as Calvinists thought of feelings of divine withdrawal as God's temptation and trial of his children, Patrick asserted the Christian was to be "content ... with our driness and barrenness of spirit, with our dullness and want of vigour ... merely out of submission to God ... because he thinks not fit to give us the pleasure of being wholly without them."[43] Towards the end of *Advice to a Friend*, he stated more explicitly that such feelings might in fact be caused by the "with-holding, in a great measure, of that strength and power which was upon us from the Holy-Ghost, to raise and elevate us to an high pitch of love, activity, and joy in well doing."[44] Such withholding precipitated a natural cycle of emotional deflation: "For as the help of that doth lift us up above our selves, so, when it much abates, we are apt to fall as much below our selves; and to be surprised with sadness and dejection of spirit, to see our selves so strangely changed."[45]

Patrick had argued in *A Friendly Debate* that true feelings of divine withdrawal could only be caused by some voluntary omission or act of sin. He nowhere equated feelings of dullness themselves with actual divine abandonment, but in *Advice to a Friend*, Patrick expanded considerably the interpretive possibilities of such feelings. The strength and power of the Holy Ghost "may be denied to us for several causes":

---

41   Patrick, *Advice to a Friend*, 161–4.
42   Ibid., 104–5.
43   Ibid., 248.
44   Ibid., 316–17.
45   Ibid., 317.

either because we have not improved it so well as we might; or because our Lord sees that our Nature cannot bear always such extraordinary motions; or that he may make us more sensible of his favours, and raise their price and value in our esteem; or that he may try our strength, as a Mother lets go her hold of the Child to make it feel its Feet; or that he may thereby bow our wills more absolutely to his, and break our self-love, which desires nothing but pleasure; or that he may prove whether we will love him for himself, and not for the delicate entertainments which he gives us; or for some such cause unknown to you and me, and every body else.[46]

Consolations of these kinds were very familiar in Calvinist circles, where such spiritual lessons were pitted against the fearful thoughts of damnation many of the godly seemed all too ready to entertain, as also against an impatience with divine benevolence and Providence some found difficult to control. Patrick does not speak at all of reprobation; his Arminian theology does not make it much of a pastoral concern. But, like the Calvinists, he was concerned in his counsel to stay impatience and complaint with these spiritual insights into the desertions of the Holy Ghost. As he posed the question to his cure: "shall we not yield submission quietly, to a thing for which there may be so many reasons; and those not at all to our prejudice, but to our profit?"[47]

The call to submit to such feelings was in part therapeutic and consolatory. Patrick warned against letting melancholic feelings open up onto intensive self-criticism: "*[b]e content to be dull sometime, and able to do nothing as you would; and yet do not think the worse of your self for it.*" To think otherwise would only aggravate the melancholy:

> [I]f it do stir up any suspicions in your mind, of you do not know what fault; yet never bluster at your self, but with a calm and gentle spirit suffer this distemper. Look upon your self as sick, and think that it is not good now to stir any humours. And therefore strive not too much with your self … when you are thus melancholy; for that will but cast you more into it. You will be the sooner eased, if you do as well as you can; and add not a greater load to your spirit, by your own fretful thoughts at this untoward indisposition.[48]

When even this "never-failing remedy" failed, and "you find your Dulness and backwardness to your Duty, at any time, continue so long and increase so much, that you are afraid there is danger in it, and it may prove pernicious to your Soul," Patrick recommended that the individual "then go and *take counsel of your spiritual Physician*, to whom I would have you open your case, as plainly and fully as you can." The mind suffering from melancholy is in such cases in need of better judgment to guide it: "He may help you to distinguish between your fears and real dangers; between your weakness and your wilfulness; between your laziness and your caution; between your bodily and your spiritual infirmities."[49]

---

46 Ibid.
47 Ibid., 246.
48 Ibid., 240.
49 Ibid., 202.

Patrick thus thought that melancholic feelings quite naturally led pious souls to question their devotion and righteousness, and he intimated further that this avenue of reflection was in some measure correct. According to Patrick, melancholy raised above all the issue of the extent to which the believer relied on feeling rather than will and reason in their spiritual exercises. But he insisted that such probing was to be pursued cautiously, in consultation with an expert, and individuals were not to jump to conclusions about the spiritual meaning of their feelings. For the most part, the religious concern and anxiety provoked by feelings of dullness would dissipate if the individual correctly appreciated the role that his body played in the practice of piety and properly took care of his "animal spirits."

Some of these cautions echo the consolatory techniques of Calvinist practical divines, who sought to show the despairing individual that, in light of the promises of the Gospel and the evidence of grace in their life, their despair was unfounded. And where the patient was unable to grasp onto this hope, English Calvinists used the idea of melancholy to explain their recalcitrant despair. But this use of the idea of melancholy was fundamentally different than the analysis of religious melancholy Patrick developed. English Calvinist ministers in the late sixteenth and early seventeenth centuries dealt with cases of religious melancholy as they did "normal" cases of religious despair, and only invoked melancholy when certain patterns of thought and behavior seemed resistant to spiritual physick. The body was thus somehow to explain the persistence of the religious melancholic's despairing thoughts, a mode of explanation which early modern medical theory supported. Patrick was giving a "longitudinal" analysis of religious melancholy which explained how more mild feelings of dullness and lethargy could develop into severe melancholy. Advanced forms of religious melancholy, in which the individual experienced feelings of worthlessness and divine abandonment, were not the product of the melancholic body as such. Rather, worry over the state of one's sorry and anxious self-examination produced these thoughts and feelings.

This is why, if we contrast a case such as that of Joan Drake to the kind of melancholy which Patrick discussed, it appears as if they are two very different and incomparable conditions. The former appears to us as a case of what we might call severe or psychotic depression, and the latter a case of mild depression, what we often call "feeling blue." But it is clear that Patrick thinks he is talking about the same kind of thing: the supposed experiences of deep despair, which were described in great detail and at great length in the vast body of "Puritan" spiritual writing, and which English Calvinist ministers had thought to be often mixed with melancholy. According to Patrick, it was this very body of writing which created the "experience" of profound and deep-rooted despair out of feelings of dullness and lethargy. Although Patrick suggested similar remedies to cases of religious melancholy as the English Calvinists, he was genuinely worried about the spiritual implications of Calvinist writing. And if he was correct in his analysis of melancholy, he had every reason to be.

In his *Instructions*, Bolton noted that lack of spiritual fervor and feeling was often the "spiritual malady" which produced questions about the presence of grace and the state of the soul in troubled souls. Bolton thus provided comfort for those who did not feel sorrow in proportion to the acknowledged grievousness of sin; for deadness of heart when there was no sensible response to prayers for the quickening of grace; for those "languishing under the heavy desolations of a spiritual desertion, and deprived of [their] former comfortable feelings of Gods favourable countenance," even though their status as redeemed had not changed.[50] But he took at face value that the lack of spiritual feeling was a *spiritual* malady rather than a feature of the human condition which the Holy Ghost sometimes allowed us to overcome, as Patrick maintained. At the same time that Bolton was consoling those whole worried over the "hardness of their hearts," he was thus reinforcing the tendency of the sufferer to read the condition in terms of the semiotics of grace. Furthermore, Bolton and others validated, even valorized, the feelings of desertion and anguish which contributed to trouble of conscience, and while they provided comfort to those troubled over their spiritual maladies, they also saw trouble of mind as evidence of the work of conscience exposing and expelling hidden sins.

For Patrick, on the other hand, a lack of feeling was never directly related to the health of our souls, although it might be used by God as a means of producing a greater degree of humility and obedience. And while genuine experiences of desertion by God did occur, Patrick was confident that they were always caused by some "provoking sin," which would be relatively clear to consciousness. Where there was no such obvious sin, there was no need to use religious trouble of mind as an opportunity to dredge up the hidden depths of the soul in search of sins to sorrow over, as late sixteenth and early seventeenth-century evangelical Calvinists asserted. Self-examination was something of a last resort, and was only to be done with an expert spiritual physician. Thus, from the perspective of Patrick, English Calvinists were consoling, and in some measure correctly, what they were at the same time provoking.

An Anglican tradition of consolation

MacDonald points to H.R. McAdoo's assertion that the practice of casuistry declined in the Church of England after 1660 as evidence for the statement that Anglican divines were unwilling to practice the kind of practical divinity popular before and during the English Civil War that had allowed for the treatment of "mental illnesses" like melancholy by counsel and spiritual comfort rather than by medicine alone.[51] Yet while the kind of Anglican moral theology and casuistry with which McAdoo is concerned seems to have been articulated in print less frequently, this should not be conflated with practical divinity. McAdoo contrasts a cool and distant eighteenth-century Deism with the ideal country parson found in George Herbert's *A Priest to the Temple* (1656), who "greatly esteems ... of cases of conscience, wherein he

---

50   Bolton, *Right Comforting*, 351–549, esp. 352, 354–5, 468, 499.

51   MacDonald, *Mystical Bedlam*, 226 n. 246; see H.R. McAdoo, *The Structure of Caroline Moral Theology* (London: Longmans, Green, 1949), 66, 96–7.

is much versed."[52] But as Donald Spaeth has pointed out, the pastoral standards of those like Herbert were still influential in the late seventeenth and early eighteenth centuries, and practical divinity was by no means abandoned, particularly when it was an arena for the competition between Anglican and nonconformist minister to win over souls.[53]

Furthermore, whereas the kind of casuistic works with which McAdoo is concerned rarely addressed the problem of religious melancholy, and then only in a rather oblique manner, the issue of religious melancholy was specifically addressed by a number of Anglican clergy in a series of published sermons and pamphlets in the late seventeenth and first half of the eighteenth century.[54] Patrick's latitudinarian colleague John Moore, Bishop of Norwich, presented a Lenten sermon to the recently enthroned Queen Mary which was afterwards published in seven editions in the following two decades under the +title *Of Religious Melancholy* (1691); the Exeter clergyman William Chilcot devoted a substantial chapter to melancholy his *Practical Treatise concerning Evil Thoughts* (1698); the famous theologian and philosopher Samuel Clarke, whose ecclesiastical career had in fact been promoted by Moore, wrote a sermon entitled "Of Religious Melancholy," which was also published several times in his collected sermons; and Edward Synge, the Archbishop of Ireland from 1716 to 1741, who was popular for his preaching and known for his works on practical piety, wrote a pamphlet devoted to the treatment of melancholy, out of pastoral concern.[55] The influential Bishop of Salisbury, Gilbert

---

52 Herbert, *A Priest to the Temple* (1652), as cited in McAdoo, *Caroline Moral Theology*, 66.

53 On the continued importance and performance of pastoral duties in the established Church of England in the late seventeenth and early eighteenth centuries, see Donald A. Spaeth, *The Church in an Age of Danger: Parsons and Parishioners, 1660–1740* (Cambridge: Cambridge University Press, 2000), 108–32, 214–22. See also Henry Dodwell, *Two Letters of Advice* (Dublin: Benjamin Tooke, 1672), 58–64 and 231–40, where Dodwell discusses the treatment of melancholy. Dodwell declares that the study of casuistry is "too much neglected, because too little experienced." But he applied this statement to Protestants in general, in contrast to Catholics, for whom the casuistic practice was instituted in the ritual of confession, and such statements can be found throughout seventeenth-century English casuistic works, both Puritan and Anglican. See Jeremy Taylor, *Ductor Dubitantium* (London: James Flesher for Richard Royston, 1660), i–ii; William Ames, *Conscience, with the Power and Cases Thereof* (London: Edward Griffin for John Rothwell, 1643), 'To the Reader,' sig. B.

54 Jeremy Taylor states that melancholy is often the root of cases of scrupulous conscience, a comment which, published in 1660, may well have been directed at believers and clergy who refused to conform to the newly established Church on grounds of conscientious objection to some of its ceremonies and practices: see *Ductor Dubitantium* 1.vi.1, 206.

55 John Moore, *Of Religious Melancholy: A Sermon Preached before the Queen at Whitehall, March VIth 1691/2* (London: for William Rogers, 1692); William Chilcot, *A Practical Treatise concerning Evil Thoughts ... especially useful for Melancholy Persons* (Exeter: Samuel Darker for Charles Yeo, John Pearce, and Philip Bishop, 1698); Clarke, "Of Religious Melancholy," Sermon 14 in Clarke, *Sermons on Several Subjects*, 7th edn. (London: for J. and P. Knapton, 1749), 10: 205–13; Edward Synge, *Sober thoughts for the*

Burnet, drew attention in his highly regarded *Discourse of Pastoral Care* (1692) to the need to minister to "sick Persons" who are "troubled of mind." And Thomas Secker, Archbishop of Canterbury from 1758 to 1768, likewise urged the clergy not to neglect the consolation of the sick, including the consolation of their dispirited delusions and anxious fears about their spiritual standing, in series of sermons in which he addressed the issue of unjustified melancholic doubts and fears in matters of faith.[56]

Significantly, except for Archbishop Synge's short pamphlet, all of these published works on religious melancholy were originally delivered as sermons, indicating that these clergy saw the condition of melancholy as an important enough pastoral concern to be addressed publicly in the pulpit; and Synge declares in his pamphlet that he intended the pamphlet for those suffering from melancholy, and had therefore made his comments brief and succinct. Exactly how popular these works were, and how many people read them is, aside from what the numerous editions of Moore's sermon seems to indicate, very difficult to tell. In any case, until at least the 1740s religious melancholy was seen by Anglican clergy themselves as a condition appropriately treated through spiritual consolation and pastoral care. It was thus not only Dissenters who "preserved the Puritan tradition of practical divinity, pastoral counsel, and consolation," as MacDonald would have us believe.[57]

Anglican works on the consolation of religious melancholy all tended to foreground the medical understanding of melancholic religious thoughts. Thus MacDonald cites Gilburt Burnet's influential *Discourse of Pastoral Care* (1692) as typical of the apparently "medicalized" Anglican approach to melancholy coming out of the critique of enthusiasm during and after the Restoration.[58] Burnet noted that some who suffered under apparent cases of the affliction of conscience were only "Melancholy hypochondriacal people, who, what through some false Opinions in Religion, what through a foulness of Blood ... fall under dark and cloudy apprehensions; of which they can give no clear or good account."[59] The fluctuation of humors, combined with a reliance on sensible feeling to measure the presence of grace in the act of prayer, created the belief that "God did sometimes shine out, and at other times hide his face," from which perception the conclusion for many was that God was angry with them. On Burnet's view, the minister was to explain to the parishioner the physiology of their condition, and Burnet, who thought that every

---

Cure of Melancholy, especially that which is Religious (London: for Thomas Trye, 1742). For biographical information on each of these writers, except Chilcot, see *The Oxford Dictionary of National Biography*, s.v. "Moore, John," s.v. "Clarke, Samuel," s.v. "Synge, Edward."

56 Burnet, *A Discourse of the Pastoral Care* (London: R.R. for Ric. Chiswell, 1692), xvi–xxx, 198–9; Thomas Secker, "On the Duties of the Sick," Sermons 41–3 in *The Works of Thomas Secker*, 3rd edn., ed. Beilby Porteus and George Stinton (Dublin: for J. Williams, 1775), 2: 183–209.

57 MacDonald, *Mystical Bedlam*, 227.

58 MacDonald, "Religion, Social Change and Psychological Healing," 118 n. 51.

59 Burnet, *Discourse*, 198–9.

clergyman should be familiar with the practice of physick, himself recommended "strong and Chalybeate Medicines."

Like Patrick, then, Burnet asserted that religious melancholy was the result of the confluence of humoral imbalance and a certain kind of understanding of spirituality, certain "false Opinions in Religion." It was the minister's duty to re-educate the religious melancholic, first making them understand the physiological source of their feelings and perspective, and then giving them the security of the true measure of spiritual condition: "They are to consider what are their Principles and Resolutions, and what's the settled Course of their Life; upon these they are to form sure Judgments, and not upon any thing that is so Fluctuating and inconstant as Fits or Humours."[60] Such a strategy is nearly identical to John Dod's attempt to persuade Joan Drake to rely on the evidences of grace in her life rather than her present feeling. To be sure, the theological understandings undergirding this therapy are different in either case: one looked to signs of grace where the other looked to moral reformation and conduct. Both, however, turned the individual away from melancholic perception towards some verifiable and substantive reality.

Burnet's advice to his colleagues thus hardly consists of a dismissal of the religious melancholic as a merely medical problem. Burnet's ideal clergyman is very involved, not just with the sufferer's body, but with their beliefs; he treats them as an individual with fears and anxieties which are to be addressed with sensitivity and attention. After recommending the use of medicine for religious melancholics, Burnet declares "yet such Persons are to be much pitied, and a little humoured in their Distemper. They must be diverted from thinking too much, being too much alone, or dwelling too long on Thoughts that are hard for them to Master."[61] Such therapies were commonplace in the treatment of melancholy, but their importance, and the importance of the conjunctive "yet" which introduces them, should not be ignored. They imply the importance of social community and the intersubjective involvement of the minister. Samuel Clarke, who distinguished as Burnet had between true and merely melancholic affliction of conscience, also asserted that although religious melancholy was "not properly and immediately of religious consideration, yet 'tis by no means to be neglected, slighted, or despised."[62] In fact, John Moore and William Chilcot had dealt with the spiritual complaints typical of religious melancholics at length in their sermons on religious melancholy. And while both Moore and Chilcot acknowledged that such feelings and thoughts were often occasioned by "the habit and constitution of the Body," both placed them as well within the context of Providential design and care.[63] Regarding blasphemous thoughts, Moore wrote:

> Do not think the worse of God for them, or accuse his Providence of want of care of you. For he might have permitted such Thoughts to have continued perpetually, or at least to have visited you much oftner, and in a more frightful manner, and all this without the

---

60   Ibid., 200–201.
61   Ibid., 199.
62   Clarke, "Of Religious Melancholy", 205–13.
63   Chilcot, *Treatise*, 219.

least diminution of his Justice ... He [is] sending these Afflictions for wise and kind Reasons; that they might be powerful Preservatives of your Souls against the hainous sins of a crooked Generation in which you live ... that they might lessen your Inclinations to the Enjoyments of this Life; that they might deaden your Appetites to sensual Pleasure, and take your hearts off of the perishing Goods of the World, which can afford you small satisfaction so long as your Minds are haunted with these black Thoughts.[64]

But while there were thus certain continuities with the Calvinist pastoral tradition, there were also crucial divergences. Two important elements of English Calvinist spirituality were abandoned by these Anglican divines in their understanding and treatment of melancholy: the suggestion that states of extreme religious fear and sorrow evidenced the grace of God in moving the soul to repentance; and the attempt to heal melancholic trouble of mind through the self-examination and the confession of sin appropriate to the affliction of conscience. Restoration Anglicans continued to emphasize the need for godly sorrow. Patrick wrote in a vein similar to Downame when he urged the grieving to "[t]urn thy sorrow for thy friend into sorrow for thy sin. Remember that thy tears may be due to some other thing, and the cure of that will cure all thy other griefs. If thou art a Christian, then it is thy duty to mourn neither for one thing nor other, but only to bewail thy self. Let the dead bury the dead (as our Saviour said) do thou presently follow the Lord with tears."[65] But melancholic feelings, analyzed by Patrick and others at their point of origin as organic vital disturbances rather than feelings of fear and sorrow *per se*, were seen as trials sent by God to sharpen the soul's humility and obedience. As such, they might expose a certain amount of weakness and sin, but they were not regarded by Anglicans as proper occasions for godly sorrow, nor were they cases of the affliction of conscience.

Separating religious melancholy from the affliction of conscience was clearly not an abandonment of the care of the melancholic soul; it was rather a line of thought and mode of treatment developed by Patrick and others for therapeutic reasons. The nonconformists, Patrick had argued, generated religious melancholy with their emphasis on religious feeling and experience as signs of spiritual health and vitality. Indeed, it was in part precisely because the differences between nonconformist, "Puritan" spiritual therapies and Anglican approaches were deeply theological that melancholy remained of serious pastoral concern to Anglicans. Religious melancholy was to be consoled through disabusing parishioners of evangelical Calvinist notions by instilling the principles of mainstream Anglican thought as it was defined in the Restoration.

---

64 Moore, *Of Religious Melancholy*, 28.
65 Patrick, *Hearts Ease*, 228.

CHAPTER FIVE

The "Puritan Tradition"?
Nonconformist Practical Divinity
and the Critique of "Enthusiasm"

The last chapter opened by noting that the critique of "enthusiasm" was launched by both Anglican and Dissenting anti-Calvinists. One of the most important of the Dissenting anti-Calvinist critics was the influential Presbyterian minister Richard Baxter. Baxter strongly objected to Patrick's portrait of the nonconformist in *A Friendly Debate*, because of its polemical tone and because it conflated the various kinds of nonconformists into one rather caricatured type. Indeed, although he was a nonconformist, Baxter was also an anti-Calvinist critic who had important ties with members of the established Church, including some of the latitudinarians. He attempted throughout his career to articulate a position on salvation that moved away from some of the key assumptions and conclusions of Calvinist theology, and provided a critique of nonconformist spiritual sensibilities similar to Patrick's. His theological orientation entailed a significant departure from the evangelical Calvinist approach to the care and consolation of melancholy found in late sixteenth and early seventeenth-century works. In some ways, it was even less sympathetic towards the religious melancholic than Patrick's.

This is not how Baxter has usually been portrayed. Baxter was immensely interested in the treatment of melancholy, touching on the issue in several of his many pastoral writings and devoting an entire sermon to the subject in 1682, which was published in a collection of sermons in 1683 and posthumously republished alone in 1713 and again in 1716.[1] That his work was seen as useful and important in the treatment of melancholy is evidenced as well by the Reverend Samuel Clifford's 1716 publication of a collection of the discussions of melancholy found throughout his voluminous published work.[2] (Curiously, this particular publication

---

1   Baxter, *The Cure of Melancholy and Overmuch-Sorrow by Faith and Physick*, Sermon 11 in Samuel Annesley, ed., *A continuation of morning-exercise questions and Cases of Conscience Practically Resolved by Sundry Ministers, in October 1682* (London: by J.A. for John Dunton, 1683), 263–304; *Preservatives against melancholy and over-much sorrow, or, The cure of both by faith and physick* (London: for Joseph Marshall, 1716); *Preservatives against melancholy and over-much sorrow, or, The cure of both by faith and physick* (London: W.R., 1713).

2   Richard Baxter, T*he Signs and Causes of Melancholy: with directions suited to the case of those that are afflicted with it. Collected out of the works of Richard Baxter by Samuel*

shows up in the library of John Munro, physician to the Bethlem Hospital, who tended on the whole to be rather hostile towards nonconformists and their style of spiritual physick for the mentally troubled.[3]) Thus, Michael MacDonald points to Baxter as evidence for the continued "Puritan" tradition of spiritual physick among the Restoration Dissenting communities.[4] Other scholars have identified Baxter as typical of Dissenting thought and expression in his emphasis on emotion in spiritual life.[5] And Baxter placed himself in the pastoral tradition of Perkins, Bolton, Dod, and Sibbes, referring to their work with respect and admiration.[6]

But although Baxter was influenced by earlier Puritan ministers, he treated melancholy in a manner fundamentally different than had the English Calvinist ministers to whom he looked back. He was markedly more cautious as to the valuation of religious feeling and emotion, and much less ready to accept cases of melancholy as mixed with genuine spiritual affliction. Indeed, like Spira's critics and "profane" Renaissance wits, he used the idea of melancholy to dismiss supposed experiences of spiritual abandonment as disease rather than celebrating them as moments of favored chastisement. Furthermore, he argued that melancholic disease itself was less a providential affliction than a state of mind caused by sinful worldly desire and disappointments. Baxter recognized that true spiritual affliction could result in melancholy through psychosomatic influence, but he thought that in most cases, the language of desertion and withdrawal and the complaints of spiritual lassitude were used by melancholic individuals to feed self-pity and arouse sympathy, even admiration, among members of the religious community who valued the expression of these religious experiences as markers of godliness and spiritual depth. Religious melancholy was indeed worldly sorrow transformed in godly sorrow, as Perkins and Bolton had envisioned; but according to Baxter, it was mired in false consciousness and bad faith.

While Baxter was apparently valued nationwide for his work with the melancholy, his was not the only pastoral approach in Dissenting circles. The London Presbyterian minister Timothy Rogers knew of Baxter, but articulated a very different mode of consolation in two works of pastoral advice published in the early 1690s. Rogers was himself melancholic, and his writing was based on his own experience of religious despair; but he is important for reasons beyond the fact that

---

Clifford (London: S. Cruttenden and T. Cox, 1716).

3   Jonathan Andrews and Andrew Scull, *Undertaker of the Mind: John Monro and Mad-doctoring in Eighteenth-century England* (Berkeley, CA and Los Angeles, CA: University of California Press, 2001), 294 n.12.

4   MacDonald, "Religion, Social Change and Psychological Healing," 110–12.

5   Rivers, *Reason, Grace and Sentiment*, 1: 89–162, esp. 125–6.

6   On Baxter's comments on Dod, Bolton, and others, see *Reliquiae Baxterianae* (London: for T. Parkhurst, J. Robinson, J. Lawrence, and J. Dunton, 1696), 1: 5–6; *The Right Method for Settled Peace of Conscience, and Spiritual Comfort in 32 Directions* (London: for T. Underhil and F. Tyton, 1653), 151, and the preface, "To the poor in spirit"; cf. Rivers, *Reason, Grace and Sentiment*, 1: 100.

he provides for the historian a "first-hand" account of religious melancholy.[7] First, Rogers believed that God was in some sense truly hiding his face from those who felt abandoned by him. He did not make the distinction Patrick had between true feelings and merely misguided interpretations of bodily feelings. Moreover, he made use of the doctrine of imputed righteousness in comforting those who felt abandoned by God in a way which, as critics such as Baxter pointed out, reinforced the primacy of feeling in the Christian life. But, second, there are also important departures from the late sixteenth and early seventeenth-century approach to religious melancholy in Rogers' consolatory works, and because Rogers generally wrote in the idiom of earlier evangelical consolations, these are all the more significant. Rogers did not stress the idea that melancholic spiritual affliction should be treated by scouring the soul and excoriating the sinful self. That the soul was sinful was taken for granted, but Rogers did not seem to think that a procedure of "Puritan" self-examination was appropriate in healing melancholic affliction. Rogers' treatment of godly sorrow is more consolatory than prescriptive in tone. Third, Rogers acknowledged, more explicitly than had late sixteenth and early seventeenth-century evangelicals, that religious melancholy was produced by a specific theologically based interpretation of certain kinds of feelings and experiences, that their spiritual meanings were not given in the feelings and experiences themselves.

Richard Baxter: the sin of melancholy

Baxter was raised and educated in the English Calvinist religious tradition; both his spiritual experiences and his pastoral concerns were deeply influenced by it. A significant portion of Baxter's prodigious output addressed the worries of the godly over the assurance of salvation. His own youthful encounter with godliness had the familiar contours of doubt and anxiety concerning his estate. As Baxter recorded the experience many years later in the *Reliquiae Baxterianae* (1696), he was "long kept with … the Questionings of a doubtful Conscience" provoked by "the Calls of approaching Death" – "a violent Cough, with Spitting of blood, &c., of two years continuance." The young Baxter was troubled with one of Bolton's "spiritual maladies": he could not find in his own conversion experience the stages of preparatory Grace traced in the writings of certain ministers; his "*Grief* and *Humiliation* was no greater," but he "could weep no more for this" lack of feeling; and "*Education* and *Fear* had done all that ever was done upon my Soul, and *Regeneration* and *Love* were yet to seek." He agonized that sins committed "*deliberately* and *knowingly*" after his conversion betrayed an absence of saving grace, from which he drew the conclusion that "if these proved that I had then *no Saving Grace*, after all that I had felt [in conversion], I thought it unlikely that *ever I should have any*" – a worry no doubt fostered by the many works that described the great extent to which the reprobate could be graced without ultimately receiving saving grace. He wondered

---

7   Useful biographical information on Rogers can be found in *The Oxford Dictionary of National Biography*, s.v. "Rogers, Timothy."

also "at the senseless hardness of [his] heart, that could think and talk of Sin and Hell, and Christ and Grace, of God and Heaven, with no more feeling: I cried out from day to day to God for Grace against this sensless Deadness: I called my self the *most hard hearted Sinner*, that could *feel* nothing of all that I knew and talkt of."

Reflecting late in life on these feelings, Baxter stated:

> I still groan under this as my sin and want, yet I now perceive that a Soul in Flesh doth work so much after the manner of the Flesh, that it much desireth sensible Apprehensions; but Things *Spiritual* and *Distant* are not so apt to work upon them, and to stir the Passions, as Things present and sensible are....and that the Rational Operations of the higher Faculties (the Intellect and Will) may without so much passion, set God and Things Spiritual highest within us, and give them the preheminence, and subject all Carnal Interest to them, and give them the Government of the Heart and Life: and that this is the ordinary state of a Believer.[8]

Baxter records that he was helped in his affliction of conscience by "the Reading of many Consolatory Books," and he attributes his life-long concern with practical divinity to his own search for spiritual comfort in the pastoral writings of Sibbes, Dod, Perkins, and others.[9] He would have encountered in this body of practical divinity the caution against putting too much emphasis on feeling because it was fleeting, an unreliable indicator of grace. Baxter also records that "that part of *Physicks* which treateth of the Soul" was one of his early and formative scholarly interests.[10] The use of seventeenth-century natural philosophical ideas of the soul to understand and evaluate religious experience is evident in Baxter's reflection in his *Reliquiae* and throughout his theological and practical writing. He consistently down-played the importance of feeling in spiritual life, noting that it was dependent to a large degree on the condition of the body, and emphasized instead the performance of moral and religious duty, effected through the power of the will and grounded in a clear understanding of the covenant of faith, as the substance of the Christian life.

Baxter was thus skeptical of assurance of election too easily raised by "high raptures and feelings of comfort" where there was little evidence the reformation of character.[11] And he was also deeply critical of the doctrine of imputed righteousness and its concomitant spiritual posture of resting in Christ where it was preached to the exclusion of recognizing the importance of obedience to the Gospel's precepts. According to Baxter, this opened the way to the licentious antinomianism he had witnessed among the more radical Ranter elements of the New Model Army in the 1640s. Baxter did not hesitate to make the case that the performance of works was in fact a condition of entering into the covenant of grace through which God justified the sinner and imputed to him Christ's perfect righteousness. As Baxter defined it early on in his *Aphorismes of Justification* (1649), faith is when a sinner, after realizing

---

8　　Baxter, *Reliquiae*, 1: 6–7.
9　　Ibid., 1: 4–5, 8.
10　Ibid., 1: 6.
11　Baxter, *Right Method*, 152, 227.

his own unrighteousness before the Law and subsequently learning of the message of grace through Christ, "doth hereupon believe the truth of this Gospel ... and do accordingly rest on him as their Saviour, and sincerely (though imperfectly) obey him as their Lord, forgiving others, loving his people, bearing what sufferings are imposed, diligently using his means and Ordinances, and confessing and bewailing their sins against him, and praying for pardon; and all this sincerely, and to the end."[12] Baxter includes in this definition the spiritual posture of resting in Christ as Savior, but it is all but displaced by the detailed emphasis on the moral performance the act of faith involved.

Thus, although Baxter insisted that humans did not merit grace through their moral performance, and that it was in fact God who bestowed the grace necessary for covenanting moral obedience, he emphasized the active role of the human will in obeying the commandments of Christ as the central component of faith.[13] Baxter was departing significantly from the theology of earlier English Calvinists, according to whom the human will was entirely passive. From another point of view, however, he was in effect defining doctrinally what English Reformed ministers had long asserted in pastoral practice: that true saving faith manifested itself in sanctification; that it was not simply in passively observing, but also in actively maintaining the steady resolve of the will in the work of godliness that the only comfortable grounds of assurance could be found. This is why Baxter could place himself in the tradition of the Elizabethan and early Stuart evangelical Calvinist practical divines. And, as for earlier Calvinist divines, the importance of emphasizing works in the definition of justifying faith was for Baxter partly pastoral. Baxter declared in *The Right Method for Settled Peace of Conscience* (1653) that the principal act of faith was the "understandings belief of the truth of the Gospel, and the Wills acceptance of Christ and Life offered to us wherein." This, he argued, was an improvement on what he took to be the prevailing understanding of faith, as a "resting on Christ for salvation." Affiance is "not the principal act, nor that wherein the very life of justifying faith doth consist: but only an imperate following act, and an effect of the vital act (which is consent, or willing, or accepting Christ offered) for it lieth mainly in that which we call the sensitive part, or the Passions of the soul."[14] The sensitive part of the soul was, as Baxter pointed out in his *Reliquiae*, that which was least in our control. To rely on affiance for assurance was to expose one's perception of assurance to the inconstancy of the passions and to the fluctuations of bodily fluids and animal spirits.[15]

---

12   Baxter, *Aphorismes*, 279–80, as cited in Rivers, *Reason, Grace and Sentiment*, 1: 137.

13   On Baxter's theological views, see the nuanced discussion in William M. Lamont, *Richard Baxter and the Millennium: Protestant Imperialism and the English Revolution* (London: Croom Helm, 1979), 135–40; 149–50.

14   Baxter, *Right Method*, 52–3.

15   Ibid., 152.

Harbored in the high valuation of feeling as evidence of grace was thus the eminent danger of disconsolation and despair, which Baxter himself had experienced. Sensibility to sin and a spiritual rebirth which consumed the emotions were indeed to be sought after; in the *Reliquiae*, Baxter regarded his own passionlessness as both his "sin and want."[16] But he took his spiritual sensibility to be an indication of the temperature of his body, spiritually significant only as the body's hindrance of the soul's godly longing, not as a measure of the working of grace in the higher faculties of reason and will which was the substance of Christian faith. Addressing himself to the worry, often voiced by those troubled in conscience, "that I grow not in grace," Baxter responded:

> They think that more of the life and truth of Grace doth lie in Passionate Feelings of Sin, Grace, Duty, etc., in sensible Zeal, Grief, Joy, etc., and do not know that the chief part lieth in the Understanding's estimation, and the Will's firm Choice and Resolution. And then they think that they decline in Grace, because they cannot weep, or joy so sensibly as before.[17]

In *The Poor Mans Family Book* (1674), Baxter asserted that this error was in fact a temptation of the devil: "he will make you think that all Religion lieth in striving to *weep* and *break your heart more*" and "that your conversion was not true, because you had no more brokenness of heart for sin." Baxter anticipates the astonished response: "Sir, You make me admire to hear you! Can such motions of holiness come from the Devil?" To which he replies: "*overdoing* is the *undoing of all*."[18] This is strongly put, and it shows clearly why he was so interested in treating religious melancholy. Theological criticism of cherished nonconformist opinions was in fact combat with the devil over souls.

The undoing Baxter thought was encouraged by the devil was examined most fully in his 1682 sermon on melancholy and "over-much sorrow," addressed originally to a London audience and published a year later. Baxter drew there the familiar picture of the individuals who, in order "to be the best Christians," "are most in Doubts, and Fears, and Sorrows, and speak almost nothing but uncomfortable Complaints." Such people "never fear *overmuch Sorrow* till it hath *swallowed them up*." To warn and to prevent, Baxter set out what defined an excess of religious trouble of mind. Sorrow and trouble of mind were too much, he argued, where reason, which should stop the passions from dwelling on "perplexing Subjects, or turn them to better and sweeter things," "hath no power against the Stream of troubling Passions." The passions of the troubled soul pull against recalling the "Matters of unspeakable Joy which the Gospel calleth us to believe":

> [I]t is wonderful hard for a grieved troubled Soul to believe anything that is matter of Joy; much less of so great Joy, as Pardon and Salvation are. Though it dare not flatly give God

---

16   Baxter, *Reliquiae*, 1: 6.

17   Baxter, *Right Method*, 470–71.

18   Baxter, *Poor Man's Family Book* (London: R.W. for Nevill Simmons, 1674), 183–4.

the Lie, it hardly believes his free and full Promises, and the Expressions of his readiness to receive all penitent returning Sinners. Passionate Grief serveth to *feel* somewhat contrary to the Grace and Promises of the Gospel; and that *feeling* hinders *Faith*.[19]

The afflicted "thinks not of things as they are, but as his Passion represents them, about God and religion, and about his own Soul and his actions." Thus, the over-sorrowful tends to regard all that they read and hear as making out "against him: every sad Word and Threatning in Scripture, he thinks meaneth him as if it named him." He cannot maintain the hope in the Gospel, "which is the Anchor of the Soul": "Fain would such have *Hope*, but they cannot. All their thoughts are suspicious and misgiving, and they can see nothing but danger and misery, and a helpless state."[20]

This reads like a classic evangelical portrayal of a case of conscience. But Baxter was not using it to warn of the terrors of conscience and the need for thorough self-examination and sorrow for sin, but rather to warn that too often sorrow for sin was excessive, perverting the correct order of the faculties on which a healthy Christian temper depended. Late sixteenth and early seventeenth-century evangelical Calvinists thought that there might be some melancholy mixed up in such extreme spiritual suffering; in Baxter's *A Christian Directory*, on the other hand, the language expressing desertion and forsakenness itself is represented as merely a symptom melancholic disease.[21] Baxter's comment on the famous case of Francis Spira is particularly illuminating. "The reading of *Spira*'s case causeth or increaseth Melancholy in many; the ignorant Author having described a plain Melancholy, contracted by the trouble of sinning against Conscience, as if it were a damnable despair of a sound understanding."[22] For the older cohort of divines, Spira's was a classic case of an afflicted conscience, illustrating its enormous emotional torment.[23] Baxter accepted it as an afflicted conscience, but aligned the emotional distress of the condition with melancholy rather than with the afflicted conscience itself. As he argued in *The Cure of Melancholy and Overmuch Sorrow*, much spiritual trouble proceeded from melancholy alone, or was self-induced by erroneous beliefs about the emotional temper of the Christian life, which could lead to melancholy. Of the apparently many individuals with mental trouble who sought him out,[24] Baxter declared in *The Right Method* that although such trouble might be caused by "some cherished corruption that breedeth and feedeth the sad uncomfortable state," "six or

---

19   Baxter, *Cure of Melancholy*, 10.

20   Ibid., 11.

21   Baxter, *A Christian Directory, or, A Summ of Practicall Theologie* (London: Robert White for Nevill Simmons, 1673), 262.

22   Ibid.

23   See MacDonald, "Narrative, Emotion and Identity." See also, for example, Perkins, *Treatise tending unto a declaration*, 378; Bolton, *Right Comforting*, 85.

24   "I know not how it came to pass," Baxter records in his autobiography, "but if men fell melancholly, I must hear from them or see them (more than any Physician that I know)"; *Reliquiae*, 2: 85.

ten to one" suffer from melancholy.[25] He urged his readers to distinguish between spiritual trouble proper and "those sorrows that come from your Spleen," insisting that the spiritual comforts of the treatise applied only to those who were genuinely troubled from "sins and wants in Grace," rather than the melancholic, or those who suffered from "discontenting afflictions in worldly affairs."[26]

Baxter thus refused to allow the melancholic to masquerade as spiritually afflicted. In a passage of advice to melancholics in the *Reliquiae*, Baxter warned:

> that Tears and Grief be not commended inordinately for themselves, nor as meer Signs of a Converted Person: And that we call Men more to look after *Duty* than after *Signs* as such … so you will call them much more to the Love of God, and let them know that that Love is their best sign, but yet to be excercised on a higher Reason, than as a *sign* of our own Hopes … [T]oo many of late have made their Religion to consist too much in the seeking of these [signs] out of their proper time and place, without referring them to that Obedience, Love and Joy, in which true Religion doth principally consist.[27]

A theological language which emphasized certain kinds of feeling as the signs of grace encouraged the spiritual hysterics of over-much sorrow by both encouraging and sheltering a weakness of reason. As Baxter noted, melancholy naturally made an individual prone to exaggerated fear and sorrow, but theological and pastoral error could be precipitating causes, pushing the soul with a weak governing power into a condition of uncontrollable sorrow and anxiety.[28]

Baxter's approach in melancholic cases was to fortify a weak reason with pastorally sound theological arguments and strategies for regulating emotion. Thus, although Baxter told the melancholic that "you may as well expect that a good Sermon or comfortable words should cure the falling sickness, or palsy, or a broken head, as to be a sufficient cure to your melancholy fears," in *A Christian Directory* he had several pages of advice for controlling melancholic thoughts."[29] Here and elsewhere, much of the counsel Baxter offered in order to "allay the symptoms" of melancholy[30] recalled his efforts to bring emotional balance to a Calvinist tradition led astray by erroneous conceptions of the acts of faith and grace. Baxter advised the melancholic not to overvalue "*the passionate part of duty, but know that Judgement, Will and Practice, a high esteem of God and holiness, a resolved choice, and a sincere endeavour are the life of Grace and duty, when feeling Passions are but lower uncertain things.*"[31] His arguments against melancholic thoughts themselves consisted of summarizing some of the main points Baxter argued against his

---

25 Baxter, *Right Method*, 282–4.

26 Ibid., 7.

27 Baxter, *Reliquiae*, 2: 86.

28 Baxter, *Cure of Melancholy*, 18.

29 Baxter, Right Method, 8; see also Baxter, *God's Goodness Vindicated, for the help of such (especially in Melancholy) as are tempted to deny it* (London: for N. Simmons, 1671), 3–4.

30 Baxter, *Right Method*, 9.

31 Baxter, *A Christian Directory*, 266.

theological opponents. Against the doctrine of limited atonement, that Christ died only for the elect, Baxter asserted that the covenant of grace was offered to all who believed in the truth of the Gospel and maintained a sincere intention to "Holiness of heart and life." Election was, from this point of view, not ascertained but asserted in action and will: "He who hath this Grace and desire, may know that he is elect; and the making of our *Calling* sure by our *Consenting* to the holy *Covenant*, is the making of our *Election* sure."[32]

Late sixteenth and early seventeenth-century evangelical Protestant therapy had stressed the importance of an authoritative figure who could guide the soul. Baxter also insisted, in this case to ministers hesitant to take on cases of conscience, that souls need a "Master and a Pilot."[33] His advice to the melancholic is, after persuading them that something is amiss with their mind, to entrust their case to a reputable minister and "believe him, and be ruled by him, rather then by your crazed self."[34] He also retained many of the kinds of therapies advocated by the late Elizabethan and early Stuart ministers and evidenced in the narrative of Mrs. Drake. He advised that the melancholic be busy, and to "always be in some pleasing *cheerful Company*, solitariness doth but cherish musings." This was the case even for prayer: public was to be preferred over secret prayer. To those who could not use "that reason and power that is left" to control blasphemous thoughts suggested by the devil, by turning thought away from them or otherwise diverting the mind in activity and company, Baxter recommended that the melancholic confide in a friend who may help to redirect the mind and emotions. In addition to frequent arguments for the "Infinite Love and Mercy" of God, Baxter urged the caregivers that if there was "any lawful thing that will please them in speech, in company, in apparel, in rooms, in attendance, give it them." "A great part of their cure lyeth in *pleasing* them, and avoiding all displeasing things as far as lawfully can be done." He noted also that "its a useful way if you can to engage them in comforting others, that are deeper in Distresses than they: For this will tell them, that their Case is not singular, and they will speak to themselves, while they speak to others."[35]

Baxter's critique of religious melancholy shared many of the same points as Patrick's, but Baxter went far beyond Patrick or any of the later Anglicans by providing an alternative assessment of melancholy's spiritual importance that pointed not just to incorrect theological belief but also to sin. Patrick traced the religious despair of the nonconformist to general feelings of deflation, which he admitted to be a common experience in the practice of piety, both among conformists and nonconformists. Baxter wrote that "the disease in some few beginneth with over-stretching thoughts and troubles about things spiritual; but in most that I have met with (ten to one), it beginneth with some worldly cross, loss or trouble, which grieveth them, and casteth

---

32 Ibid., 264.
33 Baxter, *Right Method*, 518–19.
34 Baxter, *The Cure of Melancholy*, 291.
35 Ibid., 291–5.

them into troublesome anxieties and cares."[36] Yet "were nothing *over-loved*, it would have no Power to torment us." The root of the majority of melancholic cases is the sin of too much love of the body and of the world; and "there is yet more Sin in the root of all, and that is, it sheweth that our *Wills* are yet *too selfish*, and not subdued to a due *Submission* to the *Will of God*." Anxieties and cares over worldly losses thus evidence a sinful impatience, for "it is presupposed that God trieth his Servants in this Life with manifold Afflictions, and Christ will have us near the Cross, and follow him in submissive patience." Furthermore, such impatience shows that, as we are not content with the "lowest State," we are not sufficiently humbled for our sins; and that there is still a great deal of unbelief in God's "wisdom, all-sufficiency and love." The root of melancholy, Baxter concludes, "is a Conjunction of many Sins, which in themselves are of no small Malignity," adding the ominous warning that "were they the predominant bent and habit of Heart and Life, they would be the Signs of a graceless State."[37]

The move to blame the melancholic for their condition had always been available to the Protestant religious tradition we have been discussing. It was to some extent latent in the moral philosophical approach to melancholy articulated by those like Burton. In the context of a psychology which took the heart as the physical organ of the passions, their exercise was seen to excite the entire "animal economy," disturbing its normal function, sometimes to pathological degrees.[38] Thus Burton relayed the collected evidence in the several chapters on the passions in the *Anatomy*, detailing how sorrow, fear, shame, disgrace, envy, malice, hatred, anger, covetousness, vainglory, pride, and joy could, among other perturbations of the mind, all be counted as causes of melancholy and madness.[39] Earlier evangelical writers had warned against a spiritual sorrow unaccompanied by grateful joy. As Bolton cautioned: "Thou maist, by the unsettledness of thy heavie heart unnecessarily, unfit and disable thy self for the duties and discharge of … thy callings."[40] They had also warned against an excess of sorrow for things of the world. Drawing from Proverbs 17:22, Bolton echoed the moral philosophical anatomy of sorrow: "It dries the bones, consumes the marrow, chills the blood, wastes the spirits, eates up the heart, shortneth life, and cutteth off too soone, from the day of gracious visitation."[41] Others drew attention more directly to melancholy. Downame, in stressing the need to "become in all things subject to the will of God … in the denying of our selves and our owne wills," noted that Christians should "mortifie our melancholike discontent by a true faith,

---

36 Baxter, *God's Goodness Vindicated*, 5.

37 Baxter, *Preservatives* (1716), 28–32.

38 On the details of the physiology, see Babb, *Elizabethan Malady*, 1–20, 102–27, and Anderson, *Elizabethan Psychology*. On the six non-naturals, see L.J. Rather, "'The Six Things Non-natural': Origins and Fate of a Doctrine and a Phrase," *Clio Medica* 3 (1968): 337–47.

39 Burton, *Anatomy*, I.ii.III.iv–xiv: 298–348.

40 Bolton, *Right Comforting*, 297.

41 Ibid., 192. See also Burton, *Anatomy*, I.ii.III.v: 300.

which will perswade us that that estate is best for us, in which God hath placed us."[42] The preacher Thomas Cooper wrote that the devil takes the "occasion by outward crosses to plunge the minde into immoderate sorrow, and so procures melancholicke and fearefull thoughts."[43]

In spite of this moralizing of sorrow, however, the sin attaching to inordinate affection did not frame the understanding and treatment of melancholy in late Tudor and early Stuart pastoral works. From the available evidence, it does not appear that in ministering to the melancholy as cases of spiritual or demonic affliction, or even, as in Burton, as cases for the moral philosopher, it was important to search out the specific blame attaching to their condition. Bolton's point was to channel sorrow of any kind into spiritual sorrow for sin, and Cooper followed him in this, reiterating his valuation of melancholy's potential to contribute to contrition and godly sorrow.[44] Melancholy was an important opportunity to reflect on sinfulness, but did not itself become a condition stigmatized by sinfulness; it was more dangerous as an occasion of the temptation to despair, sinfully disbelieving the goodness of God, but it did not itself reflect the indulgence of sinful thoughts. If those in the blindness of grief were to "bring the parts wounded to some certain object and matter of their trouble" and so to the "confession of some especial, secret and several sin," it was nowhere suggested that that sin was precisely their immoderate sorrow.[45] On the contrary, worldly sorrow and melancholy provided a tremendous energy for the affliction of conscience.

But one does not find Baxter recommending that melancholic or worldly sorrow be used for lamenting sin. Rather, he suggests that spiritual sorrow and desolation may in fact mask sinful, worldly sorrow. "Though there be too much of other Causes in it, yet if any of it be for Sin," the popular conventions of godly behaviour and speech allowed sorrow to be cultivated and cherished "as a necessary Duty," expressed in doubts, fears, and uncomfortable complaints. Furthermore, Baxter argued, this inflated emotional rhetoric could be used by the melancholy and sorrowful to elicit sympathy for a condition which was in fact their fault, but for which, in religious language of election, reprobation, and the signs of grace, they could be figured as the sorry victims of divine decree. Where Baxter defended the melancholic against the imputation of blame for the blasphemous and despairing thoughts incident to the disease, it was in order that the afflicted "may no[t] by Error cherish their Passions or Distress," taking them to be signs of a gracelessness and reprobation deserving pity. But if the melancholic thoughts themselves were not to be attributed to the sufferer, chastisement, not comfort, were the proper remedies for the sorrowful:

Too may Persons in their Sufferings and Sorrows, think they are only to be pityed, and take little notice of the Sin that Caused them, or that they still continue to commit, and too

---

42 Downame, *A guide to godlynesse* (London: F. Kinston for Philemon Stephens, 1629), 357.

43 Cooper, *Sacred Mysterie*, 184.

44 Cooper, *Government of Thoughts*, 189–90, 200.

45 Greenham, *A most Sweete ... Comfort*, sig. Fij.

many unskilful Friends and ministers do only comfort them, when a round of Chiding and Discovery of their Sin should be the better part of the Cure ... this would do more to cure some, than words of Comfort, when they say as *Jonah, I do well to be angry*, and think that all their denials of grace and distracting Sorrows, and wrangling against God's Love and Mercy are their Duties, it's time to make them know how great Sinners they are.[46]

Women, melancholy, and the critique of "enthusiasm"

One of the individuals who attempted to seek out Baxter because of his reputation with melancholic cases was the nonconformist Mrs. Hannah Allen, whose autobiographical narrative of her severe religious melancholy was posthumously published as *A narrative of God's gracious dealings with that choice Christian Mrs. Hannah Allen ..., reciting the great Advantages the devil made of her deep melancholy, and the triumphant victories, rich and sovereign graces, God gave her over all his stragems and devices* (1683). As the title indicates, Allen's story is cast in very similar terms to that of Joan Drake, and indeed her melancholy originated, like Drake's, in worldly disappointment. Allen writes that she was "much inclined to Melancholy, occasioned by the oft absence of my dear and affectionate Husband." After eight years of marriage, Mr. Allen "dyed beyond Sea," in 1662. Allen "began to fall into deep Melancholy, and no sooner did this black humour begin to darken my soul, but the Devil set on with his ... Temptations."[47] Allen struggles for several years with deep despair before she gradually emerges from her melancholy. She herself does not comment on the cause of her melancholy, though she prays for "Self-denial and patience to wait upon [God], and submit to him; and let him do with me what he pleaseth."[48] But interpolated without attribution into her autobiography is a third-person account by "a Minister," which relates a specific pastoral visit he paid to her, concluding with this warning: "From his Observation of the ground of her Trouble, he advises all Christians to mortifie inordinate Affection to lawful things."[49]

In the case of Mrs. Drake, published thirty-six years earlier, Joan Drake's melancholy was clearly understood to be the result of worldly discontentment, but only her great desire for the feeling of assurance was moralized, and this as dangerous, not sinful. The narrator saw in Joan Drake's case a story of God's mercy in delivering one of his children from her spiritual suffering, not an instance of punishment for excessive emotion. The anonymous preface to Hannah Allen's story emphasized similarly that the story was a narrative of the spiritual trials and

---

46 Baxter, *Preservatives* (1716), 39.

47 Allen, *A narrative of God's gracious dealings with that choice Christian Mrs. Hannah Allen (afterwards married to Mr. Hatt) reciting the great advantages the devil made of her deep melancholy, and the triumphant victories, rich and sovereign graces, God gave her over all his stratagems and devices* (London: John Wallis, 1683), 8–9.

48 Ibid., 16.

49 Ibid., 39–40.

temptations of a godly woman given over to demonic persecution, who, by the grace of God, was able eventually to overcome them. This is how Hannah Allen portrays her own suffering, though had she actually been able to see Baxter, she might found out "how great a Sinner she was."

The anonymous warning in Hannah Allen's *Narrative* and Baxter's critique of religious melancholy can be seen as part of a wider shift during the Restoration towards a greater emphasis on the need for reason to control the emotions in the spiritual life. Importantly this emphasis on a piety strictly regulated by reason was often articulated in terms of the proper hierarchy and roles of men and women. As historians of gender have helpfully illuminated, the Restoration of 1660 was not only a political restoration of the monarchy; it also inaugurated the reassertion of male power and authority, which many saw as disrupted and challenged during the religious and political upheaval of the Civil War and the Commonwealth. During the 1640s and 1650s, some women had entered the previously prescribed arena of public debate and polemic, expressing their own opinions on political and theological issues in print and by petition to Parliament. Furthermore, among groups such as the Quakers women were permitted to speak in Church meetings, and many of the most politically outspoken and incendiary Quaker prophets were women. Thus, the Restoration of Charles II was expressed by many of his supporters in terms of the restoration of a patriarchy, and the social and political disorder of the previous two decades was perceived as the result of the subversion of the proper gender hierarchy by disobedient and disorderly women. Traditional gender roles were reasserted and enforced even among the Quakers, and the more enthusiastic expression of religious devotion came to be seen by both Anglicans and Dissenters as a feature of women's emotional nature and a threat to the natural order.[50]

The connection between heightened religious experience and women was present in the present in pre-Civil War evangelical notions of gender. The emotional nature of women was seen as a source of potential disorder, particularly as according to common demonological notions, their weakness made them the fitter instrument for the designs of the devil. In 1645, likely in reaction to the public agitation of some women for an ecclesiological system of independent and autonomous congregations, the minister John Brinsley published a sermon on 1 Timothy 2:14 in which he argued that women have, in virtue of their weakness and infirmity, "a natural aptitude, and inclination ... to be deceived," which the devil used to good effect in choosing to tempt Adam through tempting Eve.[51] Women were thus associated with both separatism and heresy, which many establishment churchmen perceived as attempts to overturn

---

50   See the summary treatment in Susan Kingsley Kent, *Gender and Power in Britain, 1640–1990* (London: Routledge, 1999), 16–27. For more detailed treatments of various of these aspects, see Mack, *Visionary Women*; Anne Laurence, "A Priesthood of She-believers: Women and Congregations in Mid-seventeenth-century England," in Sheils and Wood, eds., *Women in the Church*, 345–63, and Patricia Crawford, *Women and Religion*.

51   John Brinsley, *A Looking-Glasse for Good Women* (London: John Field for Ralph Smith, 1645), 4. 1 Timothy 2:14 reads: "And Adam was not deceived, but the woman being deceived was in the transgression" (KJV).

male power and authority.[52] But at the same that their experience was to be policed by male reason, late sixteenth and early seventeenth-century evangelical piety as a whole was profoundly oriented towards the pursuit of a sensible, "living" faith. It was only when female heresy and power became more than simply a notional threat satisfactorily contained by complementary relationships between godly ministers and devout women and was perceived to have spilled out into massive disorder and tumult that the value of women's contribution to piety as a whole sharply declined in the minds of male authorities. After the Restoration, an emotional mode of piety was seen by many as more fitting for women than men, and even then in need of close policing, rather than exemplary for both sexes.

This transition can already be seen in the difference between the two editions of the Mrs. Drake narrative. Although the text of the story is the same for both, the 1647 edition is accompanied by a note from John Downame recommending it as "a singular antidote to preserve others in her condition, from being plunged into and quite swallowed up with deep despaire." The title announces a story of affliction and saving grace, and the epigraph is Psalms 66:16: "Come and heare, all yee that feare God; and I will declare what he hath done for my soule." The title of the 1654 edition, however, notes the "power and severe Discipline of Satan" and gives a very different epigraph: "I saw Satan like Lightning fall from Heaven" (Luke 10:18). In both cases, the narrative points to the activity of the Devil in Joan Drake's affliction, but in 1654, framing her affliction put her suffering as a whole in a very different light, aligning her with disorderly and enthusiastic sectaries rather than with the godly. This is made clear by the anonymous preface:

> I look upon the great part of this Nation (at present) in the condition of this afflicted Gentlewoman, purely *possessed* and *captivated* by an *encleane spirit*, which makes them *foam at the mouth*, and to rave and rage horribly against Gods ministers who endeavour their good. But they [God's ministers] hope … by their patience and perseverance … to tame these poor *Lunaticks*, and *charm* their fiercenesse, and bring them to their right temper and frame of mind again: so that they shall … crave pardon for their Extravagances, and give them humble thanks for their patience, in bearing with them in their *transports & frenzie.*[53]

The language throughout the preface is much less consolatory than it is militant. Joan Drake's ministers used the "artillery" of prayer and the "battring Engin" of fasting to rid "Joan Drake … of her imperious Governor, and uncivil Tutor." Joan Drake herself is represented as entirely passive in all of this spiritual warfare, and tellingly, the recommendation from Downame is absent in the 1654 edition.

No mention is made here of Joan Drake's melancholy. But John Brinsley had noted that one reason for the ease with which women were deceived by the devil was woman's "*dislike of*, and *discontentednesse with her present condition*." "A discontented spirit is a forge and Anvile fit for Satan to forge and hammer anything

---

52   Crawford, *Women and Religion*, 119–27.
53   *Mrs. Drake* (1647), "To the Christian Reader."

upon that is evil," he warned.[54] Baxter developed this line of thought more fully in his critique of religious melancholy, which became at this juncture a critique of nonconformist *female* piety. Consistently throughout his writings, he drew attention to the alleged natural weakness of women's reason, aligning their natural mental constitution with melancholic disease. Thus, he asserted that women in particular tended to rely on feeling and sensation for the spiritual comfort, and were thus more vulnerable to being disturbed by spiritual disconsolation rather than soldiering on with the more rational security available in theological argument. He also held that women and melancholic individuals were particularly prone to suffer from religious disconsolation, because both lacked the measure of reason sufficient to enable clear theological and spiritual insight and to combat the influence of feeling and the passions on spiritual perception.[55] But as we have seen, Baxter insisted that to cultivate godly sorrow at the expense of reasoned hope and sound understanding was to allow oneself to be deceived by the devil. Furthermore, precisely because of their weakness of reason, women were prone to develop cases of melancholy: among the "principal causes" of melancholy Baxter listed "a *weak Head* and *Reason*, joyned with strong *Passion*: which are oftest found in Women, and those to whom it is natural."[56] Women were thus naturally more inclined than men to sinful worldly grief, which often developed into melancholy, but which apparently pious women sinfully cherished in the form of over-much religious sorrow. Baxter's assumptions about female nature were entirely consistent with late sixteenth and early seventeenth-century ideas of gender and piety. But his emphasis on the authority of reason in the spiritual life and his concomitant de-emphasis of feeling had exposed the language of popular nonconformist piety as altogether suspect, and combined with the logic of the gender ideology Baxter shared with his contemporaries, they had exposed religious melancholy as a particularly female vice.

Baxter appears to have been the first to identify women explicitly with melancholy in this manner. His statements appear before the emergence in the eighteenth century of the medical discourse on "sensibility," in which women were represented as more prone to emotional upset and so to a range of nervous disorders, including various forms of melancholy. Nervous sensibility was a complex and ambiguous concept, pointing to the dangers the passions posed to the body but at the same time celebrating the emotional sensitivity and wit which nervous sensibility enabled and which were qualities of women in particular.[57] There was no such ambiguity for Baxter. Female melancholy pointed unequivocally and solely to female weakness, irrationality, and the consequent sin of excessive worldly passion. Behind Baxter's much-vaunted reputation as a minister skilled in dealing with cases of religious melancholy and affliction of conscience was a man with a strongly condemnatory, even cynical,

---

54 Brinsley, *Looking-Glasse*, 8.

55 See Baxter, *Right Method*, 152, 227.

56 Baxter, *A Christian Directory*, 314; *Preservatives* (1716), 30, 77; *Cure of Melancholy*, 294.

57 See page 154 below.

attitude towards those who claimed to suffer from such spiritual complaints. Baxter insisted that the language of spiritual feeling was a chimera and a smoke-screen, that the vocabulary of the afflicted conscience was used by weak women to hide sinful passion from the view of the godly community and from conscience itself.

Timothy Rogers: rewriting Calvinist consolation

After an absence of several years, some time in 1690 Timothy Rogers felt well enough to rise to the pulpit of the Dissenting Presbyterian congregation at Crosby Square, Bishopsgate in London, where he had previously served as one of the evening lecturers. As the congregation well knew, his absence was the result of melancholy, which had incapacitated him for the work of the ministry. He informed them that evening that by the grace of God he had recovered, and he devoted his first series of sermons to the understanding and consoling of sickness, applying the spiritual insight he had gained in his own experience. These sermons were published in 1691 as *Practical Discourses on Sickness and Recovery*. In the Epistle Dedicatory, addressed to two gentlemen who had provided a welcome retreat for the melancholic minister at their country estates, Rogers noted that he had relayed in these sermons only "some part of my Affliction": "I have not here insisted on that, which was the Trouble of my Trouble, my spiritual Distress, my Anxieties and my Fears, which were vastly afflicting to me than my bodily Pains, which yet were both sharp and long." "I do purpose," he continued, "to publish some others hereafter, that shall both contain an account of the Distresses of my Soul, and also some Directions to those that are long afflicted, and more especially to Melancholy People, to whose Case there is very little said by those who have long been so themselves."[58] *His Discourse Concerning Trouble of Mind and the Disease of Melancholy* was published that same year.

Like the Elizabethan and early Stuart divines, Rogers was quite conscious of the fact that in addressing the issue of melancholy trouble of mind, he was in the territory of medicine. He acknowledged Greenham's wisdom in recommending the use of both the physician and the minister in cases of melancholic spiritual affliction. Baxter had gone beyond this bare recommendation and provided in his tract on melancholy medical remedies and pharmaceutical recipes; he was confident, indeed dogmatic, that physick was the only proper cure for melancholy even where it was expressed (mistakenly) as an afflicted conscience. But Rogers showed a great deal of reservation about the efficacy of medicine. "I pretend not to tell you what Medicines are proper to remove it, and I know of none," he declared flatly.[59] His pessimism about the medical cure of melancholy proceeded from his own experience. As he recorded in the *Practical Discourses*: "I have often found the Insufficiency of all things that have been prescribed, and that they have not given me the least Ease in

---

58   Rogers, *Practical Discourses of Sickness and Recovery* (London: for Thomas Parkhurst, Jonathan Robinson, and John Dunton, 1691), xxviii–xxix.

59   Rogers, *A Discourse Concerning Trouble of Minde and the Disease of Melancholy* (London: for Thomas Parkhurst and Thomas Cockerill, 1691), iii–iv.

my violent and sharp pain; and how what I have taken with a design to help me has increased my Disease and made it more painful."[60]

The lesson he drew from his experience of physick's failure was that "*God only was my Physitian and my Deliverer*," a belief which broadened into the assertion that God was inescapably sovereign over every event of sickness and recovery.[61] His sovereignty was revealed "in the large difference which his Providence makes amongst those persons whose outward Circumstances seem to be much alike:"

> One sick man by the use of some mixtures or applications immediately recovers, and another that with most exact observation takes the same physick, consumes his days in tedious Sorrows, and, in the flouds of his own Tears, is carried mourning to the Grave.[62]

Rogers acknowledged that at least part of the inefficacy of medicine derived from the fact that medicine is, "like all other Humane Sciences, full of Imperfection," and he added, always would be. The increase of knowledge would at the same time reveal the great compass of our ignorance. And even with improved knowledge, its application might always be hindered through the complication of diseases, or faulty or hasty medical judgment. Rogers' conclusion, that without God, "not all the Cordials in the World can for one moment stay the departing Life," was thus enforced by his rather cynical view of the state of the medical art. He asserted that many physicians, too, are "so sensible" of the need for God's intervention that "they frequently tell you that by the blessing of God they hope to do you good."[63]

The experience of illness in general was represented by Rogers in a profoundly religious light. The inaccurate prognostics of the doctors demanded that true hope be placed in the preparation of the soul for death; and it was this hope for a blessed afterlife, established on faith in the promises of the Gospel, which provided the means of submission to the will of God in affliction. As Rogers put it, one could only submit to disease if there were a "prospect of advantage by it, either in this or the next world; for no man can possibly submit to be forever miserable."[64] Furthermore, Rogers noted that disease was, along with trouble of mind itself, closely bound to sin in its origin. From Adam and Eve's first sin, Rogers declared, "we may derive all our miseries; both the pains and sicknesses that afflict our Bodies and the fears and terrors that overwhelm our Souls."[65] Sin continued to act as both a reminder of the fallenness of the world and an immediate means of divine punishment: "What an abundance of diseases are at his beck, what an abundance of Arrows are in his quiver, what an abundance of sins do we commit which cause him to bend his bow, and provoke him to set us up as marks of his displeasure?" Rogers stressed the vulnerability of the human body, descending to the particulars of God's intervention

---

60 Rogers, *Practical Discourses*, 36–7.
61 Ibid., 36–7, 40–41.
62 Ibid., 13.
63 Ibid., 35.
64 Ibid., 27.
65 Rogers, *Discourse*, 3.

in an example with which he was all too familiar: "he can by letting loose any one Humour in your bodies make you a burden to yourselves, and to be weary of a world in which you can no longer live as you us'd to do."[66]

It was in part precisely because melancholy was a disease like any other that Rogers thought spiritual consolation to be particularly appropriate and timely for cases of melancholy. His declared intention in writing the *Practical Discourses* was to present to the public a work for the benefit of both those whose trouble of mind was the result of reflection on their physical affliction, as well as those for whom it was a symptom of the disease of melancholy.[67] Diseases and afflictions of all kinds could cast the soul into trouble over spiritual questions. Indeed, he understood his own case of religious melancholy as rooted in a series of physiological disturbances. In the account of his illness he gave in the *Practical Discourses*, Rogers relayed how the "ill habit of Body that had for some years attended" him at length flared "to a most formidable height." As a result, it seems, his "Sleep departed quite away … upon which there immediately followed a general Weakness and decay of Spirits, a general Listlessness, and a total Indisposition; and by feeling of this I had a strong Impression in my Mind, that I should very speedily die." It was this thought which caused a great deal of fear: "I thought I was immediately to go to the Tribunal of God … what a strange prospect that is, and what a mighty Change it causes in a Man's Thought." There followed many months of "restless Pain and amazing Thoughts": "all was hideous Darkness, Woe and Desolation with me."[68]

Rogers' account of his experience thus confirms Patrick's diagnosis of religious melancholy as a condition produced by the confluence of bodily unease and a certain framework of religious beliefs embedded in the catch-phrases of nonconformist language. In the *Practical Discourses*, Rogers registered the whole of his illness experience in a spiritualized language, drawing throughout on biblical texts to represent his suffering as the result of God's abandonment and displeasure:

> *I said with* Hezekiah, Isa. 38.12,13. Mine Age is departed, and is removed from me as a Shepherd's Tent … He will cut me off with pining Sickness: from day even to night wilt thou make an end of me: I reckoned till morning, that as a Lion, so will he break all my Bones.[69]

As in the pastoral and consolatory texts of the late Tudor and early Stuart period, even references to physical symptoms were expressed and perceived through a biblical language of affliction: "for many Months I could not breath without a mighty Pain, and as soon as with Difficulty I had breath'd, every Breath was turn'd into a Groan, and every Groan was big with a very deep sorrow. *I was weary with my Groaning … All Night made I my Bed to swim, and watered my Couch with Tears.*"[70] The

---

66   Rogers, *Practical Discourses*, 23–5.
67   Ibid., xxviii–xxix.
68   Ibid., 149–60.
69   Ibid., 152.
70   Ibid., 154.

italicized portion is a paraphrase of Psalms 6, which begins "O LORD, rebuke me not in thine anger, neither chasten me in thy hot displeasure/Have mercy upon me, O LORD, for I am weake: O LORD heale mee, for my bones are vexed/My soule is sore vexed: but thou, O LORD, how long?/Returne, O LORD, deliver my soule: oh save mee, for thy mercies sake" (KJV).

In the *Discourse concerning Trouble of Mind*, Rogers made the spiritual aspect of his affliction more explicit than these biblical quotations. Chapter 4 of Part 3 is entitled "*Shewing what dreadful apprehensions a soul has, that is under desertion; and in several respects how very sad an[d] doleful its condition is, from the Author's own Experience.*" In this "weeping, stormy night" the soul is "overwhelmed with continual thoughts of the Holiness, and Majesty and Glory of the Lord," but it does not "think of him with any manner of delight:" "*The deserted soul ... does look upon God as its enemy*; and as intending its hurt and ruin by the sharpness of his dispensations." Those enveloped in this spiritual night regard any grace which they previously evidenced as mere hypocrisy. The individual "feels his heart hardened at present, and concludes that it was never tender; finds himself at present listless and indisposed, and concludes that he never had any true life and motion." Their conclusion is that the are both apostate and reprobate. They cannot bring themselves to see that Christ can be savior to them, since they regard themselves as faithless. They are terrified by their conscience, which "discharges a thousand accusations against him for his guilt," and "when God sets on peculiar impressions of his wrath, and it falls upon the naked soul with its scorching burning drops, there is not then one quiet thought, nor one easie moment, all is amazement, confusion and wo[e]." With God seemingly against them, nothing else can bring comfort or pleasure; the mind is completely possessed by its sadness and fear, and it can no longer bear outward afflictions with godly patience. The soul becomes hopeless and despairing, easy prey for the devil's malicious confirmation of the feeling of abandonment.

As Rogers framed his illness experience in the *Practical Discourses*, and as he implied in the title of Chapter 4 in *A Discourse Concerning Trouble of Min*d, his spiritual anxiety and terror were caused by his sense of being given up by God to a mortal physical affliction. Thus, although he was afflicted with melancholy, his spiritual affliction itself was not melancholic. In Chapter 5 of Part 3, he explicitly defended against the objection that "[y]*ou make a great of noise and bother about desertions, and God's forsaking of the soul*; and it is nothing in the world but *Fancy* or *Imagination*, and the whimsies and the fumes of Melancholly." Rogers began his refutation of this accusation by declaring that "[i]t is no new thing for us to hear such Language from Atheistical and Prophane People."[71] On the other hand, Rogers acknowledged that melancholy was a disease which attacked the imagination. He cited Baxter's observation that, since the disease was lodged in the animal spirits, the physiological organ of thought, counsel and persuasion drove melancholic fears away only temporarily. But where Baxter took this as confirmation of the need for physick, Rogers characteristically urged his readers to seek the divine intervention

---

71 Rogers, *Discourse*, 370.

which alone made recovery possible, though apparently with the help of godly counsel and comfort, read or heard:

> My advice to such is, That in the use of such things as they find to yield a natural refreshment to their spirits, they would look up to God, who can make the Winds and Storms to cease, and make that unquiet agitation that is in the Blood and Humours, to be still again; and when he shall be pleased to give you the rest of night, and the clearness and activity of your natural spirits, then your troublesome and uneasie thoughts, by the help they will then receive by reading or advice, will wear away."[72]

His answer to the profane ridicule of the atheist was thus that "they know not the ways of God and his dispensations" and "will not search into the Methods of his Government."[73] This assertion was of immense significance – and quite contentious – in the context of the late seventeenth century, for it smeared those who critiqued the perceptions of the religious melancholic as delusional with the accusation of atheism. Moreover, it moved the ground of the discussion to a doctrine an array of Christian thinkers still routinely invoked: the doctrine of God's Providence.[74] From the perspective of the providence of God, Rogers was arguing, melancholy was under the government of God like any other disease and could be therefore understood and perceived like other diseases as being used by him for divine purposes. To a large extent, then, it did not really matter whether spiritual affliction was melancholic or not. It was the experience of the affliction itself, and the value it had for the struggle to deepen faith and sanctify the soul, which mattered. That the suffering could at some level be said to be only in the imagination was irrelevant, Rogers declared: "[t]o grant them for once, that it is Imagination, it is not the less tormenting because it is so; for a Man that strongly imagines himself to be miserable, is trully miserable; if a man think himself unhappy, he is so, whilest that thought remains."[75] The important point, however, was that the melancholic thought remained as long as God saw fit. Rogers was making much the same point that Greenham had urged his cures to recognize, that melancholy was to be thought of as an occasion, but not a cause, of spiritual affliction.

The consolation and counsel Rogers provided to those in spiritual trouble of mind in the *Discourse* were familiar. Rogers looked back to Greenham, Bolton, and Dod with admiration and gratitude for their writing on the affliction of conscience, and he iterates the insistence found in the narrative of Mrs. Drake on the need for the gentle and patient treatment of the melancholy. Unlike the late Tudor and early Stuart Calvinists, however, he was not at all concerned to apply thoroughly the cleansing purgative of the Law, but upbraids "[t]hose that under the Characters

---

72   Ibid., 146.

73   Ibid., 370.

74   See J.C.D. Clark, *English Society 1660–1832*, 2nd edn. (Cambridge: Cambridge University Press, 2000), 30, 87–8; Roy Porter and Dorothy Porter, *In Sickness and Health: The British Experience, 1650–1850* (London: Fourth Estate, 1988), 169–70.

75   Rogers, *Discourse*, 370.

of Ambassadors of the Gospel of Peace, do nothing but thunder out the Law to a wounded and a troubled Soul." These "shew they are unlike to the Jesus whom they would seem to represent; and they shew that they have in such matters very little skill, and no experience at all; neither do such do as they would be done by in the like case." Lesions were not to be cleansed but soothed: "There is a sort of balsome in compassionate and gentle words; tho' they do not fully perform a Cure upon our wounds, yet they make the pain and the smart less; whereas a rough and sour carriage does exasperate and heighten them, and is but the pouring of oyl into the flame."[76] Such had been said before, most famously perhaps by Greenham and Richard Sibbes. But it was always given as a counterbalance to the rigorous invocation of the necessary terrors of the Law, and this is absent in Rogers. He likely knew his audience well enough. Baxter had complained that those driven to religious melancholy by the preaching of damnation were drawn into mistakenly thinking that this preaching applied to them, whereas it applied to truly unrepentant sinners.[77] Rogers realized, as Baxter perhaps did not, that his nonconformist audience and readership was already converted, and needed consolation, not judgment.

Rogers' primary concern was to disabuse the afflicted of the notion that they are under the wrath, or eternal condemnation, of God. If they feel God's anger, he assured, his anger is but for a moment. God has bound himself in covenant to care for and uphold the elect, Rogers argued; and his tenderness and mercy towards his own are well attested by Scripture.[78] In fact, what appeared to the afflicted as anger was benevolent and reasoned correction.[79] But the comfort provided by knowing that affliction was chastisement and correction rather than a mark of divine wrath could only be had through the assurance that one was elect, that one had faith. This was intended by Rogers to be consoling: "Faith quiets the Soul, by directing it to consider the Nature, the Promise, and the Word of God; it takes away the sowreness of our thoughts, whereby we are apt to conclude that God is of a furious and implacable Nature; that he will never be reconciled, or have to do with Creatures so mean and so sinful as we are."[80] But Rogers took the substance of faith to be the acceptance of Christ's imputed righteousness, and as Patrick and Baxter had pointed out, such a view seemed immediately undercut Rogers' attempts at consolation.

Rogers fell back on the familiar concession that "these desires of holy Men after God, do not always burn with an equal Flame; for in Desertions, in some very perplexing Difficulty, or in great bodily indisposition and sickness, they are damped, and cannot usually be so quick so chearfull, and so sensible as at other times."[81] It was indeed no small consolation for the melancholy that "there is no question, but God will make allowances for our weakness; and the groaning after him by one under the

---

76 Ibid., 82.
77 Baxter, *Right Method*, 392–3, 395–6.
78 Rogers, *Discourse*, 22.
79 Ibid., 27.
80 Ibid., 100–101.
81 Ibid., 295–6.

power of a disease, may be as grateful to him, as a long continued Prayer by one in health."[82] But Rogers also emphasized at length that the absence of sensible delight in piety was the direct consequence of God's desertion, the withdrawing of divine favor rather than a weakness or natural condition of the physiological mechanism. Whereas for Patrick, the feeling of spiritual listlessness and languor was perceived primarily through the mechanism of the body, for Rogers, the sensations of the body were themselves indications of divine intention. The displeasure of God was manifested in the "fear and sadness" which "damp and contract our spirits," and his favor could, in a similar fashion, be felt in the liveliness of the spirits.[83] As Rogers understood it, melancholy was merely one manifestation of God's withdrawal among others, such as physical diseases and feelings of abandonment produced immediately. Rogers encouraged his readers to pray that God would not afflict them with diseases which affected the mind, and encouraged the convalescent melancholic to be careful of a relapse of spiritual affliction.[84] But he was not concerned with either errors of physical regimen, or with problems in the government of the emotions, but with sin in general.

Implicit in Rogers' writing is thus the idea that religious melancholy is a species of the afflicted conscience, a form of God's chastisement visited for the same reasons as other forms of "loving punishment." But the point remains only implicit; he did not encourage the melancholic to search his soul to discover "some secret, especial and several sin," as Greenham did.[85] Furthermore, the guilt attaching to personal sinfulness did not exhaust the reasons Rogers gave for the feeling of the loss of God's favor and the sadness, fear, and anxiety which ensued. Rogers seemed aware that such an experience occurred even where the individual was as above reproach as one could be in terms of Calvinist anthropology, and he gave several alternative understandings of God's reasons outside of punishment for affliction. These were comprised mainly of the ends, rather than the causes, of affliction. Affliction made us more dependent on God; the "remembrance of that horror, pain and smart" will cause us to exert ourselves to greater lengths in avoiding sin; it should cause us to value Christ, who has taken on himself the burden of God's wrath, as well as to value more highly the grace which delivers us from the torment of damnation; and finally, spiritual affliction "discovers more clearly to us the corruption and defilement of our nature."[86]

Rogers argued that there was a certain propriety in the feeling of sorrow brought by affliction: "Among all the other excellent appointments of Providence, this is one, That there should be a time to weep, *Eccles.* 3.4." It was excellent because as "an imperfect passion," it was created by God not "for itself, but for some higher use ... so Sorrow is made for Joy, and Joy is the end of Sorrow; and God, we may be sure,

---

82   Ibid., 88.
83   Ibid., 223–7.
84   Ibid., 421–43, and Rogers, *Practical Discourses*, 136.
85   See page 62 above.
86   Rogers, *Discourse*, 151–71.

will have his end." The point is quintessentially Augustinian. Rogers was arguing for the importance of a purifying godly sorrow as the only solid basis of a lasting joy. But he also argued that sorrow was appropriate to a world which, marred by sin, was a vale of tears. He described, with no small eloquence and pathos, the full range of human misery, from death and disease to losses of fortune and livelihood, from weariness from constant labor and care to "the variety of intricate Opinions, the many involutions of Controversies and Disputes, which are apt to whirl a Man about with a Vertigo of contradictory possibilities."[87] It was, he insisted, simply folly to "expect to find nothing in [the life of man] but what is pleasant."[88] Misery resulted from the fall, of course; Rogers' point was that since humankind has sinned, humankind must suffer. This recognition of human and worldly sorrow, which was at the same time harsh and sympathetic, looked back to those like Downame who, sensible of the force of worldly grief, used it to mark spiritual truths. Ultimately, too, Rogers was drawing melancholy into the trajectory of godly sorrow, affirming the importance and redemption of grief in the light of heaven and the life ever after.

Sorrow was to be one of the main constituents of the Christian temper, Rogers argued, a claim which throughout the seventeenth century had elicited the criticism of the godly that they *discourage men from all Religion*" by making it "such a mournful business." "The servants of God do not have such light and frothy spirits as others," Rogers admitted. "They do not indeed always mourn, but even when they rejoice, 'tis with a serious and solid Joy." Yet there was much to be serious and sorrowful about:

> Their own Sins, and the fear they have of sinning, and concern they have for the sins of others, cause them to walk softly. The many Miseries to which they are obnoxious, and the many that they see the Church of God groaning under, keep them from innumerable Follies, from many lightnesses and Vanities in Conversation, which others do no scruple; tho frequently when their Countenances are grave, their Hears are full of the most lively joys.[89]

Those who, on the other hand, sought to "drink sorrow away" and "not perplex [their] minds with melancholly thoughts" could not cheat the coming night of eternal misery.[90] The sorrow and fear of melancholy, if it could be shaped as religious experience and sanctified by seeing it as Providential, was a burden appropriate to the Christian's life on earth, and useful to the work of salvation.

Importantly, these were consolations of a sorrow which Rogers recognized as undesirable and distressingly painful; the spiritual insights of melancholy were dearly bought. Rogers' understanding of godly sorrow was thus very different from that which prevailed in nonconformist circles. Rogers emphasized the trajectory of godly sorrow towards joy, whereas the nonconformists Baxter criticized tended

---

87 Ibid., 317–31.
88 Ibid., 333.
89 Ibid., 383.
90 Ibid., 372.

to take sorrow as an end in itself since it provided a sign of grace and salvation. Rogers was attempting to find meaning in an experience he clearly would rather have forgone. The love of God, he noted in his description of the "fruit of a livelier Faith," could from a philosophical point of view be described as "an eager desire of absent amiable Good," which "raises an agreeable Sensation ... in the Natural Spirits."[91] This was clearly more desirable than the dampened spirits of the melancholic, and Rogers does not console spiritual affliction by dressing it up as a sign of the soul's sensibility towards feelings of repentance, as had Bolton. Sorrow and melancholy are seen by Rogers as facts of the fallen human condition, painful but useful. Melancholy revealed to the often reluctant soul the vanity of worldly existence. Rogers' godly sorrow does not consist in "Puritan" self-excoriation; it is indeed rather more philosophical, closer to Moore's consolation of blasphemous thoughts. God sends such afflictions for "wise and kind Reasons," Moore wrote: to "lessen your Inclinations to the Enjoyments of this Life; that they might deaden your Appetites to sensual Pleasure, and take your hearts off of the perishing Goods of the World."[92] For Rogers, the illness experience imparts to the tractable soul a sober and "realistic" view of human existence and encourages reflection on God as the source of human happiness.

Rogers' treatment of melancholy as a disease which, like other diseases, tended to precipitate reflection on the soul's standing with God protected against the dismissal of the specifically spiritual concerns of the melancholic as symptoms of their disease. A variety of sickness and disease could generate spiritual concern; melancholy was a divine affliction which generated such spiritual concern in a more terrifyingly inescapable fashion. As the Anglican Archbishop Thomas Secker put it several decades later, "every indisposition is a Call from Heaven, and some are very loud ones."[93] Rogers was thus claiming for the treatment of melancholy the role of consoling and healing which had long been a duty of the priest. As he put it a sermon published in 1684 as *Consolation for the Afflicted; or the Way to Prevent Fainting under Outward or Inward Trouble*: "The vast numbers of the Sick, the Melancholy, the Desolate, and the Mourning, require at the Hands of all a great deal of pity, especially theirs, who by their Character and Office are obliged to tender the Welfare of Souls, of which I have the honour to be one."

He went on in this sermon to say that, as he was treating of "the Disease of fainting" (a disease of murky clinical definition, but suggesting some form of melancholy), "I could have made a great noise with *Syncope, Leipothymia*, and *Deliquium*, and other Physical Words." But, he declared, "it belongs to my office not to have recourse to the Dispensatory, but to the Bible," a point he repeated a little later: "I appear here not as a Doctor, but as a Divine, not as a healer of your Bodies, but as a Reliever

---

91   Ibid., 295–6. In the *Practical Discourses*, Rogers cited Dr. Walter Charleton's *A Natural History of the Passions* (1674), which was by and large a popularization of the works of Réné Descartes and Thomas Willis on the passions: see *Practical Discourses*, 147.

92   See page 102 above.

93   Secker, Sermon 42 in *Works*, 2: 185, 192–3, 203.

of your Souls, and a Helper of your Faith."[94] Rogers drew heavily in this sermon on the then current natural philosophy of the emotions and the animal spirits to understand why we "faint" under trouble.[95] He noted that *a natural Weakness of the Body ... is ... a cause of fainting under trouble*." Again, this was not far removed from Patrick's understanding of religious melancholy as discouragement arising from the body's listlessness and languor. Here also was Rogers' most secularized treatment of melancholy: "If you are naturally *Melancholy*, and fearful, by healthful diet, and innocent diversions, you may at first keep under that obstinate humour."[96] But the exercise of faith, rather than the advice and precepts of philosophy, gave the only solid basis of tranquility. Hope, he noted, displaying his familiarity with Willis' physiological ideas, "puts the Blood into a Brisk Circulation, it recruits their Spirits, and gives them new Heart," and according to Rogers, only a certain kind of hope could perform the cure: "Oh! How quieting a thing is Hope in the Word of God...it is a plant that grows in Jerusalem, and not in Athens." He then repeated that melancholy, once it had progressed to a "raging and unconquerable" pitch, could not be cured "by Argument and Consideration," but "only by that power which is omnipotent." To be sure, the melancholy were to "begin the cure in [their] own minds." But "tormenting Passions and Cares," which only "fret and gall our own spirits," were to be remedied through the exercise of faith rather than reason or the therapies of diversion.[97]

This was to put Baxter's connection between excessive passion and melancholy in a therapeutic rather than condemnatory light, as had late sixteenth and early seventeenth-century divines. Rogers had none of Baxter's sharp-edged skepticism about the sorrow of the godly. From Rogers' point of view, it was entirely natural and understandable that pious souls would feel abandoned by God in times of outward affliction, as well as in times of melancholic trouble of mind. This, after all, had been his own experience. And his illness experience had revealed also that the art of medicine held much less promise for the cure of melancholy than those like Baxter seemed to think, whereas sympathetic and kind consolation was of the utmost importance to the afflicted soul. Rogers' ultimate message was that sickness of the body could only be endured if its meaning was sought in terms of the ultimate ends of human existence.

Put in this light, it is clear that the general approach of Rogers to the problem of melancholy shared a broad common ground with that of the Anglicans, even if it diverged in emphasis, doctrine and, to a lesser degree, in tone. For Patrick, struggling with the weight of the body was a spiritual problem, to be overcome by Christian humility and forbearance. Archbishop Synge's advice to melancholics in his Sober thoughts for the Cure of Melancholy (1743) echoed Rogers' "Puritan" warnings

---

94 Rogers, *Consolation for the Afflicted; or the Way to Prevent Fainting under Outward or Inward Trouble* (London: for Thomas Parkhurst, 1694), Preface, 10–11.

95 Ibid., 12–14, 16, 26–7, 64–6.

96 Ibid., 68.

97 Ibid., 64–6.

against using pleasurable diversion to cure melancholy. "Some Persons think to drive away all *Melancholy*, by giving themselves up to what we call Diversions," he noted; "such as Hunting, Stage-plays, Balls, Dances, Musick, or any Thing that may, for the present, raise their Spirits (as they express it) and stir them up to Mirth." But even if these were innocent, they were ultimately ineffective against melancholy. A life spent avoiding melancholy in such pursuits took the individual away from "doing that Good in the World, of which God has made him capable." Then, "when, by sickness or old Age, he comes to lose the Relish of these diversions, and begins to reflect how foolishly and unprofitably, or it may be wickedly, he has spent so great a Part of his precious Time ..., he will certainly find his *Melancholy*, his Sorrow and Anguish of Mind, to be much increased." And this more terrible melancholy of regret was irremediable.[98] While acknowledging the physiological nature of melancholic disease, Synge pulled away from treating the problem of melancholic emotion in a purely secular manner, instead placing medical regimen and cure within the context of the proper spiritual ends of human life. Synge was not advocating the practice of piety as the best therapy for melancholy, as Rogers seemed to recommend; he was, however, noting the general importance of spiritual and moral health to psychic well-being and guiding the attention of the melancholic from his preoccupation with avoiding melancholic feeling to the necessity of his Christian duties.

---

98 Synge, *Cure of Melancholy*, 6–7.

CHAPTER SIX

From Religious Despair to Hypochondria: The Languages of Melancholy Transformed

The previous two chapters have displayed how difficult it is to characterize adequately the differences between the various pastoral approaches to the treatment of melancholy articulated before and after the Restoration. As the contrast of Baxter and Rogers shows, not all Dissenters spoke with the same voice; and even Rogers, who is closest in tone and substance to the late sixteenth and early seventeenth-century practical divines, displays significant departures from Elizabethan and Jacobean models. On the other hand, while I have suggested that something of a distinct Anglican *consolatio* emerged after the Restoration, it is arguable that, to a degree, the Anglican approach is continuous with the Calvinist past in certain of its practical aspects.

Certainly, it seems too sweeping a generalization to speak of the treatment of melancholy as being secularized in the late seventeenth century, as Michael MacDonald and others have done. But such a claim is not without some insight either, and to examine only pastoral texts on melancholy would give a rather skewed perspective on the issue. Situating these texts in the context of their reception and use would help provide a richer picture of the treatment of melancholy in the "long" eighteenth century. Unfortunately, Anglican works on religious melancholy have left very little historical trace beyond their publication, and, to an extent, the same is true of Dissenting practical works. But it is not unreasonable to suggest that Anglican pastoral texts seemed to be responding to their audiences' use of religious language to understand and express their melancholic feelings, and this would seem to show that to some extent practical divinity was still sought out by sufferers. Moreover, we can assume that these sufferers were comprised of a generally educated reading public, and not simply of the lower classes, for whom, according to MacDonald, spiritual and demonic perceptions of mental illness survived as a feature of popular culture.[1] In confirmation of the continued cultural importance of religious consolation for melancholic emotion, we can turn as well to James Boswell, who exclaims in his popular column in *The London Magazine*: "How blessed is the relief which [the

---

1 MacDonald, "Religion, Social Change and Psychological Healing."

melancholic] may have from the divine comforts of religion!"[2] On the other hand, there are several eighteenth-century voices which eschew altogether the use of religion in the treatment of melancholy. The essayist Thomas Gordon wrote: "When one is under the strong Influence of [the spleen],[3] I know not whether a rigorous Application to Religion be adviseable; since it is the Nature of it to fill the Head with Fanaticism, or the Mind with Despair."[4] Similarly, when the eighteenth-century poet William Cowper first began to suffer from severe feelings of despair and turned to the religious poetry of George Herbert for consolation, "a very near and dear relation" advised Cowper "to lay him aside, for he thought such an author was more likely to nourish my melancholy than to remove it."[5]

Such views had been circulating since at least the Elizabethan period, and it would be ill advised to extract from them a representation of the dominant eighteenth-century perspective on religion and melancholy. In the case of Dissenting practical divinity, however, it is possible to trace more clearly a history of an increasingly problematic and unpopular cultural status, in part because Dissenting practical divinity remained a flashpoint for broader social fears and a continued target of cultural censure and criticism. The Dissenting experience and treatment of religious melancholy articulated by those like Timothy Rogers was becoming repugnant not only in terms of the Restoration shift of theological sensibility; it also offended the emerging concern with polite and polished taste and social affability. This was felt within parts of the Dissenting community itself, and it appears that Dissenting practical divines moved away from Rogers' pastoral style as a result, policing more carefully the channeling of melancholy into godly sorrow and religious despair.

The result was that moderate Dissenting pastoral styles ended up converging with, and indeed drawing on, the Anglican approach, but as I have argued above, the Anglican approach itself cannot be properly described as a secularizing of mental trouble of mind. This depends, of course, on what is taken to constitute secularization. In their study of the cultural and social history of suicide, MacDonald and Terence Murphy define the term "secularization" to mean "the rejection of belief in the frequent and potent intervention of the supernatural in the natural world."[6] This approach to the notion of secularization is simply too narrow, however. I would suggest that "secularization" can be more productively talked about as the limiting of frameworks explaining and assigning meaning to natural and human events in terms relating only to natural and human causes and entities. This way of talking about secularization makes room for taking seriously late seventeenth and early

---

2   Boswell, "On Hypochondria," no. 34, December 1780, in *The Hypochondriack*, 2: 45–6.

3   The terms "the spleen," "the vapors," "hypochondria," and "hysteria" broadly designated a similar condition, but were not quite interchangeable: see page 151 below.

4   Gordon, *The Humourist: Being essays upon Several Subjects* (London: for W. Boreham, 1720), 13.

5   Cowper, *Adelphi*, in *The Letters and Prose Writings of William Cowper*, ed. James King and Charles Ryskamp (Oxford: Clarendon Press, 1979), 1: 9.

6   MacDonald and Murphy, *Sleepless Souls*, 6.

eighteenth-century Anglican consolations of melancholy as deeply spiritual, but it addresses as well the issues MacDonald and Murphy point to in their definition of secularization. There is indeed at this time a remarkable shift in cultural mentality regarding the presence of the supernatural in the human and natural world, a shift which forms a central part of the history of melancholy. Talk of the devil rather suddenly disappears from pastoral language used to console melancholy around the time of the Restoration, in both Dissenting and Anglican works. Scholars have proposed various explanations for this shift, none of them entirely satisfactory. I suggest here that it has a great deal to do with the turn towards less passional and agonistic spiritual expression and experience, and with the post-Calvinist de-emphasis of religious despair as a moment of signal spiritual importance.

As we will see, Rogers stressed in his defense of "affectionate" Dissenting spiritual language that the expression of melancholic suffering was somehow therapeutic. It would not be inappropriate to imagine for ourselves the figure of the melancholic at this particular moment in the history of English experience. No longer finding that melancholy was indeed a moment of religious despair, placing the suffering individual between God and the devil and calling for expressions of torment and of hope, and in any case severely censured for any such moves to express their emotion in rhetorical terms adequate to their inner torment, melancholy was a condition in need of a language. And although it is difficult to trace the extent to which the censure of religious and demonological expression acted as a cause, it seems to have found just such a language in the medical discourse on hypochondria and hysteria. I will argue in the next chapter that the reinvention and popularization of medical discourse on the melancholic condition did not entail the disappearance of moral philosophical or religious approaches; but the language of hypochondria and hysteria did mark out a distinct way of talking about melancholic emotions, and its popularization can be accounted for both in terms of the psychological and social needs of the melancholy in the cultural context of the late seventeenth and early eighteenth centuries, and also in terms of new demands placed on the medical profession.

This chapter gives a series of brief analyses of several specific strands in the history of the ways in which melancholy has shaped and expressed: the demonological, the "affectionate" evangelical, and the medical. There are some suggestive links between these individual strands, and together they are indicative a shift in the expression and treatment of melancholy and in the experience of the melancholic condition itself. This shift falls along, and is indeed a central part of, the broader contours of changes in Augustan cultural sensibilities about social behavior and the correct conduct of speech and emotion.

The devil dissolved in his bath

One of the more remarkable moves to mute demonological talk in treating melancholy occurs in Timothy Rogers' *Discourse Concerning Trouble of Minde*. This is remarkable for at least two reasons. First, Rogers was explicitly interested in melancholic religious affliction, and as we have seen, there was a long tradition associating the devil with melancholic thought and behavior. Secondly, whereas very early in the seventeenth century the established Church had, partly for political reasons, shied away from treating cases of trouble of mind through the Protestant methods of exorcism, those in the Dissenting circles generally did not. This is certainly clear in the Mrs. Drake narrative. And the Baptist Hannah Allen, who herself perceived that she was possessed by Satan, reported in her posthumously published autobiographical account of the religious melancholy she suffered during the 1660s that she was told by some friends "of some that were possest with the Devil, and by Prayer dispossest."[7] As Michael MacDonald points out, Restoration Dissenters used the practice of exorcism and dispossession to discredit the established Church, just as "Puritans" like John Darrell had earlier in the seventeenth century.[8]

But Rogers explicitly cautions against invoking the idea of the devil too often in spiritual comfort and consolation. To be sure, he had no doubts but that the devil often took advantage of the condition of melancholy to throw "in his Bombs, and his fiery Darts." "To amaze us more when we are compassed with the Terrors of a dismall Night," he continued, "he is bold and undaunted in his Assaults, and injects with a quick and sudden malice a thousand monstrous and abominable thoughts of God, and which at the same time seem to be the motions of our own minds, and so do most terribly grieve and trouble us." Yet after his vivid description of demonic affliction, Rogers concluded with a warning: "I would not have you to *bring a Railing Accusation against the Devil*, so as to attribute to him a thousand things, wherein he has no hand at all."[9]

This cautionary conclusion comes close to the Anglican position, which MacDonald characterizes as strongly secularist in tendency. MacDonald quotes Archbishop of Canterbury John Tillotson as a particularly prestigious and influential example of the reticence among clergy of the established Church to acknowledge demonic affliction. On the idea that the devil interjected despairing and blasphemous thoughts into the people's minds, Tillotson wrote: "I chuse rather to ascribe as much of these to a bodily distemper as may be, because it is a very uncomfortable consideration that the devil hath such an immediate power upon the hearts of men."[10] This is perhaps the reason why Tillotson's colleague John Moore made no mention of the demonic in discussing blasphemous thoughts in his sermon *Of Religious Melancholy*, although he did account for them as within the realm of Providential affliction.[11]

---

7   Hannah Allen, *Narrative*, 54.

8   MacDonald, *Mystical Bedlam*, 228–9.

9   Rogers, *Discourse*, xv.

10   John Tillotson, *The Works*, ed. Thomas Birch (London: J. and R. Tonson, 1752), 2: 532. MacDonald cites this passage in "Religion, Social Change and Psychological Healing," 118.

11   See pages 101–2 above.

Some continued to affirm to their parishioners the hand of the devil in melancholy thoughts, in a less cautionary way than Rogers. The conforming clergyman William Chilcot was quite clear about the origin of the melancholic and despairing thought that "*God* hath *rejected* thee":

'Tis a Strategem of the accursed Enemy of our peace, who takes advantage (perhaps) of the weakness, and tenderness of thy Spirits, caus'd by some *Bodily Disposition* or other, to inject *dreadful* Thoughts; representing Almighty GOD as an implacable Judge, endeavouring to make him seem the same to us, that he is to himself.[12]

Richard Baxter concurred with Chilcot:

In almost all [cases of melancholy] I perceive, besides their Disease, that a malignant Spirit, by advantage of it, doth agitate them incessantly against God and Jesus Christ, and against themselves, as he acteth Witches to do mischief to others. I know that the Disease it self is, to the Imagination, as disquieting as a Dislocation or Lameness is to a Joint: But there is some malignant Spirit that driveth it so importunately to Mischief.[13]

But Baxter, who was taken by many to be the Dissenting expert on the consolation and cure of religious melancholy, rarely mentions the devil in his practical therapeutic work. Indeed, this statement occurs as a piece of evidence for the presence of demonic power in the physical and human world. Baxter's demonology is articulated on the level of theory and argument, not within the context of the practice of healing souls. And Chilcot nowhere mentions the Protestant exorcism of prayer and fasting for the cure of demonic thoughts, instead stressing the need to overcome disconsolation through sound theological understanding, "Religious and Cheerful conversation," and the mortification of immoderate worldly desire. This last "cure" he explained along Baxterian lines: "how remote soever *Covetousness* may seem from *Despair*, the *former* doth frequently conduce to the *latter*."[14]

The views of Rogers and Baxter all seem to confirm a certain disenchantment of the early modern worldview, a "waning of the spirit-drenched cosmos," in Roy Porter's phrase.[15] But it is questionable whether we can talk about Restoration English culture in these terms. As Simon Schaffer has pointed out, such prominent Restoration intellectuals as the Cambridge philosopher and theologian Henry More and the divine Joseph Glanvill were insisting on the importance of proving, through the experimental scientific apparatus of credible testimony, the presence of spirits in Restoration England as a way of defending against the atheistic uses of the mechanical natural philosophy they themselves favored. Against those who would attempt to use natural philosophy to close off the natural world from the influence of spirit – the "Saducees," in Glanvill's phrasing – More, Glanvill, and Robert Boyle insisted that

12   Chilcot, *Treatise*, 235.

13   Baxter, *The Certainty of the World of Spirits* (London: T. Parkhurst and J. Salisbury, 1691), 171.

14   Chilcot, *Treatise*, 251–8.

15   Porter, *Mind-forg'd Manacles*, 78–9.

experience, even when controlled by the strictures of experimental validity which constituted laboratory investigations as credible, proved otherwise.[16]

Thus, although the medical theory of melancholy had been used to discredit the spiritual claims of some evangelical Protestants from as far back as the late sixteenth century, there was in the second half of the seventeenth century a revival of interest in the idea of melancholy as a spiritual medium. As Simon Schaffer argues: "In 1649, at the establishment of the Commonwealth, Henry More explained the hypocrisy of the self-styled 'godly' party by 'childish humours, and melancholic impressions upon their disturbed spirits.' But in the later 1660s ... More's ally Glanvill offered a humoral account of possession exactly to raise its spiritual status."[17] Glanvill was seeking to marry natural philosophy to demonology, and the signs of the influence of the demonic were once again mapped onto the symptomology of humeral imbalance. Where diseases like melancholy had been used by those like Walker, Deacon, and Jorden to exclude recourse to the supernatural in accounting for human behavior, to Glanvill and others they suggested a point of weakness exploited by the devil. Indeed, a physician as eminent, respectable, and skeptical as Sir Thomas Browne testified during a witch trial in 1664 that the victims of the accused were indeed bewitched, that "the devil in such cases did work upon the bodies of men and women upon a natural foundation," and that physical disorder itself could be "heightened to a great excess by the subtlety of the devil."[18]

The use of natural philosophy as a means of explaining how spirits worked in the world was entirely conventional early modern demonology, which took as one of its basic assumptions that the devil could only work through the laws of nature, rather than *super*naturally, since the laws of nature had been established by God himself.[19] And yet the sustained interest in melancholy as the devil's bath did not

---

16 Simon Schaffer, "Godly Men and Mechanical Philosophers: Souls and Spirits in Restoration Natural Philosophy," *Science in Context* 1 (1987): 55–85, esp. 72–3; Stephen Shapin and Simon Schaffer, *Leviathan and the Air-pump: Hobbes, Boyle and the Experimental Life* (Princeton, NJ: Princeton University Press, 1985), 209, 314–15, and T.H. Jobe, "The Devil in Restoration Science," *Isis* 72 (1982): 178–95. See also John Henry, "The Matter of Souls: Medical Theory and Theology in Seventeenth-century England," in Roger French and Andrew Wear, eds., *The Medical Revolution of the Seventeenth Century* (Cambridge: Cambridge University Press, 1989), 87–113.

17 Schaffer, "Piety," 176–7. Glanvill argued that melancholic imbalance was one of the sources of the demonic powers of witches: see Glanvill, *A blow at modern sadducism* (London: E.C. for James Collins, 1668), 20. The quote from More is from a letter from More to Samuel Hartlib, 30 December 1649, as cited in Alan Gabby, "Cudworth, More and the Mechanical Analogy," in Ashcraft, Kroll, and Zagorin, *Philosophy, Science and Religion*, 114. This view of More's is also expressed in his *Enthusiasmus Triumphatus*.

18 Thomas Howell, *Collection of State Trials* (London: Hansard, 1810), vol. 6, 697, as cited in Schaffer, "Piety," 174.

19 See Stuart, *Thinking with Demons*, and his "Demons and Disease: The Disenchantment of the Sick, 1500–1700," in Marijke Gijswijt-Hofstra, Hilary Marland, and Hans de Waardt, eds., *Illness and Healing Alternatives in Western Europe* (London: Routledge, 1997), 38–58.

translate into the use of demonology as a therapeutic discourse. Andrew Scull has suggested the need to pay attention to the institutional and disciplinary setting of "disenchantment," arguing that the critique of enthusiasm acted in concert with the more specialized medical study of the mad beginning in the late seventeenth century – Scull singles out Thomas Willis in particular – and with the increased separation of mad people from the rest of society in private and public madhouses to force out demonological explanations of and therapies for conditions like melancholy.[20] But given the nature of early modern demonology, there is, at least *prima facie*, no reason why the medical study of melancholy and other forms of madness led to secularized concepts and treatments. Indeed, Thomas Willis' physiological analysis of the sensitive soul was used by Richard Gilpin in his *Daemonologia Sacra, or, A Treatise of Satans Temptations* (1677) to show that even if the devil did not have power directly over immaterial souls, his ability to manipulate physical matter gave him "*a nearer access* to our Passions than every one is aware of." In fact, the devil's possession of minds could be understood from within the category of "obsession":

> Our Passions, in their workings, do depend upon the fluctuations, excursions and recursions of the Blood, and animal Spirits, as *Naturalists* do determine: Now that Satan can make his approaches to the *Blood* and *Humours*, and can make *alterations* upon them, cannot be denied, by those that consider what the Scripture speaks in *Jobs* case: for if he could afflict *Job* with *grievous Boils*, 'tis plain he disordered and *vitiated* his Blood and Humours … and these were much more than the disorderly Motions of Blood, Spirits or Humors which raise the passions of Men.[21]

Gilpin was a Dissenting minister, well known both for his pastoral concerns and for his medical advice. In 1676 he obtained a medical degree at Leyden to legitimize his *de facto* medical practice, and he wrote his medical dissertation on hysteria, one of the diseases which, under various names, had been used both to dismiss cases of demonic possession as purely physiological on the one hand, and to elucidate the means whereby the devil worked in nature on the other.[22] As Jonathan Westaway has pointed out, Gilpin was, like More and Glanvill, clearly interested in using natural philosophy to prove to skeptics and atheists the presence of spirits in the natural world. But Westaway has also noted that the title of Gilpin's treatise is somewhat misleading, since it is "above all a manual of puritan self-examination."[23] Thus, Gilpin consistently aligned demonic temptation with the temptation to sin more generally. He drew on the moral philosophical writings of René Descartes, Antoine LeGrande, and the English divine Edward Reynolds to argue that the senses dress up worldly objects in irresistible garb, while the imagination "doth more towards

---

20   Scull, *The Most Solitary of Afflictions*, 175f.

21   Gilpin, *Daemonologia Sacra, or, A Treatise of Satans Temptations* (London: J.D. for Richard Randel and Peter Maplisden, 1677), 307.

22   See Jonathan H. Westaway, "Gilpin, Richard (1625–1700), *nonconformist minister and physician*," *Oxford Dictionary of National Biography*.

23   Ibid.

perswasion, by its *insinuations*, than a *cogent Argument*, or *rational Demonstration*." But this was to show the reasons "we have ... to suspect that [the devil] may have ways of Deceit and *Imposture* upon our *Senses*," which he uses to stir up "the corrupt principle" of the flesh within us.[24]

This gives us a hint as to why demonological therapies fell increasingly out of favor in the latter half of the seventeenth century. In Gilpin's treatise, demonic temptation shaded into the "normal" temptation to sin harbored in our fallen nature; the devil and the sinful flesh became closely aligned, and from the experiential point of view, were all but indistinguishable. This reading is confirmed by Baxter's *The Certainty of the World of Spirits* (1691). Baxter's primary aim in writing this work was to assemble evidence, against atheists and anti-supernaturalist skeptics, for the reality and continued intervention of spiritual beings in the natural world. He included in his list of stories many cases of physical demonic possession, but drew attention away from these more dramatic instances of demonic activity towards the more mundane forms of evil, which, he argued, were all the more insidious and revealed a profound demonic possession of the mind: "O! how much more miserable is a Worldly, Proud Gluttonous, Dives, Lord, Knight or Gentleman, and sensual Youth distracted with Vain Mirth and Lust, than one Bewitcht, or Bodily only possest by Devils: and how much should the most godly be afraid of Sin and Temptations?"[25] Baxter's "demonology" here is consonant with his view of the Christian life as the endeavor to obey the moral precepts of the Gospel through the exercise of reason and will. For Baxter, those who had succumbed to the demonic temptation to sorrow "over-much" were to be dispossessed with sound theological understanding and moral upbraiding rather than prayer or fasting. The treatment of melancholy during the Restoration was not so much "secularized" as it was "spiritualized," along with the devil himself.

To be sure, Tudor and early Stuart evangelical ministers warned that Satan was especially empowered during times of emotional turbulence, and Christians were thus warned to moderate their passions.[26] Ministers thus urged individuals to take full responsibility for their thoughts and feelings, rather than blaming them on the devil. According to most Protestants and many Catholic demonologists, demonic affliction was to be understood as God's Providential means of testing and strengthening Christian virtue, and it was argued that a pious and devout life was the best and only means to combat witchcraft and demons.[27] This is the understanding imparted by Greenham when he advised a "gentlewoman troubled in minde" not to ascribe her temptations to melancholy, witchery or Satan but rather to "look steadfastly to the hand of God, surely trusting on this ... that whatsoever is done directly, or indirectly, by means or immediately; all is done and governed (by his divine providence) for

---

24 Gilpin, *Daemonologia Sacra*, 78–83.
25 Baxter, *Certainty of the World of Spirits*, 9.
26 See page 113 above; cf. MacDonald, *Mystical Bedlam*, 219–20.
27 Stuart, *Thinking with Demons*, 445–56; MacDonald, *Mystical Bedlam*, 219–20.

your good."[28] Melancholy, witchery and the demonic affliction were to be considered occasions, but not causes, of temptations to sin.

But while this tendency to spiritualize demonic impulses was to some extent already latent in the Providentialism of early modern Protestant demonology, there remained a strong tendency early in the seventeenth century to express and experience spiritual affliction in terms of the Manichean conceptual binary of God and the Devil which had sustained early modern demonological thought.[29] Michael MacDonald has thus argued that early seventeenth-century individuals often expressed emotional and moral conflict in a language which had fully absorbed the dramatic "iconography" of the medieval morality play, which depicted "the hapless Everyman as the prize in a struggle between God's angels and the devil."[30] Such representations were quite at home in "Puritan" religious discourse.[31] Moments of melancholic demonic possession were also moments potentially open to (and, in published narratives, always resulting in) the display of God's healing grace; as we have seen, Puritan discourse as a whole tended to explore the extremes of religious experience, finding the way to grace and comfort through the depths of hell and despair, all the while emphasizing a passive posture which relied only on the grace of God. God's miraculous dispensation of grace in providing, at the eleventh hour, a feeling of absolute assurance of salvation for Joan Drake is indeed the lesson comfort given in the *Mrs. Drake* narrative. And, indeed, there is evidence to suggest that those suffering from religious despair latched onto talk of the devil's power over them precisely as a way of expressing and understanding their sinfulness and resulting despair. The dissenter Hannah Allen wrote of her experience of religious despair:

> When I complained how vile I was, my Friends would tell me, *It was not I, but the Devils Temptations*, I Would Answer, No, it is from myself; I am the Devil now, the Devil hath now done his work, he hath done tempting of me; he hath utterly overcome me.[32]

The Restoration reaction to the tumultuous enthusiasm of the 1640s and 1650s stressed the need for reason and will, rather than passivity and grace, to govern the practice of piety, in part as a way of combating the despairing effects of "Puritan" spirituality. This "moral philosophical" language seems to have subsumed the language of demonology as a means of understanding, expressing and treating trouble of mind, including religious melancholy, and it did so precisely by attempting to level the

---

28   See page 62 above.

29   On the importance of binary categories to early modern demonology, see Clark, *Thinking with Demons*, Part 1.

30   MacDonald, *Mystical Bedlam*, 167.

31   Addressing the seventeenth-century French context of demon possession, Sarah Ferber notes the importance of mysticism and ecstatic forms of spirituality to the seventeenth-century rise in cases of possession and exorcism: see *Demon Possession and Exorcism in Early Modern France* (London: Routledge, 2004), Part 3.

32   Allen, *Narrative*, 54.

dangerous peaks and valleys of religious nonconformist experience: grace was not to be pursued in the sudden release from demonic spiritual temptation and suffering, but in the quiet and steady cultivation of Christian virtue and the performance of devotional duty. Despair was thus no longer a heroic moment in Christian life, a pivotal overcoming of the Christian's main adversary; it was rather in the more mundane aspects of evil that the devil was most insidiously powerful and most to be feared. Excessive emotional disturbance was thus not simply an occasion for more specifically demonic forms of temptation, such as despair, but was often the main substance of demonic temptation.[33] Talk of the devil disappeared from the treatment of melancholy because despair, while it remained one of the central temptations associated with melancholic affliction, was no longer considered to be a kind of spiritual touchstone. Practically speaking, the advice, exhortation, and consolation given to someone like Joan Drake, thought to be demonically afflicted, was often the same as that proffered by Restoration practical divines to the religiously melancholy. Late seventeenth and early eighteenth-century melancholics seemed to have struggled with the same kinds of blasphemous and despairing thoughts as their late sixteenth and early seventeenth-century counterparts. But the doubts of a Joan Drake were now seen strictly in terms of Providential trials and natural psychophysiological cycles of feeling rather than in terms of an active enemy. The age of possession was over; an age of self-possession had arrived.

The connection between an evangelical, passional style of piety which emphasized the centrality of despair in religious experience and the discourse of therapeutic demonology, which began to break apart under the popularization of more "rational" models of piety, is further confirmed by a comment of Timothy Rogers'. The reason Timothy Rogers urged healers of the melancholic not to mention the devil was not only that many evils tended to be incorrectly ascribed to the devil; Rogers also thought that there was considerable therapeutic benefit to keep silent about the devil's "Bombs, and fiery Darts":

> [I]f you be speaking in every Action of Melancholly persons, that it is from this Evil Spirit, you will, as it is easie to fix any sort of direful Impressions on such as are overcome with fear, persuade them, it may be, at length, that they are possest, and that all that they do, is from him, when at the same time they are pained in every part; and then finding themselves unable to get out of their distress, your Discourses plunge them very low in misery.[34]

Rogers was suggesting that the language of demonology, when used as a therapeutic device, actually produced "possessed" behavior by aggravating melancholic thought and perception. While Rogers was no anti-enthusiast, he here advocated a view on nonconformist demonic despair which resonates with Baxter's. Rogers, like Baxter, wanted to avoid exacerbating feelings of despair, and thus suggested that talk of the

---

33 Gilpin, *Daemonologia Sacra*, 304–7.
34 Rogers, *Discourse*, xv.

devil be avoided; but Baxter suggested that an intensifying of despair was precisely what the nonconformist sought.

Archbishop Tillotson had used a tantalizingly vague word in arguing against the idea that the devil could interject thoughts directly in the human mind. Such an idea was "uncomfortable," he wrote. We could do worse than take him at his word. If we were to take seriously Rogers' comment as a therapeutic insight, we would be faced with the credible possibility that the disappearance of the terms of popular demonological psychology which represented mental suffering as demonic affliction was not, as MacDonald would have it, in one of the closing lines of *Mystical Bedlam*, "a disaster for the insane," but was in fact an improvement, and was encouraged precisely for the benefit of the insane.[35] In any case, this appears to have been the belief which informed at least some clergymen and ministers, who none the less remained firmly committed to the pastoral care of the melancholic soul.

Politeness and religious despair

Rogers was by no means an anti-Calvinist critic of enthusiasm, but whether he intended to or not, he replicated the concern expressed by those like Baxter and Patrick about the tendency of nonconformist language to cause and exacerbate melancholic madness. Indeed, Restoration writing on melancholy as a whole continually raised the issue of the interaction between melancholic feeling and the languages used to express and describe such feelings, and the crucial difference between Rogers' consolation of melancholy and Patrick's turned precisely on the issue of the language. Patrick advised the melancholic to desist from expressing their melancholy in spiritualized complaint and argued that the nonconformist language of the afflicted conscience dangerously and usually needlessly fanned feelings of physical and emotional lethargy and dullness into a full-blown melancholy. His analysis recognized that such feelings did seem to suggest some loss of God's grace, but he insisted that to think of this spiritual state in terms of God's abandonment was precisely the cause of more intensified forms of religious melancholy. Rogers' analysis of religious melancholy affirmed that the experience of spiritual affliction was an interpretation of bodily affliction, but he insisted that it was the correct interpretation since even bodily disease was providentially inflicted and healed by God alone. He also agreed that in all physical afflictions, "we ought in patience, in an humble and a quiet silence to possess our souls, and to approve of all the dispensations and the works of God." But he went on to argue at length that we might hold our souls calm even where we were driven by the intensity and magnitude of our grief to express it in complaint:

[F]or how it is possible for us not to manifest our sense of grief, even in doleful expressions, I know not: When a Man is under a burthen that he cannot bear, or when he is in sharp pain, 'tis natural for him to groan and to sigh; 'tis a thing that cannot be helped. It would

---

35 MacDonald, *Mystical Bedlam*, 230.

be … a needless labour, to advise people under great affliction, and spiritual distress, not to complain; for say what we will, they cannot but complain … Our blessed Lord himself, in the days of his flesh, when his suffering encreased upon him, *offered up prayers with strong crying and tears* … And in the pain of his inexpressible agonies on the Cross, he cryed out with a loud voice, *My God, my God, why hast thou forsaken me?* … There are some natural, unavoidable expressions of grief and sorrow which are consistent with that waiting and dependence upon God.[36]

As we have seen in Rogers' description of his own case, these "natural, unavoidable expressions" consisted of the speech of the afflicted conscience, culled from the cries of biblical saints on whom God had turned his back and hidden his face. Thus, according to Rogers, the language of the afflicted conscience was an entirely appropriate way in which to express and experience grief and pain. Furthermore, "natural" and "unavoidable" did not mean "moderate." He wrote in the Preface to the *Discourse* that he sought to describe the suffering of the reader with all of the power and force of his inner experience; his descriptions were in fact expressions, conveyed with as much "spirit and passion" as he could muster:

Tho' I have not in the following Book given such a particular relation of my Troubles, as perhaps the Readers may expect; yet I desire them to take notice, that where ever I speak of inward distress, as by a third person I there speak what I my self have felt. It is an observation of the Readers of St. *Cyprian*, that through all his Writings almost every word doth breath *Martyrdom*; his Expressions are full of spirit and passion, as if he had writ them with his blood, and conveyed the *anguish of his sufferings into his Writings*: If I had had the judgment and Pen of so Eloquent a person, I might have much better described the sadness of my case; but I am sure nothing in the world could fully express it, it was so terrible, and the greatness of the danger does heighten the mercy of *God my deliverer*.

In championing an emotionally heightened rhetoric of spiritual affliction in the consolation of melancholy, Rogers turned out to be on the losing side of the debate. This cannot be attributed solely to criticisms like those advanced by Baxter and Patrick. Rather, Rogers' spiritualized expression of melancholy became a matter of distaste in a culture increasingly concerned with pleasing and convivial self-presentation. One of the complaints which Restoration Anglican writers had lodged against the nonconformists was that they were impolite. Divines such as Benjamin Whichcote insisted that politeness was the necessary companion of a religious life correctly regulated through reason, whereas if imagination dictated religious belief, the result was an unsociable dogmatism. The Restoration High Church Anglican Samuel Parker branded nonconformist Baptists, Presbyterians, and Independents as "the rudest and most barbarous people in the World," "morose and churlish Zealots" of "morose and surly Principles," who had "brought into fashion a … Grace without good Nature, or good Manners."[37] The opposition of grace to good nature and manners

---

36   Rogers, *Discourse*, 117–18.

37   Samuel Parker, *Discourse of Ecclesiastical Politie*, ii–iii, iv–viii, xx, xxviii–xxix, 74, as cited in Laurence E. Klein, *Shaftesbury and the Culture of Politeness: Moral Discourse and*

in this vitriolic polemic was a succinct summary of the Anglican representation of the fundamental difference between the theology of the established Church and that of the Dissenters. Politeness demanded of individuals that their behavior, speech, and conduct be gratifying to the company and conversation of others; and they demanded a similar pleasantness of the arts and sciences, and of divinity itself, if they were to become subjects worthy of conversation and study in cultured social circles. The Dissenter, Restoration writers inferred, was preoccupied with himself and with his feelings and perceptions, while the Anglican was virtuously sensitive to the perceptions and feelings of others. Anglicans saw the nonconformists' refusal to agree to participate in the national Church a dangerously seditious elevation of individual "principle" over the good of the social body, and continually linked up Dissent with what they saw as the "Puritan rebellion" against Charles I, which had terminated in Civil War and the execution of the King himself.

The ideals of politeness were not unique to the late seventeenth century. As scholars such as Anna Bryson have pointed out, they grew in part out of the ideals of Renaissance civic humanism: good breeding and correctness in conduct were seen as an aspect of the cultivation of the virtues which would enable the gentleman courtier to serve well the commonwealth. In the late seventeenth century, with the growth of urban centers and, in particular, the creation in London of public spaces whose primary use was the practice of gratifying self-presentation and sociability, the discourse on sociability and politeness became detached from civic humanist ideas and became a central constituent of the self-image and social practices of the elite.[38] And the Restoration characterization of the nonconformist "Puritan" as impolite further cemented this self-understanding. Barbarous "Puritan" culture was what the urbane English gentry understood themselves as having overcome in their cultural and moral advance into more refined forms of sociability.[39] The Third Earl of Shaftesbury, Anthony Ashley Cooper, who was one of the most important popularizers of politeness in the eighteenth century, wrote of the "*Moroseness, Selfishness, and Ill-will*" of the Calvinist Dissenters, and he represented the ethic of politeness as a corrective to ostensibly divisive nonconformist sensibilities. Joseph Addison identified the temper of the "Puritan" as fundamentally melancholy when he poked fun in *The Spectator* at English culture "about an age ago," where "it was the fashion ... for every one that would be thought religious ... to abstain from all appearances of mirth and pleasantry, which were looked upon as the marks of

Cultural Politics in Early Eighteenth-century England (Cambridge: Cambridge University Press, 1994), 164.

38   Norbert Elias, *The Civilizing Process: Sociogenetic and Psychogenetic Investigations*, trans. Edmund Jephcott, ed. Eric Dunning, Johan Goudsblom, and Stephen Mennell (Oxford: Blackwell Publishers, 2000); Anna Bryson, *From Courtesy to Civility: Changing Codes of Conduct in Early Modern England* (Oxford: Clarendon Press, 1998).

39   See Bryson, *Courtesy to Civility*, 181–6, 215; Klein, "Politeness," 874.

a carnal mind." "The saint was of a sorrowful countenance," he continued, "and generally eaten up with spleen and melancholy."[40]

Addison relayed a story of an interview the Independent minister Thomas Goodwin conducted for a position at the college where he was head in the 1650s. Carried out in "chamber hung with black," Goodwin, with "religious horror in his countenance," asked the candidate nothing about "what progress he had made in learning," but about "how he abounded in grace":

> His Latin and Greek stood him in little stead; he was to give an account only of the state of his soul, whether he was of the number of the elect; what was the occasion of his conversion; upon what day of the month and hour of the day it happened … The whole examination was summed up with one short question, namely, "Whether he was prepared for death?"[41]

Addison was making the same connection that Restoration critics had made between an obsessive concern about the signs of grace and an unsociable and melancholic temperament. States of extreme fear and sorrow were in fact the currency of conversation and sociability among the nonconformists, according to Baxter and Patrick; Addison argued that cheerfulness and good humor rather than sorrow and melancholy were the true emotional expressions of the Christian religion. Evangelical ministers had long insisted that their preaching and practice did not conduce to melancholy; now melancholy had become a name for what they had seen as a sober and godly life.

Rogers was keenly aware of the emerging milieu of polite writing and conduct, and was eager to show that the Dissenting tradition should not be so easily dismissed as barbarous and unrefined. He admitted that "I could in the composing of the following Book have used a little more exactness, had I set my self studiously to do so, and by that means it might have been more pleasant to the Reader." His self-conscious defense of his ability to polish his writing signaled his awareness of new standards of writing and speaking which put a premium on a style which was pleasing to the audience. He was well aware, he asserted, "that the age in which we live is very curious and critical, and that the *English Language* has been within a few years greatly improved," and with this in mind, he had endeavored to omit any "bombast" from his writing, to avoid "a neglected and a careless manner," and write instead with "plainness and clearness." None the less, Rogers' *Practical Discourses* was dismissed in the reviews published in the *Athenian Gazette* and *The Works of the Learned* as cant, the term of criticism so often applied during the Restoration to

---

40   Anthony Ashley Cooper, Earl of Shaftesbury, ed., *Select Sermons of Dr. Whichcot* (London: for Awnsham and John Churchill, 1698), sig. A6r, as cited in Klein, *Shaftesbury*, 32; Addison, *The Spectator*, no. 494, in *Works*, ed. Richard Hurd and Henry G. Bohn (London: George Bell and Sons, 1892), 4: 10.

41   Ibid.

Dissenting language.[42] The review in *The Works of the Learned* apparently struck a raw nerve. In a sermon published a year after the *Practical Discourses*, Rogers invoked "sense and good-breeding" against what he saw as the unfair and prejudiced criticisms of the reviewers, asserting that "the Dissenters know a little what belongs to Sense and good Language, too."[43]

Rogers would continue throughout his career to reflect on the place of Puritan language in modern culture. In a preface to the collected works of the respected nonconformist minister Thomas Gouge, Rogers stated, again somewhat apologetically: "Here is not indeed the Finery, the Sauce and the Garnish with which the Masters of Modern Eloquence treat their Readers; but here is very Seasonable Substantial Food."[44] Yet if Rogers did at times pay his respects to politeness, the preface to Gouge's *Works* was also a subtle indictment of polite learning and writing. It had long been a criticism of the ideals of politeness that it regarded only the surface of behavior, and so encouraged hypocrisy rather than real virtue.[45] Writers like Shaftesbury and Addison sought to use the language of politeness in order to cultivate virtue, attempting to persuade their readership that "good-breeding" in fact demanded the polish of a person's character, not simply of social personality.[46] For his part, Rogers stressed the substantiality of Gouge's language, contrasting this with merely pleasing ornamentation: "His Language is as he himself was, very Grave and Modest, substantially Good, and not full of Shew and Ostentation."

Indeed, Rogers implied that those who could not appreciate such good Christian writing were indeed themselves spiritually unfit: "the Table is spread and the Provisions healthful, if their Appetite and Taste be good."[47] In the *Discourse*, Rogers defended for therapeutic reasons his choice to put aside the canons of refined taste and the aim to please. Making his words more polite and aesthetically appealing would "not so well have served my design," he argued:

---

42   *The Supplement to the Third Volume of the* Athenian Gazette (London: for John Dunton, n.d.), 31; Jean Cornand de Lacroze, *The Works of the Learned; or, An historical account and impartial judgement of books newly printed, both foreign and domestick* (London: for Thomas Bennet, 1691/92), November, 152.

43   Rogers, *Fall not out by the way* (London: for John Dunton, 1692), Epistle Dedicatory.

44   Gouge, *The Works of the late Reverend and Pious Mr. Thomas Gouge* (London: Thomas Braddyll, 1706), sig. A3.

45   See Bryson, *Courtesey to Civility*, 201.

46   See Anthony Ashley Cooper, Earl of Shaftesbury, *Soliloquy, or, Advice to an Author*, in *Characteristics of Men, Manners, Opinions, Times, etc.*, ed. John M. Robertson (London: Grant Richards, 1900), esp. Part 3, 1: 182–234; see also Carey McIntosh, *The Evolution of English Prose, 1700–1800: Style, Politeness, and Print Culture* (Cambridge: Cambridge University Press, 1998), 15–16; Laurence E. Klein, "Politeness and the Interpretation of the British Eighteenth Century," *Historical Journal* 45 (2002): 868–98; his *Shaftesbury*, and his "The Third Earl of Shaftesbury and the Progress of Politeness," in *Eighteenth-Century Studies* 18 (1984–85): 186–214.

47   Gouge, *The Works of ... Thomas Gouge*, sig. A3.

[F]or according to that old saying ... A Physitian that can remove the disease, is more welcome to the sick than one that can talk finely about it, but do him no good; and if the Cure be performed, 'tis no matter tho' the potion was not extreamly sweetned. I purposely avoided all pretence to a regular smoothness of stile, because that the Ears of the people in great affliction, are not so tender and so delicate as theirs are, who are in health.

Rogers was not only suggesting that smoothness of style was a mere ornament, which those possessed of grief would simply not perceive; he was stating that it was actually ineffective.

Rogers did not spell out precisely why this was so, why the ears of the suffering needed a rougher, less polished manner of address. But as we have seen, Rogers was concerned in his consolatory writing to find a language commensurate with the inner agony of those suffering from the affliction of conscience, a suffering which was ultimately beyond expression. He indicated in the preface to Gouge's *Works*, the power of Gouge's writing lay in representing "Religion ... to the life." Therapeutically, then, descriptions of spiritual suffering with "expressions ... full of spirit and passion" represented to the melancholic reader his or her own suffering, but in a context which linked up the agony of despair to the recognition of God's great mercy and grace. It attempted to transfigure the language of complaint exhibited by the sufferer into a sacred language embedded in a soteriological trajectory and shared by a community of faith.

But a language which had its origin in groaning complaint and the expression of disturbing emotion was bound to breach the standards of polite conduct. As the Scottish philosopher Adam Smith later pointed out in his codification of the acceptable limits of sociable emotional expression, the articulation of strong emotion, and particularly of grievous emotion, was generally repugnant for others.[48] Rogers' writing was, in the parlance of the day, much more "affectionate" than the norms of politeness could allow.[49] A language which had once framed and articulated the identity of the godly individual and which was because of this an important medium of social exchange for the melancholy and unafflicted alike became the subject of caricature. In polite society, religious melancholy was the name not for a compound of spiritual affliction and physical disease, but for the very emotional temper which Dissenters like Rogers thought marked those with a healthy concern for their soul. Eighteenth-century medical treatises on melancholy, by way of defending religion against scoffers, declared that the religious melancholy had more melancholy in it than true religion; as Dr. George Cheyne put it, "there is at bottom little solid piety."[50]

---

48   Smith, *The Glasgow Edition of the Works and Correspondence of Adam Smith, Volume 1: The Theory of Moral Sentiments*, ed. D.D. Raphael and A.L. MacFie (Oxford: Clarendon Press, 1976), 1.2.1.5; 1.2.5.3, and 1.3.1.10 and 15.

49   On emotion and the literary style of the Restoration nonconformists, see Keeble, *Literary Culture*, 240–62.

50   Cheyne, *An Essay of Health and Long Life* (London: for George Strahan and J. Leake, 1724), 157.

Rogers registered, at a relatively early date, the tensions developing within the Dissenting tradition in relation to the high valuation post-Restoration culture put on polish and refinement, in which the display of sentiment was trimmed in a manner intended as pleasing for others. In 1730, addressing the worry of many Dissenting ministers that interest in the Dissenting faith was declining in England, Strickland Gough argued that the remedy was to become more polite. Gough recognized that many of the objections to Dissenting religion were in fact criticisms of the "aukwardness and unpoliteness of our Preachers." He noted as well "how often have we been insulted by the Church-party, for what they stile the *cant* of preaching." Many "people of wit and politeness grew asham'd" of the Dissenting style, or lack of style, "and chose a more *graceful* way of religion." But Dissenting ministers appeared to be blind to this loss, Gough inveighed. They too often bowed to the tastes of the people to please the congregations which gave them employment, which was a grave mistake, since "the people not usually know wherein oratory, strength of speech, the art of persuasion, &c. consist, and therefore 'tis vanity in such to pretend to be judges of them." "[T]he being pleas'd, which they generally insist so much upon, seldom arises from any thing but some oddness that hits their peculiar humour, and is not from any view to edification at all ... I wish I could deny that, amongst us, they generally fall into the falsest and lowest taste imaginable." For the minority whose humors were so tickled by bad taste, Puritan language had driven "as many away from us," Gough lamented. If Dissenting congregations were to survive – and it was for society's good that they, as a free and uncoerced form of religion, should survive – then "'twould be an instance of their modesty to resign up their pleasures to the general notions and judgment, for then there could be no general objections against them; thus a man would mortify his inclinations to sensual pleasure, for the good of society."[51]

Gough was adopting a position similar to that of Glanvill and the latitudinarians on the rhetorical nature of Puritan speech, except that where the latitudinarians had emphasized a form of speech governed by reason, Gough opposed the canons of good taste upheld in polite society to the forms of rhetoric governed only by the base sensuality he attributed to Dissenting taste. Presumably, these canons of good taste were more appropriate vehicles for the truth, as the latitudinarian's plainness of speech had been for reason. He was also asserting, with Addison and Restoration Anglican critics, that dissenters lacked the quality of cheerfulness so important to the religious temper: "A mixture of reverence and cheerfulness is the true spirit of devotion. There is too little of the one in some places, and too little of the other among us." An "affected gravity, that has nothing in it manly and chearful" was the sentiment governing the Dissenting personality, Gough declared.[52]

In response to Gough's *Enquiry*, the minister Philip Doddridge insisted that if the arts of politeness were to be studied, it was not to be at the expense of the "practical

---

51 Gough, *An Enquiry into the Causes of the Decay of the Dissenting Interest* (London: for J. Roberts, 1730), 33, 41.

52 See ibid., 33, 39–40.

religion, and vital holiness" wherein the essence of the Dissenting interest lay. He argued that for all the polish and refinement of the new generation of preachers, their sermons lacked the spiritual depth which was alone necessary for effective preaching: "without suspicion of flattery, I can congratulate the rising generation of ministers among us, with the great improvements they have made, in the method and style of their performances. But if the form and order of them is better, I am afraid the temper of our minds is worse." The sermons of the century reviled for its impoliteness were more effective than those of the ministry's recent innovators, precisely because of the spiritual zeal of the late sixteenth and early seventeenth-century English Calvinists. To be sure, the "regular charm of reasoning," "propriety of thought or of expression," "elegance of language," and "decency of address" were not to be abandoned by the modern minister, Doddridge asserted: "'Tis what he owes to himself, and to the politer part of his audience." But Doddridge argued that the ultimate source of the power of effective preaching was the indwelling of the Holy Spirit: "If the *Holy Ghost dwelleth in us*, and assists us, we shall lead and guide spiritual worshippers, in presenting seasonable and proper petitions to GOD, and the divine warmth and fervency of our own souls, will be a means to kindle the like holy fire in theirs."[53]

Doddridge thus cautioned against dismissing the taste of "the people" in favor of polite learning and presentation. What pleased the people was in fact an important indicator of source of the Dissenting interest:

> [T]he generality of the Dissenters, who appear to be persons of serious piety, have been deeply impress'd with the peculiarities of the gospel-scheme. They have felt the divine energy of those important doctrines, to awaken, and revive, and enlarge the soul; and therefore they will have a peculiar relish for discourses upon them. So that if a man should generally convince himself to subjects of natural religion, and moral virtue, and seldom fix on the doctrines of Christ, and the spirit, and then perhaps treat them with such caution, that he might seem rather to be making concessions to an adversary, than giving vent to the fullness of his heart on its darling subject, he would soon find, that all the penetration and eloquence of an angel, could not make him universally agreeable to our assemblies.

Doddridge was making much the same point that Rogers had made in preferring the impoliteness of affectionate rhetoric above efforts to improve the smoothness of his style. It was pastorally much more important to write and preach with the spiritual vivacity imparted through experience than to bow to polite taste, because it was precisely such experiences which provided the basis for the Dissenting community of faith. According to Doddridge, to abandon nonconformist language was to devalue the experiences that had drawn individuals into Dissenting congregations in the first place; according to Rogers, it was to abandon the melancholy in their suffering. Doddridge thus went on to defend the "experimentall preaching" which those like

---

53 Doddridge, *Free Thoughts on the Most Probable Means of Reviving the Dissenting Interest* (London: for Richard Hett, 1730), 9.

Patrick had criticized, arguing that the moral exhortation typical of latitudinarian preaching was foreign to the Dissenting interest:

> Many of our people have pass'd thro' a variety of exercises in their minds, relating to the great concern of eternal salvation. And they apprehend that the scripture teaches us to ascribe this combat to the agency of Satan, and the corruptions of our own heart on the one hand, and the operations of the holy spirit of God on the other. It is therefore very agreeable to them, to hear these experimental subjects handled with seriousness and tenderness ... it grieves them when these subjects are much neglected, and gives them the most formidable suspicions if one word be dropt which seems to pour contempt upon them, as if they were all fancy and enthusiasm.[54]

Doddridge added, in parentheses, "with which it must be granted, they are sometimes mix'd." Isabel Rivers has pointed out how Doddridge and his colleague Isaac Watts sought to mediate between the extremes of enthusiastic religion and the shallowness of polite culture, casting an appeal to the emotions they thought to be an important basis of the practice of religion into polite and reasoned forms. As Rivers argues, the result of this effort was sometimes that the experiences of the pious were treated "in a coolly objective manner" and at other times that the polite audience was put off by distasteful and rationally insubstantial religious rhapsodies.[55] Apparently, *pace* Doddridge, the Dissenting minister did need to fear "that a prudent regard to" the arts of politeness would "spoil his acceptance with the people," and conversely, that their disregard would jeopardize his relation to the educated and cultured.[56]

Both Gough and Doddridge evidence the fact that many Dissenters continued to favor affectionate language in framing their religious experience. And, as scholars have pointed out, Methodist ministers such as John Wesley and George Whitfield insisted that certain cases of alleged madness were actually cases of spiritual trouble of mind.[57] In the extremely popular *Rise and Progress of Religion in the Soul* (first published in 1742), Doddridge wrote vividly about the feelings of sorrow, terror, guilt, and anxiety that inevitably came upon the soul during the conversion process, and the despair and terror which sometimes occurred when God "hid his face" from the believer afterwards.[58] And in 1749, in the wake of a series of religious revivals in the Presbyterian parishes of Kilsyth and Cambuslang in Scotland, the Reverend James Robe published his *Counsels and comforts to troubled Christians*, which followed the seventeenth-century evangelical understanding of the work of conversion and sanctification, as well as in their forms of consolation and comfort.

---

54 Ibid., 19–20.

55 Rivers, *Reason, Grace and Sentiment*, I, 197.

56 Doddridge, *Free Thoughts*, 22.

57 Andrews and Scull, *Undertaker of the Mind*, 75–93; MacDonald, "Religion, Social Change and Psychological Healing," 111–25.

58 Doddridge, *The Rise and Progress of Religion in the Soul* (Exeter: Henry Ranlet, [1742] 1794).

Out of these various eighteenth-century religious movements, the Methodists were the most likely to treat melancholy through treating the affliction of conscience, particularly in view of the continued insistence of Wesley and his colleagues on the continued reality of demon possession in cases of melancholy. Doddridge, although he provided religious consolation for individuals who were possibly suffering from a combination of melancholy and spiritual affliction, was careful to foreground the need to discriminate between melancholy and the affliction of conscience. In *The Rise and Progress of Religion*, he began his address to the individual suffering under feelings of religious despair and disconsolation by urging them to "carefully inquire whether your present distress does indeed arise from causes which are truly spiritual; or whether it may not rather have its foundation in some disorder of body." Directly contradicting Rogers' arguments regarding the withdrawal of God's presence through natural afflictions, Doddridge continued:

> Why should God be thought to have departed from us, because he suffers natural causes to produce natural effects, without interposing by miracle to break the connexion? When this is the case, the help of the physician is to be sought rather than that of the divine, or at least, by all means, together with it; and medicine, diet, exercise, and air, may, in a few weeks, effect that which the strongest reasonings, the most pathetic exhortations or consolations, might for many months have attempted in vain.[59]

Clearly, Doddridge continued to allow room for spiritual consolation during melancholic trouble of mind, as did the Anglican ministers discussed in the previous chapter. But his assessment of the efficacy of medicine is vastly more optimistic that Rogers', and his understanding of the connection between natural causes and God's Providence is consequently very different as well. The failure of medicine had indicated for Rogers that his suffering was a spiritual matter, that he was directly under the hand of God; the efficacy of medicine indicated to Doddridge that the process was, even if Providentially allowed, more straightforwardly natural. In addition, Doddridge, who had emphasized in his reply to Gouge the importance of powerful and affectionate rhetoric and developed such a style in his own writings, dismissed out of hand the efficacy of "pathetic exhortation" in these cases.

The point was made explicitly in reference to Rogers' work on melancholy in the Reverend Job Orton's preface to the Dissenting minister Benjamin Fawcett's *Observations on the Nature, Causes and Cure of Melancholy; especially of that which is called Religious Melancholy* (1780). Orton wrote that "some Tract of this kind was much wanted, as the subject hath been only touched upon occasionally by most practical writers; and those few, who have written directly upon it, especially Mr. *Timothy Rogers*, have handled it so largely and in so confused a method, that their books are not so proper to put into the hands of the melancholy and dejected."[60]

---

59   Ibid., 283–84.

60   Job Orton, Preface, in Benjamin Fawcett, *Observations on the Nature, Causes and Cure of Melancholy; especially of that which is commonly called Religious Melancholy* (Shrewsbury: J. Eddowes, 1780), iii.

In Fawcett's work, as in Baxter's, the phrases of complaint which Rogers had argued were not only natural, but therapeutic and consoling, appeared as clinical indications of melancholic disease: they were not expressions of the individual's actual spiritual condition, but symptoms of their physical disease.[61]

It should be emphasized, of course, that the pastoral consolation of melancholy did not disappear, but was reinvented within the canons of polite style. Although he cited Richard Baxter extensively, Fawcett did not replicate Baxter's apparent move to exclude the melancholy from religious consolation. Fawcett quoted Samuel Clarke in arguing that the care of the soul was important in ministering to the melancholy: "though it is not properly and immediately of religious consideration, yet 'tis by no means to be neglected, slighted, or despised," and significantly, Fawcett's *Observations* draws not only on previous works but also on many instances of pastoral experience. Similarly, in a letter to "a Lady, under dejection of mind on religious account," Fawcett's teacher Doddridge urged her to consider the weakness of her ailing body, but directed much of his advice to the improvement of her mind.[62]

But, at least within the tradition of moderate Dissent, it was Baxter's effort to distinguish sharply between humor and genuine spiritual experience and to deny the language of spiritual complaint to the melancholic which carried the day, and perhaps also in the practice of pastoral care more generally. Rogers' *Discourse Concerning Trouble of Mind* can in an important sense be considered the last of the consolations of melancholy using the language of religious experience that had been articulated by late sixteenth and early seventeenth-century English Calvinists. What makes Rogers' writing even more significant was his self-consciousness as a "Puritan" who lived in an age of politeness and who, to a certain extent, accepted its values. His self-consciousness is testimony to the fact that if spiritual complaint was still a language of melancholy and a forum for its consolation, the "fanatick times" were indeed over. Rogers' *Discourse* was republished in a second edition in 1706, and again in 1708 by Thomas Parkhurst and his associates. These publications can be taken to show some measure of positive reception of Rogers' approach, likely among the moderate Dissenting community whose writings Parkhurst handled and promoted.[63] In addition, *Mr. Timothy Rogers' Advice to the Friends of the Melancholy*, a version of the preface to Rogers' *Discourse*, appeared again in 1749 as an appendage to Robe's *Counsels and Comforts*. But there are, so far as I have been able to discover, no other references to Rogers' *Discourse* in published works until Orton's disapproving comment in 1780. Nor are there any other works like it for the remainder of the eighteenth century. In 1708, the year in which the

---

61   Fawcett, *Observations*, 26–7.

62   Doddridge, "To a Lady, under dejection of mind on religious account," 25 June 1745, in *Letters to and from the Rev. Philip Doddridge* (Shrewsbury: J. and W. Eddowes, 1790), 329.

63   Parkhurst published a variety of works, pastoral, theological, and polemical, by Presbyterian and Congregationalist clergy such as Richard Baxter, Matthew Mead, John Howe, Edmund Calamy (both son and father), and Matthew Henry, among others.

Discourse was last published in full, Rogers was forced to retire from the ministry for good, and he suffered, in literary silence, from hypochondriac melancholy until his death in 1728. While the pastoral care of melancholy continued, the language of the afflicted conscience, which had been so important in the work of consolation in the seventeenth century, had been largely silenced in pastoral circles. A crucial element of the evangelical Protestant therapeutic language of the late sixteenth and early seventeenth centuries gradually disappeared from the mainstream Dissenting vocabulary.

Rewriting melancholy: medical theory in polite society

Late in 1681, the great English physician Thomas Sydenham published his famous letter to Dr. Cole on the disease of hysteria, which was to become the *locus classicus* of eighteenth-century medical texts on the subject. The "hysterick passion," as it was sometimes called, was notoriously difficult to diagnose and to treat because of the range of its symptoms, which the inexperienced physician often mistook for "symptoms … from some Essential Distemper of this or that part, and not from an Hysterick Disease." Sydenham wrote that "a Day would scarce suffice to reckon up all the Symptoms belonging to Hysterick Diseases, so various are they, and so contrary to one another, that *Proteus* had no more shapes, nor the Chameleon so great Variety of Colours." Thus, hysteria could manifest itself in apoplectic and epileptic fits, headaches, violent vomiting, heart palpitations, diarrhea, and back pains. Hysteric patients "sometimes belch up ill Fumes as often as they eat," and they are tormented in their sleep by nightmares.

Amidst this tormenting physical pain emerges another, more familiar set of behaviors and complaints. Sydenham rounded out the symptomology of hysteria by adding that "the Sick is oppressed by a dreadful Anguish of mind, and wholly despairs of Recovery; which dejection of Soul, and as it were a certain Desperation, as certainly accompanies … this kind of Hysterick Diseases as the Pain and Vomiting above-mentioned":

> [T]heir minds are worse affected than their Bodies, for an incurable Desperation is mixt with the very Nature of the Disease, they are very angry when any one speaks never so little of the hopes he has of their Recovery, easily believing that they undergo all the Miseries that can befall a man, foreboding the most dreadful things to themselves, entertaining in there [*sic*] restless and anxious Breasts upon small occasions and perchance for none at all, Fear, Anger Jealousy, Suspicions, and worse passions of the mind, if any can be worse, abhorring all Joy, Hope, and Mirth.[64]

---

64   *Dissertatio Epistolaris* (1681/82), trans. as *An Epistolary Discourse to … Doctor William Cole, concerning … Hysteric Diseases* in *The Whole Works of that Excellent Practical Physician Dr. Thomas Sydenham*, trans. John Pechy (London: for Richard Wellington and Edward Castle, 1696), 441–6.

There is no mention of religious anxiety, but someone like Joan Drake or Timothy Rogers is easily recognizable here. Ironically, so is Richard Baxter, but in a different way. Baxter insisted in his autobiography that although his "Catarrh and Cough" and his fear of contracting consumption led in his youth to a fear of death and damnation, he was "never overwhelm'd with real Melancholy": "My distemper never went so far as to possess me with any inordinate fancies, or damp me with sinking sadness." But he asserted this in spite of the fact that "the physicians call'd it the hypochondriack melancholy" (and he consulted over "six and thirty" physicians). Hypochondriac melancholy exhibited a range of symptoms similar to hysteria, including its irritability, peevishness, and melancholy as well as many of the physical pains, and it was, like hysteria, extremely difficult to isolate and treat.[65] Indeed, Restoration physicians such as Sydenham and Thomas Willis, both of whom eschewed the traditional notion that hysteria was caused by vapors rising from the womb, thought that hysteria and hypochondria were female and male variants of the same type of disorder in the nervous system's "animal spirits," and this idea became medical orthodoxy throughout the eighteenth century.[66] But hypochondriac melancholy was traditionally thought to be partly an affliction of the imagination, and the hypochondriac was thus ridiculed for exaggerating, if not imagining, their pains.[67] Reflecting on his chronic pain, Baxter writes towards the end of his life that he had "lain in above Forty Years constant Weaknesses, and almost constant Pains. My chief Troubles were incredible Inflamations of Stomach, Bowels, Back, Sides, Head, Thighs, as if I had been daily fill'd with Wind. So that I never knew, heard, or read of any man that had near so much." "Thirty Physicians (at least) all called it nothing but Hypochondriack flatulency," he added indignantly, a diagnosis Baxter suspected was intended to relieve his worry that he suffered from kidney stones, and so relieve his distress. But the hypochondriac diagnosis led instead to Baxter's humiliation: "I became the Common Talk of the City, especially the Women; as if I had been a melancholy Humourist, that conceited my Reins were petrified, when it was no such matter, but meer Conceit. And so while I lay Night and Day in Pain, my supposed Melancholy (which, I thank God, all my Life hath been extraordinary free from) became, for a Year, the Pity, or Derision of the Town."[68]

In the description of Joan Drake's case, although her indigestion and "vaporish" headaches are mentioned, her long struggle is over spiritual matters. Timothy Rogers expressed his condition in similar terms. Baxter, on the other hand, was able to console his spiritual doubt and anxiety, but his body became a life-long source of worry and preoccupation. He was constantly consulting physicians and trying new medical and dietary regimens in order to cure his body. And it was figures

---

65   Burton, *Anatomy*, I.iii.II.ii: 472.

66   Willis, *Souls of Brutes*, in *Works*, 105, 112–3, 146–7, 192–4; Sydenham, *Epistolary Discourse*, in *Works*, 446.

67   Burton, *Anatomy*, I.iii.II.ii: 474.

68   Baxter, *Reliquiae*, 1: 9–10; 3: 173–4; cf. the insightful discussion of Baxter's case in Wear, "Puritan perceptions of illness," 91–9.

such as Baxter who were to become increasingly familiar in eighteenth-century England, both as subjects of medical care and attention and as subjects of raillery and ridicule; as the language of spiritual affliction fell out of favor, beginning in the late seventeenth century, the language of the hypochondriac became increasingly pervasive and increasingly contentious. In his essay *Of Health and Long Life* (1681), Sir William Temple relayed an anecdote of "an ingenious Physician, who told me in the Fanatick Times, he found most of his Patients so disturbed by Troubles of Conscience, that he was forced to play the Divine with them before he could begin the Physician."[69] Temple, like Restoration critics of "Puritan" enthusiasm, clearly thought of the "Puritan" age as over. On the other hand, he commented in his essay on the recent "epidemic" of hysteria and hypochondria, known in popular language as "the vapors" and "the spleen." Hypochondriacal disorders, Temple wrote, "employ our Physicians, perhaps more than other Diseases."[70] Sydenham remarked in 1681 that "Hysterick Diseases, at least those that go under that Name, are half ... the Chronical diseases," accounting for one sixth of all physical diseases in general.[71] Later medical writers were to repeat and embellish his statistics in emphasizing the rampancy of cases of hypochondria. In his widely read text on hypochondria and hysteria entitled *The English Malady* (1733), Dr. George Cheyne generously extended the diagnosis of the illness that had become identified with the English character to include almost one third of the population.[72]

The hypochondria diagnosis came to occupy a central place in eighteenth-century consciousness. When James Boswell entitled his weekly column in the *London Magazine* "The Hypochondriack," he was invoking a concept and a condition which had become part of the language of everyday experience, social interaction, and personal reflection. Popular remedies for hypochondria and hysteria were advertised in the pages of polite journals; collections of songs were marketed as cures for the spleen and the vapors; poetic reflection turned to analyzing and exploring the crippling disease; well-to-do patients flocked to fashionable spa towns such as Bath, where taking the waters was urged as a cure and where popular physicians like Dr. George Cheyne developed their successful practices; and characters succumbing to hysteric and hypochondriac symptoms peppered the novels of Samuel Richardson, Henry Fielding, Tobias Smollet, and others.[73]

---

69   Temple, *Of Health and Long Life*, in *The Works of Sir William Temple*, 2nd edn. (London: for Benjamin Motte, 1731), 1: 288.

70   Ibid., 1: 282–3. The essay was written in the 1680s and first published posthumously in 1701.

71   Sydenham, *Epistolary Discourse*, in *Works*, 440.

72   Cheyne, *English Malady*, 34–42; see also Richard Blackmore, *A Treatise of the Spleen and Vapours* (London: for J. Pemberton, 1725), iii–iv.

73   See, for example, *The merry musician, or, A cure for the spleen* (London: for J. Walsh, 1716); *Jordan's elixir of life and cure for the spleen, or, A collection of all the songs sung by Mrs. Jordan* (London: for William Holland, 1789); *A collection of merry poems ... proposed as a pleasant cure for the hyp and the spleen* (London: T. Boreman, 1735); Anne Kingsmill Finch, Countess of Winchelsea, *The Spleen, A Pindaric Poem* (1709), in *Selected Poems*,

In many ways, the language of hypochondria came to occupy a similar position in relation to English melancholy as the language of the afflicted conscience did in the late sixteenth and early seventeenth centuries, but in a reversed fashion. Sydenham drew attention, in a rather understated way, to the possibility that the epidemic of hypochondria might be partly due to misdiagnosis of the disease. The point was taken further by critics throughout the eighteenth century, who continued to cast suspicion on hypochondriacs, arguing that hypochondria was little more than a set of theatrical behaviors and inflated complaints, deceivingly scripted in medical language. Many dismissed hypochondria as "merely" melancholic discontent, caused by insufficient control over the passions but masked by the language of hypochondria and hysteria. Thus, hypochondriac patients complained throughout the eighteenth century that the reality of their illness was dismissed, and that the "hyp" was a term of derision.[74] It was no mistake that Molière's *Le malade imaginaire* (1673) was entitled *The Hypochondriack* in its eighteenth-century English translations.[75]

On the other hand, prominent physicians enlisted to defend vigorously the reality of hypochondriac illness against such dismissive perceptions. Sir Richard Blackmore wrote that "the Spleen and Vapours are, by those that never felt their Symptoms, looked upon as an imaginary and fantastick Sickness of the Brain, filled with odd and irregular Ideas; and accordingly they make the Complaints of such Patients the Subject of Mirth and Raillery."[76] The point of Blackmore's detailed analysis of the physiology of hypochondriac illness was to correct, through irreproachable natural philosophical principle and investigation, the "great Mistake" that constituted the hypochondriac as "an Object of Derision and Contempt" in the opinion of those who did not suffer from the disease. When Blackmore published his treatise on hypochondria in 1724, Dr. Bernard Mandeville and Dr. John Purcell had already published treatises outlining the physiological causes and the real organic nature

---

ed. Denys Thompson (Manchester: Carcanet Press, 1987); Alexander Pope, *The Rape of the Lock* (1714), in *The Poems of Alexander Pope, Volume 2: The Rape of the Lock and Other Poems*, ed. Geoffrey Tillotson (London: Methuen/New Haven, CT: Yale University Press, 1962), 4–5: 182–212. On the rise in hypochondriac disease and the popularity of the spa, see Anita Guerrini, *Obesity and Depression in the Enlightenment: The Life and Times of George Cheyne* (Norman, OK: The University of Oklahoma Press, 2000), 105; more generally, see Moore, *Backgrounds*, 179–243. On the prevalence of medical remedies for hypochondria, see G.S. Rousseau, "Psychology," 204. On nervous disorder in novels, see Mullan, *Sentiment and Society*, and Raymond Stephanson, "Richardson's 'Nerves': The Physiology of Sensibility in *Clarissa*," *Journal of the History of Ideas* 49 (1988): 267–85.

74   On the ridicule and suspicion voiced by some in regards to the hypochondriac patient, see Porter and Porter, *In Sickness and Health*, 203–10.

75   Molière, *The Hypochondriack* (London: for John Watts, 1732); *The Hypochondriack*, trans. James Miller and H. Baker (London, 1755).

76   Blackmore, *Treatise*, 97; Bernard Mandeville, *A Treatise of the Hypochondriack and Hysterick Passions* (London: Dryden Leach and W. Taylor, 1711), 199. Mandeville's *Treatise* was republished in a revised edition in 1730 under the title *A Treatise of the Hypochondriack and Hysterick Diseases*, 2nd edn. (London: for J. Tonson, 1730).

of the spleen and the vapors. Other physicians soon followed suite: within the first half of the century, Nicholas Robinson, George Cheyne, and William Stukeley all published medical treatises on hypochondria which used the latest principles of natural philosophy to elucidate the pathology of the spleen and the vapors in a popularized form, and more were to follow later in the century.[77]

Furthermore, just as English Calvinist physicians of the soul argued that religious despair was a sign of spiritual sensitivity to sin, few eighteenth-century physicians failed to note that hypochondria distinguished the sufferer as a privileged and rightful member of polite society, marked out from the lethargic stupidity of the unpolished laboring masses by the "sensibility" and quick wit that a delicate and refined nervous system imparted to the mind.[78] This translated the ancient notion of the connection between genius and melancholy into eighteenth-century medical language: a more finely textured nervous system provided elevated mental ability at the same time that it increased the danger of mental collapse from nervous disorder. Novelists such as Samuel Richardson extended these ideas about the psychological implications of the delicacy of the nervous system to the operation of moral feeling as well, making sensibility the basis of such virtuous qualities as compassion and benevolence.[79] More cynically, the French essayist and sometime resident of London Jean-Bernard Le Blanc noted in his commentary on hypochondria in his *Lettres sur l'Anglais* (1745): "This disease is called the disease of the sensible and witty people; and this is a sufficient reason that I am not surprized at the progress it has made in an age when every body pretends to good sense and wit."[80] Thus, in spite of a continued level of ridicule of the hypochondriac patient's melancholic complaints, it is arguable that medical language and theory became the dominant mode of analyzing and expressing hypochondriac melancholy throughout the eighteenth century. As Boswell put it in 1782: "There is too general a propensity to consider *Hypochondria* as altogether a bodily disorder. I lately got from France a very ingenious little treatise upon it, which

---

77   Cheyne, *English Malady*; Nicholas Robinson, *New System of the Spleen, Vapours and Hypochondriack Melancholy* (London: A. Bettesworth, W. Innys, and C. Rivington, 1729); William Stukeley, *Of the Spleen* (London: for the author, 1723). See also Jonathan Andrews, "'In Her Vapours … [or] Indeed in Her Madness'? Mrs. Clerke's Case: An Early Eighteenth-century Psychiatric Controversy," *History of Psychiatry* 1 (1990): 125–43.

78   Blackmore, *Treatise*, 24, 89; Cheyne, *English Malady*, 36–7; Guerrini, *Obesity and Depression*, 123, and for other examples, Mullan, *Sentiment*, 205–10. See also Walter Charleton, *A brief discourse concerning the different wits of men* (London: R.W. for William Whitwood, 1669), 78–81.

79   On Richardson and eighteenth-century ideas of sensibility as genius and as a moral quality, see Stephanson, "Richardson's 'Nerves'": 267–85. Many of the case histories that make up Part III of Cheyne's *The English Malady* are distinguished by their ingenuity and intellectual ability. Most others are described as virtuous, and of great worth and merit.

80   Le Blanc, *Letters*, 135.

professes to manage vapours in the human constitution, with the same facility that a good naturalist commands air to come and go in any material substance."[81]

Following eighteenth-century critics like Le Blanc, historians often represent eighteenth-century hysteria and hypochondria in terms of its "fashionability," pointing in particular to its importance in the "culture of sensibility" as a sign of genius and moral character.[82] But to say that hypochondria and hysteria were fashionable describes and does not explain; and the connection with sensibility is no doubt one aspect of the popularity of the hypochondria diagnosis, but it must not be overemphasized. John Mullan has argued that many of the physicians who wrote on hypochondria and hysteria exhibited a worry over the dangers of "sensibility" in causing diseased emotional and physical disturbance and sometimes precipitating madness.[83] Nor can it account for the early popularity of the language of hysteria and hypochondria: already in the early 1680s the essayist Sir William Temple was commenting on the popularity of "the vapors," and this is well before the "culture of sensibility" came into being.[84] Nicholas Jewson offers another explanation in arguing that the prevalence of hypochondria shows the extent to which eighteenth-century medical theory and treatment were dictated by the illness perceptions of patients rather than anything approaching a scientific, "objective" process of diagnosis. Physicians were dependent for their livelihood on patronage, and "when the wealthy and powerful chose to identify emotional stress with disease, practitioners accepted their definition of the situation and acted as if such maladies were real pathological entities."[85] In as much as this assumes that hypochondria was in fact a "psychosomatic" illness, this interpretation is open to objection. Moreover, it does not explain why the wealthy and the powerful would *choose* to express emotional stress with disease.[86]

---

81   Boswell, "On Hypochondria," no. 63, December 1782, in *The Hypochondriack*, 2: 236.

82   See G.S. Rousseau, "Psychology", 204–8; Roy Porter, "Rage of Party," 35–50; Porter, *Mind-forg'd Manacles*, 85, and C.A. Moore, *Backgrounds*, 192.

83   See John Mullan, "Hypochondria and Hysteria," 141–74, and his *Sentiment and Sociability*, 207.

84   On Temple, see page 164 below; on the eighteenth century's "culture of sensibility," see G.J. Barker-Benfield, *The Culture of Sensibility: Sex and Society in Eighteenth-century Britain* (Chicago, IL: University of Chicago Press, 1992).

85   Jewson, "Medical Knowledge and the Patronage System in 18th Century England," *Sociology* 8 (1974): 369–85.

86   Several critics in the "long" eighteenth century had some rather plausible explanations; see page 164–70 below. There is also evidence to suggest that hypochondriac patients fully understood their condition to be both of the mind and of the body, but declined from discussing their mental "trouble of mind" with their physician for the reason that the care of the mind was not the physician's area of expertise: see *The Complete Letters of Lady Mary Wortley Montagu*, ed. Robert Halsband (Oxford: Clarendon Press, 1966), 1: 176, as cited in Heather Meek, "Eighteenth-century Female Spleen: The Woman Writer as Diagnostician," paper presented at the annual conference of the Northeast American Society for Eighteenth-Century Studies, Fredericton, 3 October 2005. (My thanks to the author for providing me with

But the fact that physicians were dependent on wealthy patrons for their livelihood was none the less quite important in popularizing the language of hypochondria as a form of illness behavior in the eighteenth century, and we can advance this thesis without committing to any assumptions of whether hypochondria was "psychosomatic" or "real." William Temple, despite his own skepticism about the reality of "the spleen" and "the vapors," gives us a clue as to role of patronage in the pervasiveness of the language of hypochondria and hysteria in the eighteenth century. Temple thought that hypochondriacal disorders had become one of the main concerns of physicians since physicians are "fain to humour such Patients in their Fancies of being ill, and ... prescribe some Remedies, for fear of losing their Practice to others that pretend more Skill in finding out the Cause of Diseases, or Care in advising Remedies, which neither they nor their patients find any Effect of, besides some Gains to one, and Amusement to the other."[87] Temple was not being merely cynical in his suggestion that the physician was in some measure expected to entertain and amuse. Sydenham noted that hysteria was a disease which tended to attack those who pursued, or were confined to, a life free of physical labor or sport. It was thus the disease of men who "are wont to study hard," and women in general, "because kind Nature has bestowed on them a more delicate and fine Habit of Body, having designed them only for an easie Life."[88] As moralists put the matter, it was the disease of the idle, and in the eighteenth century this meant that it was seen as the disease of the increasing numbers who devoted their life to the pursuit of polite amusements. Significantly, not least important among these amusements was the display of knowledge and wit in sociable conversations on topics in natural philosophy and medical theory.[89] There is indeed evidence to suggest that the display of "Skill in finding out the Cause of Diseases" and "Care in advising Remedies" was something of a pastime for both the hypochondriac and polite society in general. Temple's comment points not to patronage *per se*, but rather to an altering cultural and social environment immensely productive of the kind of medical discourse which he thought so much amused the hypochondriac patient and encouraged his or her illness behavior.

Harold J. Cook has argued that, up until the late seventeenth eighteenth century, the office of the physician was that of a learned counselor and advisor on a range of matters relating to the government of the soul and the conduct of life, and that the authority of this office was premised on the possession of a virtuous character. In the late seventeenth century, however, this ideal was eroded by the need to sell one's practice in a competitive medical market place through advertising the efficacy of one's cure and through appealing, in appearance and behavior, to fashionable tastes

---

a copy of this paper.) This may have skewed physicians' analyses of the condition in favor of a somatic register, although many seem to be aware of the importance of emotion in causing the condition.

87   Temple, *Of Health and Long Life*, in *Works*, 2: 238.
88   Sydenham, *Epistolary Discourse*, in *Works*, 440, 447.
89   On the association of "idleness" and nervous disorder, see pages 167 and 175 below.

– to being, in other words, a commodity in polite society. This led to an increased therapeutic emphasis on "heroic" medical cures, consisting of batteries of powerful pharmaceuticals, rather than more dietetic cures. In addition, it meant engaging with the patient as something of a colleague. There was a deep interest in medical theory and knowledge among the gentry, and many expected their physician to be as much an interlocutor on matters medical as a healer.[90]

No one conveyed this better than Dr. Bernard Mandeville, in a series of shrewd, often biting, satirical observations on the contemporary medical profession and its patients in his *Treatise of the Hypochondriack and Hysterick Passions* (1711; 2nd edn. 1730). Mandeville declared in the Preface to the *Treatise* that his emphasis on the slow accretion of therapeutic insight through long and careful observation would be "swimming against the Stream in our sprightly talkative Age, in which the silent Experience of Pains-taking Practitioners is ridicul'd, and nothing cried up but the witty Speculations of Hypothetical Doctors."[91] Scholars have noted that the use of mathematics in medical theory was an important feature of early eighteenth-century medicine, stemming largely from the massive popularity of Newton's works.[92] Mandeville attributed the widespread use of a Newtonian natural philosophical idiom in medical theory to the demands of polite society:

> The Study of this Science is become fashionable, and the Knowledge of it look'd upon as a necessary Qualification that Men of Letters ought to be possess'd of, whatever Profession they are of. Some of the politest People value themselves upon being *Philomaths*; and there are Ladies, who, by the Testimony of known and able Mathematicians, are very expert in *Algebra* and sir *Isaac*'s Fluxions.

The lesson for physicians, which they had indeed learned quite well, was obvious:

> When once any Part of Knowledge comes to be in such Vogue, and cultivated as well as approved of by the *Beau Monde*, the Want of it becomes a Defect in a Man, that has been brought up at the University ... The first Step to gain Favor of the Publick is to render our selves acceptable to it; and no Point is to be gain'd among any Set of People if we will not, in some measure at least, comply with their Notions, as well as their Manners.[93]

---

90   Cook, "Good Advice, Little Medicine: The Professional Authority of Early Modern English Physicians," *Journal of British Studies* 33 (1994): 1–31; Roy Porter and Dorothy Porter, *Patient's Progress: Doctors and Doctoring in Eighteenth-century England* (Cambridge: Polity Press, 1989), 137–8, 158–9, 190–91, 197–8, and Roy Porter, "Laymen, Doctors and Medical Knowledge in the Eighteenth Century: The Evidence of the *Gentleman's Magazine*," in Porter, *Patients and Practitioners*, 283–314.

91   Mandeville, *Treatise* (1730), v.

92   The work of Anita Guerrini is especially important. See "Archibald Pitcairne and Newtonian Medicine," *Medical History* 31 (1987): 70–83, and "James Keill, George Cheyne, and Newtonian Physiology, 1690–1740," *Journal of the History of Biology* 18 (1985): 247–66.

93   Mandeville, *Treatise* (1730), 176.

The social personality and duties of the physician were, according to Mandeville, fundamentally altered in the context of polite sociability. Natural philosophical knowledge was only one of a variety of trappings that constituted the credentials of the successful society physician by developing his ability to please his patients. As Mandeville's mouthpiece, Philopirio declares:

> If you are not extraordinary in any of the Branches [of natural philosophy] I have named ... shew yourself a Scholar, write a Poem, either a good one, or a long one, Compose a *Latin* Oration, or do but Translate something out of that Language with your Name to it.

One cannot help but think here of the literary activities of Sir Richard Blackmore, whose poetic output in the early eighteenth century was prodigious. In the second edition of the *Treatise*, Mandeville drew even more attention to the need for the physician aspiring to success to integrate himself thoroughly into the world of polite sociability. Misomedon, the hypochondriac patient in Mandeville's dialogue, argues that the most important subject to be studied by the young physician was not mathematicks; rather, he must "converse with and learn the Language of the *Beau Monde*":

> His first and greatest Care should be to have his Name often mentioned among them. In order to this he should make his court chiefly to the Favourites of the Ladies, keep company with Men of superficial Knowledge, and all the great Talkers about town. Every now and then he should entertain those of his Acquaintance with something that is curious in Nature, or by the Help of microscopes, Prisms, or an Air-Pump, amuse them with some sight or other...that should be cleanly as well as diverting. For the rest, I'd have him dress well, study Politeness, and in every thing *la belle maniere*.[94]

Mandeville was not simply arguing that the physician needed to shape his personal manners and conduct according the norms and tastes of polite society; rather, he was asserting that the practice of medicine itself had become theatrical. The physician took on the role of actor and playwright, whose aims were to divert and please the imagination. As Philopirio puts it, describing the demands put by polite taste on modern medical discourse: "In some of our Modern Hypotheses there is as much Wit to be discover'd as in a tolerable Play, and the contrivance of them costs as much labour."[95]

The hypochondriac and hysteric conditions, as particularly difficult diseases to understand and treat, and indeed as controversial and dubious medical phenomena, would have provided a particularly attractive platform for theoretical theatrics. As Philopirio observes:

> I know it is a received Opinion now-a-days, that a Man of Sense who understands Anatomy, and something of Mechanick Rules, ought to penetrate into the Manner of every Operation that is performed in a Human Body, it being but a mere Machine; nay, 'tis

---

94 Ibid., 205.
95 De Mandeville, *Treatise* (1711), 89.

beneath a Gentleman, that pretends to Natural Philosophy, to be ignorant of any thing, or so much as surmise, that it should be in Nature's power to contrive a Work, for which he could not give a plausible reason.[96]

The many eighteenth-century medical treatises which analyzed hypochondria using the conceptual framework of the new mechanical philosophy for a generally educated readership can be seen as part of an endeavor to display the physician's learning in polite society. The popular medical discourse on hypochondria in the eighteenth century was in part an artifact of the practice of medicine in the context of a culture of polite sociability; the "Skill at finding out the Cause of Diseases" that Temple argued physicians used to retain the hypochondriac patient was simply one of the techniques needed by the successful physician to attract patients who expected him to be able to converse intelligently and with wit on topics of theoretical speculation. The practice of polite medicine invested the hypochondriac diagnosis with immense cultural currency, injecting it into the popular consciousness as a fashionable, polite, and serious subject.

The status of Mandeville's own *Treatise* was thus somewhat ambiguous: although the physician in the dialogue that made up the *Treatise* eschewed theoretical flights of fancy, he was astute enough to satisfy his patient's appetite for medical discourse, a therapeutic acuity through which Mandeville could broaden his own appeal to polite consumers and patients. (Indeed, Mandeville advises in his preface that interested patients contact him through his bookseller.[97]) Other medical works on hypochondria were similarly written to capitalize on popular interest in scientific and medical theory. John Purcell, for example, opened his *Treatise of the Vapours* (1702; 2nd edn. 1707) by remarking that "in all Sciences nothing now pleases the Generality, but what is altogether conformable to Modern Philosophy." And he himself clearly intended to please the generality: the subtitle of his work announced that he intended to analyze the vapors "*according to the newest and most Rational Principles,*" and he declared that while in the medical community traditional Galenic physicians still maintained a powerful voice, "those Ingenious Gentlemen who are well vers'd in Modern Philosophy, Geometry, and the structure of Mans Body, 'tis them I'd chuse to be my Judges."[98] Nicholas Robinson's *New System of the Spleen, Vapours and Hypochondriack Melancholy* (1729) was a particularly ambitious and elaborate attempt to analyze hypochondria through a detailed discussion of the "*Structure, Mechanism,* and *Modulation* of the NERVES, necessary to produce *Sensation* in ANIMAL BODIES," as his title page advertised it.

Medical theories of hypochondria were consciously crafted as sociable and polished science, often explicitly appealing to an educated female readership. Blackmore wrote:

---

96   Mandeville, *Treatise* (1730), 115.

97   Ibid., xviii.

98   Purcell, *Treatise* (1702), Preface.

I have endeavoured to convey my Sentiments to the Reader in clear and obvious Expression, not only to the Sons of Art, but to all intelligent persons, though not great Scholars, or Students in Physick; and I hope there will not appear to Persons of a competent Capacity any thing intricate or obscure, for want of significant and intelligible Words.[99]

Indeed, for all his satire of the contemporary practice of medicine in polite society, Mandeville himself choose to play the part of the society physician, writing his *Treatise* in dialogue form in order to "make what I had to say as palatable as I could to those, I had in view for my Readers." It was, he thought, a literary form "both serious and diverting, that might embellish, and yet not be too remote from the Subject.[100] In the 1730 edition of the *Treatise*, Mandeville translated the extensive Latin quotations for the benefit of the female readership. Purcell, whose book was intended for the benefit of the "fair sex," apologized for "the Impoliteness of my stile, and some hard words, which the subject render'd impossible for me to avoid," thereby submitting himself to the specifically "soft" female sensibilities which were thought to govern polite sociability.[101]

The endeavor of physicians to include women in their polite audience was part of their effort of physicians to expand their influence and fame in a society in which, in Mandeville's words, "there are Ladies, who, by the Testimony of known and able Mathematicians, are very expert in *Algebra* and Sir *Isaac*'s Fluxions." It was a recognition that medical fame was, to a certain extent, brokered by the women of polite society, who, like men, were caught up in the craze for natural philosophy.[102] Again, as Mandeville facetiously advised, the aspiring physician "should make his court chiefly to the Favourites of the Ladies." Furthermore, since "very few Women … are quite free from every Assault of this Disease," as Sydenham noted, treating of hypochondria and hysteria would have been a particularly ingratiating method of self-presentation. Anne Finch, the Countess of Winchilsea, wrote in her famous poem *The Spleen* (1709) that female hysteria accounted for "the physician's greatest gains": "his growing wealth he sees / Daily increased by ladies' fees." It was all the more profitable since the spleen "dost … baffle all his studious pains," particularly for the doctor who could, like Mandeville, Purcell, Cheyne, and others, advertise himself as a specialist in the treatment of nervous disorder, promising a cure where other doctors continually failed.[103]

---

99 Blackmore, *Treatise*, vi–vii.

100 Mandeville, *Treatise* (1730), xi. Various scholars have pointed to the importance of the dialogue in popularizing natural philosophy in the eighteenth century: see, for example, Alice N. Waters, "Conversation Pieces: Science and Politeness in Eighteenth-century England," *History of Science* 35 (1997): 121–54.

101 On the connection between femininity and polite sociability in the eighteenth century, see Barker-Benfield, *Culture of Sensibility*.

102 Elite women had long been important in ensuring professional success: see Michael Stolberg, "A Woman Down to Her Bones: The Anatomy of Sexual Difference in the Sixteenth and Early Seventeenth Centuries," *Isis* 94 (2003): 292.

103 Finch, *The Spleen*, in *Selected Poems*, 44.

Mandeville drew attention to the pleasure that the hypochondriac gained from being able to converse on medical theory and practice.[104] The hypochondriac was an avatar, perhaps even an addict, not only of medicines, but also of medical discourse and conversation. Misomedon declares of one of his former physicians: "the loss of him so much affected me, that I often thought, I could willingly have given him tripple Fees; if he could only have kept his Temper, and invented new Reasons, to sooth my fancy, tho' he had done nothing to my Disease."[105] At the end of the dialogue, Misomedon confesses a certain disappointment with the prospect of being cured: he will no longer be able to benefit from the company and conversation of the physician. Philopirio responds by pointing out that "all Hypochondriacal People are delighted with a new Physician." It is, he says, "a Symptom of the Disease."[106] Yet according to Mandeville's analysis, the pleasure of sociable conversation on topics of medical theory was one of the motivating features of modern patient-practitioner interactions more generally. The male hypochondriac represented in Mandeville's dialogue in the *Treatise* is in many ways representative of the qualities to which both men and women in society aspired and through which the popularizing physician attempted to establish his appeal: he is genteel, widely read and broadly educated; as Mandeville describes him in the Preface, he "is very talkative, loves to converse with Men of Letters, and ... seems not to want Sense or Penetration."[107] Mandeville was, like Temple, placing hypochondria directly in the territory of larger patterns of polite medical practice. Thus, while physicians wrote works of theory on hypochondria to vie for social approbation, enabling their readers to congratulate themselves on their own intelligence in digesting the latest in natural philosophy, the language of hypochondria benefited by becoming the locus of fashionable displays of knowledge, and the hypochondriac by having a surplus of theories and physicians through which to comprehend their own personal constellation of ailments.

It was thus not only that physicians' dependence on patronage produced a complicity with patients in regarding their hysteric and hypochondriac symptoms as features of a legitimate disease entity, as Jewson argues. Rather, the demands on medical practice created in the specific context of early eighteenth-century polite society offered the phenomenon of hypochondria as an attractive topic to explicate using medical theory, and this helped to popularize the language of hypochondria as a cultural illness identity more generally. Roy and Dorothy Porter note that eighteenth-century physicians resented the "residual power lodged with the laity and the degree to which they had to humour lay foibles. The public at large were medically ignorant, many doctors state or implied, yet they puffed themselves up with a simulacrum of medical knowledge, pretending to be what James Makittrick Adair called 'lady and gentlemen doctors.'"[108] But some physicians were quite clear

---

104 Mandeville, *Treatise* (1730), 45.

105 Mandeville, *Treatise* (1711), 19.

106 Mandeville, *Treatise* (1730), 379–80.

107 Ibid., xii, xiv, xvi.

108 Porter and Porter, *Patient's Progress*, 134.

about the fact that they were providing a language of illness which would in fact shape patient expressions and empower their medical judgment. In the preface to the second edition of *A Treatise of the Vapours* (1707) Purcell defended his decision to write "the history of diseases and their theory in English" by arguing that patients could thereby "learn how to make known their distemper to a Physician, which they wanted terms to express fully and intelligibly." "And certainly," he added, "it must be a very great satisfaction to the Patient, by knowing something of these matters, to judge whether the Cause the Physician ascribes of his distemper be rational; and the method of Cure be answerable to the cause he assigns."[109]

Clearly, at least some physicians were aware that they were popularizing a specific way of expressing bodily illness, attempting, perhaps, to provide more clinical definition to a vaguely defined and wide-ranging cluster of symptoms. But while medical language became an established and "fashionable" mode of expression, hypochondria and hysteria were by no means thought of as simply medical conditions. For all of the popularity of medical language, both physicians and moralists viewed hysteria and hypochondria as deeply moral and spiritual problems well into the eighteenth century, in some cases by accepting the medicalized understanding that was being built up around hypochondriac and hysteric illness behaviors, in others by rejecting the notion of hypochondria and hysteria as primarily organic disorders. It is to these moral and spiritual ways of articulating the problem of melancholy and to their eighteenth-century contexts that we now turn.

---

109 Purcell, *A Treatise of Vapours, or, Hysterick Fits*, 2nd edn. (London: for Edward Place, 1707), "To the Reader."

CHAPTER SEVEN

Curing Augustan Hysterics: Morality, Politics, and Religion

In his *Treatise*, Mandeville drew attention to hypochondria as a kind of pathological form of sociability. The hypochondriac wanted constant medical attention, as well as sympathy, for his condition, and his interactions with others revolved around his illness. Dr. Purcell rather comically attempted in his *Treatise on the Vapours* to provide a mechanical account of the social dimension of hysteria in his explanation of the crying fits of the hysteric:

> The thoughts of such persons being generally employ'd upon dismal and melancholy Subjects; the Impressions of painful Sensations are renew'd: whereupon the Soul causes all those motions in the body which were established by the Laws of the Soul's Union to it, to move *Pity* and *Compassion* to the beholders. These motions are chiefly a violent Depression of the Eyebrows and upper Eyelids, an Elevation of the under Lids: which happening together cannot but press the Glands which are situated within them, at each corner of the Eye; and thereby squeeze out of the that serous watery Humour call'd *Tears*.[1]

But such crying fits suggested to others more skeptical of the medical reality of the diagnosis that hypochondriacs and hysterics were in fact somehow more actively and intentionally *using* physical illness behaviors to express, to mask, or perhaps to legitimate and understand, emotional perturbance, and many suggested that hysteria was a ploy of specifically *female* desire. Sydenham had written that "as often as Women advise with me about this or that Disorder of the Body, the reason where cannot be deduced from the common Axioms, for finding out Diseases, I always diligently enquire of them, whether they have been disturbed in their minds, and afflicted with Grief, which if they confess, I am abundantly satisfied that the Disease must come under this Tribe we now discourse of."[2] *Pace* Sydenham, some suggested that the link between emotion and hysteric symptoms called for a moral rather than a medical analysis of hysteria.

But the medical language of hysteria and hypochondria could itself be both spiritualized and moralized. Several medical writers argued that it was ultimately sensual desire, conceived as unreasonable, disorderly, luxurious, and effeminate, which lay lie behind hypochondriac bodily disorder. This representation of nervous

---

1   Purcell, *Treatise* (1707), 124–5.
2   Sydenham, *Epistolary Discourse*, in *Works*, 446.

disorder was to be given its fullest and most popular expression in the work of Dr. George Cheyne, but with a rather surprising twist. For Cheyne fully moralized hysteria and hypochondria by reinventing the discourse on the afflicted conscience, using medical language and concepts to argue that the practice of Christianity was in fact the only means to moderate appetite; and, echoing late sixteenth and early seventeenth-century valuations of female spiritual sensitivity, Cheyne ascribed sensitivity of conscience precisely to the effeminate body.

Hypochondria, hysteria, and the "contrivances of passion"

One of the most incisive critics to explore the moral psychology of hypochondria was Sir William Temple, whose comments on the subject that can be found scattered throughout essays written in the seventeenth century and published throughout the eighteenth century in the several editions of his works. In his essay *Of Health and Long Life*, Temple pointed to the series of revolutions in illness fashion he had witnessed in his life:

> In the course of my Life, I have often pleas'd or entertain my self with observing the various and fantastical Changes of the Diseases generally complained of, and of the Remedies in common Vogue, which were like Birds of Passage, very much seen or heard of at one Season, and disappeared at another, and commonly succeeded some of a very different kind. When I was very young, nothing was so much feared or talk'd of as Rickets among Children, and Consumptions among young People of both Sexes. After these the Spleen came in play, and grew a formal disease: Then the Scurvy, which was the general Complaint, and both were thought to appear in many various Guises ... After these, and for a Time, nothing was so much talked of as the Ferment of the Blood, which passed for the Cause of all sorts of Ailments, that neither Physician nor Patients know well what to make of. And to all these succeeded the Vapours, which serve the same Turn, and furnish Occasion of Complaint among Persons whose Bodies or Minds ail something, but they know not what.[3]

What emerges here is an analysis of hypochondria very similar to Simon Patrick's analysis of religious melancholy in its sensitivity to the relationship between the physical feeling and its language of expression in producing melancholic disease. Like other diagnoses at one time fashionable, "the vapors" and "the spleen" were terms of an amazing elasticity, "thought to appear in many Guises," and were thus immediately available and immensely useful for those suffering from some form of non-specific discomfort to be able to represent their affliction as "a formal disease." In his *Observations upon the United Provinces*, Temple declared in a more condemnatory fashion that the spleen is "the Disease of People that are idle, who think themselves but ill-entertain'd, and attribute every fit of dull Humour, or Imagination, to a formal Disease, which they have found this Name for." Again, the *language* of hypochondria and its power as a diagnostic label were of central

---

3   Temple, *Of Health and Long Life*, in *Works*, 1: 282.

importance in constituting hypochondriac symptoms as a distinct form of illness, a medical condition requiring both pity and expert attention. Temple thus echoed Patrick when he described the occasion of hypochondriac behavior. Fits of "dull Humour," he wrote:

> are incident to all Men, at one time or other, from the Fumes of Indigestion, from the common Alterations of some insensible Degrees in Health and Vigor; or from some changes or approaches of changes in Wind and Weather, which affect the finer Spirits of the brain, before they grow sensible to other parts; and are apt to alter the Shapes, or Colours, or whatever is represented to us by our Imaginations, whilst we are so affected.

Temple argued that the effect of these "imperceptible" physiological changes, far from deserving to be considered as a serious medical condition, "is not so strong, but that Business, or Intention of Thought, commonly either resists, or diverts it: and those who understand the Motions of it, let it pass, and return to themselves." The hypochondriac condition itself was produced by the confluence of such feelings and a moral attitude of studied unhappiness:

> But such as are idle, or know not from whence these Changes arise, and trouble their Heads with Notions or Schemes of general Happiness or Unhappiness in Life, upon every such Fit, begin Reflections on the Condition of their Bodies, their Souls, or their Fortune; and (as all Things are then represented in the worst Colours) they fall into melancholy Apprehensions of one or other, and sometimes of them all: these make deep Impression in their Minds, and are not easily worn out by the natural Returns of good Humour, especially if they are often interrupted by the contrary; as happens in some particular Constitutions, and more generally in uncertain Climates, especially if improv'd by Accidents of ill Health, or ill Fortune.[4]

Temple himself was all too aware of the impact of uncertain climate, ill health, and ill fortune on contentment of mind. Temple's sister, Lady Giffard, wrote in her *Character of Sir William Temple* that:

> his humor [was] gay, but a great deal unequal, sometimes by cruel fitts of spleen and melancholy, often upon great damps in the weather, but most from the cross & surpriseing turns in his business, & cruel disapointments he met with soe often in … the contributing to the honour & service of his country.[5]

---

4   Temple, *Observations upon the United Provinces of the Netherlands*, in *Works*, 1: 54. There are also some interesting parallels between Temple's analysis of the hypochondria and hysteria diagnosis, and the anthropologist and psychiatrist Arthur Kleinman's exploration of the ways in which illness behaviors and cultural assumptions interact with disease entities such as depression or dysthymnia in creating culturally specific clinical profiles: see Kleinman, *Patients and Healers*; his *Social Origins of Distress and Disease*, and his *The Illness Narratives*, 40–41, 100–120.

5   Lady Giffard, *The Character of Sir William Temple*, in *The Early Essays and Romances of Sir William Temple*, ed. G.C. Moore Smith (Oxford: Clarendon Press, 1930),

Lady Giffard also records that Temple developed the gout at the age of 47, "wch he attributed to the air of Holland" and "upon wch he grew very Melancholy being then Ambassador at ye Hague, said a man was never good for any thing after it."[6] But while Temple recognized the importance of such physical factors as climate, temperament and illness in creating feelings of melancholic unease, he consistently located the problem of how to manage such feelings in a moral philosophical context, analyzing melancholy in relation to the conduct of life and of the passions. In the *Observations upon the United Provinces*, Temple noted that foreigners in the Netherlands "are apt to complain of the Spleen," but the Dutch themselves "seldom or never. Which I take to proceed from their being ever busie, or easily satisfy'd," he continued:

> This is a Disease too refin'd for this Country and People, who are well, when they are not ill; and pleas'd when they are not troubled; are content, because they think little of it; and seek their Happiness in the common Ease and Commodities of Life, or the Encrease of Riches; not amusing themselves with the more speculative Contrivances of Passion, or Refinements of Pleasure.[7]

Here and elsewhere, Temple recognized that diversion and occupation could prevent feelings of melancholy from consuming the soul. As he put it in a note in the *Heads, Designed for an Essay on Conversation*: "Men that do not think of the present, will be thinking of the past or future; therefore Business or Conversation is necessary to fix their Thoughts on the present. In the rest, seldom Satisfaction, often Discontent and Trouble, unless to very sanguin Humours."[8] But behind the admiration of the Dutch ethos Temple expressed in the *Observations* stood a philosophical reflection significantly more profound than the commonplace insight that keeping busy and occupied was effective in preventing an outbreak of the spleen. It was received therapeutic knowledge that idleness commonly gave rise to melancholy as diversion and business cured it.[9] But to be well when not ill, pleased when not troubled, and to seek happiness "in the common ease and commodities of life" – these were expressions of the Epicurean philosophy Temple found so attractive as a *mode de vivre*.

Recognizing the insight of the ancient philosophical maxim that "a Man's Happiness [is] all in his own Opinion of himself and other Things," Temple sought to determine the correct estimation of the degree of mental tranquility and bodily

---

27. The *Character* was also published anonymously in *The Works of Sir William Temple*. See *Works*, 1: 19.

6   Lady Giffard, *Character*, in *Early Essays*, 29.

7   Temple, *Observations*, in *Works*, 1: 54.

8   Temple, *Heads, Designed for an Essay on Conversation*, in *Works*, 1: 311.

9   One of the most famous lines from Burton's *Anatomy* is, of course, "Be not solitary; be not idle" (III.iv.II.vi: 494). See also Barrough, *Methode of Phisicke*, 36, and Willis, *Soules of Brutes*, in *Works*, 194.

ease that would result from the enjoyment of any given object or quality.[10] Chief among Temple's concerns regarding the conditions for happiness was the Epicurean effort to define the limits of the pursuit of pleasure. This was a problem not only of ascertaining "those Pleasures, which upon Thought we conclude are likely to end in more Trouble or Pain, than they begin in Joy or Pleasure," but of limiting the very appetite for sensual pleasure.[11] One of the fundamental insights of Epicurean moral philosophy, was, according to Temple, "to place true Riches in wanting little, rather than in possessing much; and true Pleasure in Temperance, rather than in satisfying the Senses."[12] This was precisely the moral strength of the Dutch, who were, Temple perceived, content with "the Common Ease and Commodities of Life."

According to Temple's analysis, this form of life was superior because it was sustainable. The majority of people are "busied" with the "common designs of satisfying their Appetites and their Passions," wrote Temple in his essay *Upon the Gardens of Epicurus* (1685); but the result was that they were caught up in the exertion of "making endless Provisions for both."[13] "The true end of Riches ... [is] Ease and Pleasure," Temple elsewhere observed; "the common Effect, to encrease Care and Trouble."[14] The idle – those who gave themselves more directly to the pursuit of pleasure rather than industriously applying themselves to the pursuit of wealth – fared no better. In the *Heads, Designed for an Essay upon the Different Conditions of Life and Fortune*, Temple noted that "to rich Men, the greatest Pleasures of Sense either grow dull for want of Difficulty, or hurt by Excess."[15] Temple contrasts "Mankind ... thus generally busied or amused" with the philosophers, who "have chosen what they thought a nearer and surer Way to the Ease and Felicity of Life, by endeavouring to subdue, or at least to temper their Passions, and reduce their Appetites to what Nature seems only to ask and to need."[16]

According to Temple's analysis, hypochondria was popular in part because it offered an explanation for the vague, uneasy feelings produced by the inevitable emotional deflation brought about through the pursuit of refined pleasures. But as the comparison of Dutch to English culture made clear, this was not simply a matter of individual moral character, but of national mores and ways of life; Temple's moral analysis of hypochondria was also a critique of the modern urban conditions of luxury and of the impulse to polish and refine taste and pleasure, which were becoming the central and celebrated constituents of the English elite's self-image at the turn of the century. The art forms sponsored and enjoyed in the courts of the

---

10   Temple, *Heads, Designed for an Essay upon the Different Conditions of Life and Fortune*, in *Works*, 1: 308.

11   Ibid.

12   Temple, *Upon the Gardens of Epicurus; or, Of Gardening, in the Year 1685*, in *Works*, 1: 173.

13   Ibid., 1: 172.

14   Temple, *Heads, Designed for an Essay upon the Different Conditions of Life and Fortune*, in *Works*, 1: 307.

15   Ibid., 1: 306.

16   Temple, *Upon the Gardens of Epicurus*, in *Works*, 1: 172.

sixteenth and seventeenth century became widely available in populous commercial towns in the eighteenth century, promoted and enjoyed now by the increasingly affluent population that drew its life from trade and consumption.[17] Members of polite society clamored to distinguish themselves from the common and the vulgar through displays of refinement in gastronomy and dress, and through the cultivation of an "idle" life given to the consumption of an expanding range of "pleasures of the imagination," such as novels and operas. But Temple, although he was certainly a consumer of such pleasures, thought that the explosion of hypochondriac cases indicated that such people were altogether "too refin'd." He tied a life of idleness and the pursuit and invention of more sophisticated and luxurious kinds of sensual gratification with the advance of disease in general: "all the great Cities, celebrated most, by the Concourse of Mankind, and by the Inventions and Customs of the Greatest and most delicate Luxury, are the Scenes of the most frequent and violent Plagues, as well as other Diseases."[18] Temple's analysis of hypochondria confirmed this diagnosis of civilization: for not only did the pursuit of luxury result in bodily unease, it also created a sense of mental unease which found expression in hypochondriac illness behavior, in complaint about and exaggeration of physical ailments. Thus, Temple regarded the hypochondriac condition itself as something of a contrivance of passion; being ill had itself become a form of amusement and occupation.

Temple's is a particularly nuanced analysis of the complex interaction between mind and body, language and sensation, in the production of hypochondria. He clearly regarded hypochondria and hysteria as "diseases of the soul," originating in certain beliefs and ways of life, but he was aware that there was a physiological dimension to the hypochondriac condition. Thus, while he criticized individuals "whose bodies and minds ail something, but they know not what" for using medical labels to describe their condition, his analysis also explained why medical language would be appealing in understanding and explaining vague, non-specific feelings of unease. Moralists who followed Temple were, however, much more condemnatory in tone, and on the whole more interested in drawing attention to the ways in which medical language was used very intentionally to mask moral folly. Jeremy Collier argued in a short essay "Of the Spleen," first published in 1695, that where the hypochondriac temper was the product of melancholic uneasiness, an individual could simply plead hypochondriac disease rather than admit a weakness of mind or a moral fault:

> As the Spleen has great Inconveniences, so the Pretence of it is a handsome Cover for many Imperfections. It often hides a Man's Temper, and his Condition, from breaking

---

17   See John Brewer, *The Pleasures of the Imagination: English Culture in the Eighteenth Century* (London: HarperCollins, 1997); Paul Langford, *A Polite and Commercial People: England, 1727–1783* (Oxford: Clarendon Press, 1989), 68–76; Klein, "Politeness and the Interpretation of the British Eighteenth Century," and the comments in Shaftesbury, *Characteristics*, 1: 124–5 and 2: 256–72.

18   Temple, *Of Health and Long Life*, in *Works*, 1: 279.

out to Disadvantage. For the Purpose: One Man … is severely mortified by some great Disappointment; but this must not be owned. No: The Man is impregnable, he has his Mind on a String; but no body can command a Constitution. He that has dispirited himself by a Debauch, drank away his good Humour, and it maybe raised his Conscience a little upon him, has this Pretence to guard against Censure: A civil Guesser will believe him Hypocondriacal.[19]

Collier admitted that there were genuine cases where hypochondriac melancholy was the result of disease. But he also insisted that the medical category had a social function: having entered into the polite vocabulary, it had become a very useful part of the equipment of polished self-presentation, a "handsome cover" in cases where melancholic emotion breached social expectations for the conduct of one's mind and actions. While it would be hard to see how the splenetic temper Collier described was "handsome," the hypochondriac illness label had at least rendered it "civil" – acceptable, pitiable, and to a degree even irreproachable, if not exactly respectable. According to Collier, the invocation of hypochondriac bodily illness had the remarkable power to smooth over the unpleasant edges of melancholic and peevish personality in the context of social interaction. "If he is silent and unentertaining to a Visiter, the Spleen is his Excuse, and conveys his Pride or Disaffection out of Sight," Collier wrote. "In short, the Spleen, does a great deal of Service in Conversation: It makes ill Nature pass for ill Health."[20] Melancholic moroseness and disaffection had been among the list of evils associated with the nonconformist during the Restoration, and were opposed to the allegedly polite and equable temper produced by Anglican allegiances; according to Collier, the hypochondriac melancholy label had now entered into the practice of polite sociability as a very useful and acceptable form of moral hypocrisy.

The point was made again by Jean-Bernard Le Blanc in his commentary on London life and culture written in the mid-eighteenth century, where he referred approvingly to Temple's observations on hysteria. In an epistolary essay on the vapors, Le Blanc wrote to an anonymous addressee that "the mind has its diseases as well as the body … You labour to destroy the foibles, prejudices, errors, passions, and vices of all kinds, which are the real diseases of the mind." "In the list of diseases there is one, which I think to be more your province than that of ordinary physicians," he continued: "you will easily guess I mean the vapours."[21] Following Temple, he noted that hypochondria "chooses to dwell only in the bosom of idleness and opulence: which furnishes us with the best idea of its real cause." Idleness created in persons "an uneasiness that devours them," and opulence the means to fill up "the vacant

---

19 Collier, "Of the Spleen," *Miscellanies upon Moral Subjects: The Second Part* (London: for Samuel Keeble and Joseph Highmarsh, 1695), 37–8. This essay was republished in numerous editions of Collier's moral essays throughout the first half of the eighteenth century, under the title *Essays upon Moral Subjects*.

20 Collier, "Of the Spleen," 38.

21 Le Blanc, *Letters*, 180.

hours of their lives" with the "excessive indulgence of pleasures."[22] Thus, "in the greatest part of the men vapours are nothing but violent uneasiness," which "we pity, when we ought to accuse." He did not deny that hypochondria could indeed be a condition of the body: "The soul and body act mutually and necessarily on each other." But, he declared, "I suspect that many of those who complain of [the vapors], are less sick in body than in mind; and that in general they affect more the head than the stomack or nervous system." On Le Blanc's analysis, the physical symptoms of hypochondria were generated by the prideful need to hide the moral nature of the underlying cause of hypochondriac affliction, melancholic discontent:

> I own that uneasiness is the most cruel of all distempers ... In this sense the vapoured have reason to complain: for no creatures can be more unhappy. But they will not confess that they are uneasy, for fear of discovering a fault in their mind, or an irregularity in their appetites. By the disease they affect, they surprize our pity; whereas a confession of the truth would but mortify their self-love.

Like Collier, Le Blanc argued that the cultivation of hypochondria as a social illness identity was a mechanism of human vanity mobilized to gain public sympathy for what was a private moral fault: "We derive a sort of vanity from our unhappiness, but we are always secretly ashamed of our defects. At least we had rather appear sick than foolish; and some gains of folly may possibly be an ingredient in the most part of vapours."[23] Such statements would have touched a raw nerve in the eighteenth-century self-image of an age whose advancement of the arts and sciences was thought to be accompanied by an advancement in morals and manners. Moralists such as Shaftesbury and Joseph Addison had argued that politeness and refinement of taste could be a kind of education into virtue.[24] Yet critics insisted that politeness could be just as easily pressed into the service of moral hypocrisy rather than moral improvement.[25] Most incisive among these critics was in fact Bernard Mandeville, who argued in his notorious *Fable of the Bees* (1724) that politeness was, like ancient virtue, merely a means to play on the human sense of pride in order to shame individuals into acting more sociably. But politeness, unlike strict classical republican virtue, did not demand of the individual that he "conquer his Passions, it is sufficient that he conceals them": "Virtue bids us subdue, but good breeding only requires we should hide our Appetites."[26] Moralists such as Collier and Le Blanc contributed

---

22   Ibid., 184–5.

23   Ibid., 181.

24   Klein, *Shaftesbury*, 34–47.

25   See Nicholas Phillipson, "Politeness and Politics in the Reigns of Anne and the Early Hanoverians," in J.G.A. Pocock, ed., *The Varieties of British Political Thought, 1500–1800* (Cambridge: Cambridge University Press in association with the Folger Institute, Washington, DC, 1993), 225–7.

26   De Mandeville, *Fable of the Bees, or, Private Vices, Publick Benefit*, ed. F.B. Kaye (Indianapolis, IN: Liberty Fund, 1988), 1: 72, 349–55; see also E.J. Hundert, *The Enlightenment's "Fable": Bernard Mandeville and the Discovery of Society* (Cambridge: Cambridge University Press, 1994), 178–9, 198–9.

to these indictments of the eighteenth century's polite manners and morals in their analysis of the "epidemic" of hypochondria and hysteria. The widespread use of the medical language of hypochondria was not a feature of any advancement in natural philosophical knowledge about the nervous system or the stomach, nor more generally in the refinement of wit and sensibility; instead, it provided a form of rhetoric which increased the ability of human vanity and self-love to disguise publicly "mental diseases" which would rightly bring social condemnation and shame.

Le Blanc and Collier indicated that men as well as women were at fault in this moral hypocrisy. But female hysteria was often singled out as particularly wilful and strategic. Anne Finch wrote in *The Spleen* that the vapors arose in the "imperious wife" through "o'erheated passions." The hysteric woman's "o'ercast and showering eyes" exerted the force of the spleen "upon her husband's softened heart" so that "he the disputed point must yield."[27] In Samuel Richardson's *Pamela, or, Virtue Rewarded* (1740), Mr. B. traces the married woman's vapors to the fact that upon being married, she is subject to her husband's will, and "thinks it very barbarous, now, for the *first* time, to be opposed in her will, and that by a man from whom she expected nothing but tenderness."[28] Richardson had Lovelace comment in *Clarissa* (1747–48) that a woman "can be ill or well when she pleases" in order to refuse male sexual demands. As Raymond Stephanson points out, "Lovelace's attitude toward nervous sensibility ... owes much to an older view of masculinity," on which hysteric and hypochondriac symptoms were taken as the signs of both feminine weakness and female rebelliousness rather than as the virtuous sensitivity into which Richardson and others were attempting to fashion them.[29] It had indeed been common to associate female and effeminate weakness with hysteric symptoms in the early eighteenth century, and this association remained available throughout the century, in spite of the popularization of more "sensitive" ideals of virtue.[30] In *The English Malady*, Cheyne noted that nervous distempers "in the *Sex*" were often ascribed to *Daintiness, Fantasticalness,* or *Coquetry.*"[31] And in Mandeville's *Treatise,* an hysteric patient complains of the male point of view: "I never dare speak of Vapours, the very Name is become a Joke; and the general notion the Men have of them is, that they are nothing but a malicious Mood, and contriv'd Sulleness of

---

27 Finch, *The Spleen*, in *Selected Poems*, 42. For an insightful interpretation of Finch's *Spleen* as a critique of male medical representations of the female and of female hysteria, see Desiree Hellegers, *Handmaid to Divinity: Natural Philosophy, Poetry and Gender in Seventeenth-century England* (Norman, OK: University of Oklahoma Press, 2000), 141–67. See also Meek, "Eighteenth-century Female Spleen."

28 Samuel Richardson, *Pamela, or, Virtue Rewarded*, ed. William M. Sale, Jr. (New York: W.W. Norton, 1958), 471–2.

29 See Samuel Richardson, *Clarissa* (New York: Everyman's Library, 1932), vol. 4, 91. Cf. the insightful discussion in Stephanson, "Richardson's 'Nerves,'" 277–8.

30 See Barker-Benfield, *Culture of Sensibility*, 27–36, 77–98, 104–53.

31 Cheyne, *English Malady*, 179–80.

willful, extravagant, and imperious Women, when they are denied, or thwarted in their unreasonable Desires."[32]

Alexander Pope gives us an example of a man joking about female vapors. In his poem *The Rape of the Lock* (1714), Pope represents "Affectation" as one of the "handmaids" of the Spleen, mixing in both "coquetry" and "extravagance" into the characterization of the vapors:

> There *Affectation* with a sickly Mien
> Shows in her Cheek the Roses of Eighteen,
> Practis'd to Lisp, and hang the Head aside,
> Faints into Airs, and languishes with Pride;
> On the rich Quilt sinks with becoming Woe,
> Wrapt in a Gown, for Sickness, and for Show
> The Fair-ones feel such Maladies as these,
> When each new Night-Dress gives a new Disease.[33]

And, confirming the views of the hysteric patient in Mandeville's *Treatise* that female hysteria was seen by men to involve unreasonable desire, Belinda, the poem's protagonist, is represented as falling into a raging fit of spleen over the loss of a curl of hair.

The analysis of hysteria as disappointed female desire found a place in the writing of some physicians as well. Writing in 1702 in one of the first popular English works on hysteria, John Purcell devoted a short section near the end of his treatise to discussing the need to "avoid all concerns, Anxieties, and Passions":

> For upon diligent search and enquiry, you will almost always find, that those who are troubled with Vapours, have some deep Passion or Concern upon them, which renders them Pensive and Thoughtful: Wherefore the Physician ought to consider attentively the Circumstances of his Patient, and to inform himself of her acquaintance, what may be the cause of her Concern, which having found out, he must, with the aid of Friends and Relations, facilitate to her, the means of obtaining what she desires. I know an eminent Practitioner who assured me, he has found better Effects from this Method alone, than from most other Remedies that can be prescrib'd in this Disease. Two very considerable Cures I my self saw him do in this nature; one was of an ancient Gentlewoman, who used to lye for two Months together in violent Fits, seldom being able to get the least repose; all the Remedies she had taken for two years and a half, were ineffectual; but the Doctor had no sooner found out what it was that troubled her, and put her into a way of obtaining what she so passionately desired, but all her violent Symptoms were abated to a Miracle.[34]

---

32 De Mandeville, *Treatise* (1730), 169–70.

33 Pope, *The Rape of the Lock*, 4.31–8, in *The Poems of Alexander Pope*, 2: 186.

34 Purcell, *Treatise* (1702), 155. Cf. Ilza Veith, *Hysteria: The History of a Disease* (Chicago, IL: University of Chicago Press, 1965), 147–51, who notes that the seventeenth-century Italian physician Giorgio Baglivi argued that hysteria was almost always caused by the passions of the mind. Baglivi's work was well known across Europe, and was translated into English several times in the eighteenth century.

But here the physician was treading on dangerous territory, for by prescribing "the means of obtaining what she desires" as a cure, he was potentially empowering the woman in what might be regarded by others as a struggle for power over her husband. From the moralist's perspective, this was to underwrite female sedition and disorderliness. Anne Finch, who experienced the severely restricted sphere of the early modern female will as a married woman, wryly recognized that although the woman was "armed with spleen" and the husband must at times "something resign of the contested field," it was "lordly man" who is "born to imperial sway … and woman … does servilely obey."[35] Pope has Clarissa remind Belinda that "good Humour can prevail / When Airs, and Flights, and Screams, and Scolding fail / Beauties in vain their pretty Eyes may roll / Charms strike the Sight, but Merit wins the Soul."[36] Hysteria was not be indulged, but was rather to be disciplined through virtue, and for women this meant obedience and passivity.

Writing in *The Spectator* in 1711, Sir Richard Steele had "A. Noewill" write to notify "Mr. Spectator" of Mrs. Freeman's "terrible Fit of the Vapours, which, 'tis feared, will make her miscarry, if not endanger her Life." "Therefore, sir," he continues, "if you know of any Receipt that is good against this fashionable reigning Distemper, be pleased to communicate it for the Good of the Publick." In a previous installment of *The Spectator*, "Mr. Freeman" had written to complain of his wife's imperious insistence on his remaining home with her perpetually. The lady's vapors indeed occurred when Mr. Freeman left in a coach, after a rage occasioned by his upbraiding speech to her:

> I am from this Hour Master of this House; and my Business in it, and every where else, is to behave my self in such a Manner as it shall be hereafter an Honour to you to bear my Name; and your Pride that you are the Delight, the Darling, and Ornament of a Man of Honour, useful and esteemed by his Friends; and I no longer one that has buried some Merit in the World, in Compliance to a forward Humour which has grown upon an agreeable Woman by his Indulgence.[37]

Steele was suggesting that the cure of hysteria involved the reinforcement of early modern gender hierarchy. The vaporish wife was merely the latest embodiment of figure of the disorderly woman. It appears that Steele's "cure" is at the expense of Mrs. Freeman's health, since her fit of vapors endangers her life and the life of her child. But "Freeman" is not Mrs. Freeman's name; it is her husband's. She is merely an ornament, the purpose of whose existence is to please her husband. "A. Noewill" may have been looking for a medical cure for the vapors, but as the fictional name suggests, a medical cure would merely mask the underlying problem, which is a failure of the male to assert his will over the female's.

---

35 Finch, *The Spleen* in *Selected Poems*, 42.

36 Pope, *The Rape of the Lock*, V, 31–4: 201.

37 Joseph Addison and Richard Steele, *The Spectator*, ed. Gregory Smith (London: Dent for Everyman's Library, 1966), nos. 212 and 216, 2: 131–3, 142–4.

Luxury's plague: hypochondria and commercial society

In Tobias Smollet's *Humphrey Clinker* (1771), Mrs. Bayard cajoles her husband through nervous fits of passion and tears "deeper and deeper into the vortex of extravagance and dissipation." "The family Plate was sold for sold silver, and a new service procured; fashionable furniture was provided." Mr. Bayard does not upbraid his wife for her extravagance "on the supposition that his wife's nerves were too delicate to bear expostulation."[38] It was an early modern commonplace to align luxury consumption with the female appetite, particularly as many of the new luxury commodities such as furniture and tea services were intended for the domestic sphere.[39] But the "epidemic" of hypochondria and hysteria was not interpreted by all authorities in the way Smollet does, as a female ploy. For some authorities, it pointed to the deeper problem of a society infected with luxury.

The subject of luxury had long been a moral concern in Western civilization. When Temple associated disease with luxury, he was stating an intellectual commonplace. From Plato through Aristotle to Latin legislators and Stoic philosophers, luxury was viewed as a force dangerously subversive of the proper ordering of human desires and needs. The pursuit of luxury satisfied the baser human appetites at the expense of the exercise of reason and virtue, and consequently of health and well-being.[40] These concerns about the nature of luxury and sensual appetite became central themes of discussion, critique, and polemic in the eighteenth century as English society became increasingly a commercial society, its cultural practices oriented around the trade and consumption of material goods. But early modern critics viewed many of the new forms of pleasure as corrosive of moral character. Town life drew criticism from those who saw the theater as provoking lust, and the fashionable classes that consumed the new high culture as at best superficial, at worst profoundly given over to vice, pride, and vanity.[41] And, as J.G.A. Pocock has pointed out, many late seventeenth and early eighteenth-century political writers expressed the worry that moral personality was no longer envisioned in terms of the pursuit of public virtue made possible by material independence in the form of ownership of land, as it had been in the dominant mode of Aristotelian and classical republican political thought, but rather in terms of an individual who had delegated the practice of his political freedom to others in order to involve himself in the consumption of cultural artifacts,

---

38   Smollet, *The Expedition of Humphrey Clinker* (New York: New American Library, 1960), 287–8, as quoted in Barker-Benfield, *Culture of Sensibility*, 28–9.

39   Elizabeth Kowaleski-Wallace, *Consuming Subjects: Women, Shopping, and Business in the Eighteenth Century* (New York: Columbia University Press, 1997), 57–8; Barker-Benfield, *Culture of Sensibility*, 154–214.

40   See Christopher J. Berry, *The Idea of Luxury: A Conceptual and Historical Investigation* (Cambridge: Cambridge University Press, 1994), 45–86, and John Sekora, *Luxury: The Concept in Western Thought, Eden to Smollet* (Baltimore, MD: The Johns Hopkins University Press, 1977), 29–109.

41   Brewer, *Pleasures of the Imagination*, 72–3.

both for his own pleasure and for the sake of social esteem. The citizen enamored with culture had no time for public political life.[42]

Hysteria and hypochondria figured in the context of critique of luxury as particularly damning signs of English intemperance, symptoms of a moral disease which some argued would terminate in the death of English liberties. The Whig literary critic John Dennis, in pointing to the dangerous decline in the "Publick Spirit" caused by the "Growth of the *British* Luxury," contrasted the disease-ridden gentry of early eighteenth-century England with the healthy and virtuous gentry of Henry VII's reign: "Their way of Living in the Country, their Diet, their Air, their Oeconomy, and their rural Diversions and exercises confirm'd their Healths, and improv'd their Estates, and supply'd them both with Strength of Body, and with Vigor of Mind. So that their Minds were serene, or their Passions moderate; their Distempers neither frequent nor violent, and their Children healthful [and] lively robust."[43] In lamenting the prodigious consumption of wine and liquor, Dennis pointed in particular to the "numerous melancholly Crowd of deep hysterical Symptoms" attending the rise in the consumption of wine and liquor among British women.[44] Early in the eighteenth century, the Cambridge-educated physician Peter Paxton had developed an historical argument linking the rise of luxury and progress of the arts of entertainment with vice, excess, and illness, and had specifically traced disorders such as female hysteria and male hypochondria to the "excess and irregularity" of the modern diet, which was full of "Foreign rarities" and "a variety of Liquors." "If with all these we will continue in a lazie, sedentary and unactive Life," he declared, "it can be no wonder if we bring upon ourselves an infirm habit, a wretched and unhealthful temper."[45]

The moral and political significance of the "epidemic" of hypochondria and hysteria to which critics like Dennis and Paxton pointed was made into the central device of the anonymous Whig pamphlet published after political fallout of the collapse of the South Sea bubble in 1720, entitled *Observations on the Spleen and Vapours, containing Remarkable cases of persons of both sexes and all Ranks, from the aspiring director to the humble Bubbler, who have been miserably afflicted with those melancholy disorders since the fall of the South-Sea and other publick Stocks, together with descriptions of treatments and remedies* (1721). The *Observations of the Spleen and the Vapours* went beyond the link between hysteric symptoms and irrational female tyranny, pointing instead to luxurious and disorderly desire among both men and women as the cause of hypochondria and hysteria. To be sure, the wives of ordinary tradesmen who have had to turn to stock-jobbing to earn a quick sum are represented as supporting their husbands' endeavors because of the promise

---

42   J.G.A. Pocock, *The Machiavellian Moment: Florentine Political Thought and the Atlantic Republican Tradition* (Princeton, NJ: Princeton University Press, 1975), 430–33.

43   Dennis, *An Essay Upon Publick Spirit; Being a Satyr in Prose Upon the Manners and Luxury of the Times* (London: for Bernard Lintott, 1711), 13.

44   Ibid., 15.

45   Paxton, *A Directory Physico-Medical* (London: for J. Sprint, 1707), 6–13, and his *An Essay Concerning the Body of Man* (London: for Richard Wilkin, 1701), 240–41.

of luxury goods: diamond rings, silver cups, Damask gowns, beds and easy chairs, sets of china, and silver teapots. Their fervent hopes for these promised goods, and the great impression such articles make on the female imagination, lead to a deluge of cases of the vapors in women as the stocks decline in value. But men, too, are urged in the pamphlet to moderate their desire for wealth and luxury; and the *Observations* is as much a critique of female weakness as it is of the attempt of the tradesmen to emulate wrongfully the splendor of the social elite. This is indeed part of the joke of the pamphlet, for against the myth of hypochondria and hysteria as diseases of England's upper social ranks, even the "humble Bubbler" is stricken with the disease. Where even the laborers had such fine nerves, the problem of luxury was being posed not as a problem of female desire, but of the growing effeminacy of the British nation, a term which occurs continually in other denouncements of luxury in the eighteenth century. And from this perspective, the "epidemic" of hysteric symptoms was not caused by wilful female desire subverting rational male authority, but was rather due more generally to the pursuit of material wealth and pleasure.

Nervous disorder as conscience: George Cheyne's "wounded soul"

The argument that the "epidemic" of nervous disorder was to be understood as a feature of the massive increase of trade and consumption in England was declared most powerfully for eighteenth-century audiences by George Cheyne, perhaps the most famous of eighteenth-century physicians specializing in the treatment of nervous disorder, whose works on hysteric disorders and diet went through several editions in his lifetime and after. Cheyne's descriptions and condemnations of luxury in *The English Malady* echo those of Paxton and Dennis. Paxton had written that "we ransack the *Indies* for Spices, and the most remote parts for Foreign rarities … to tickle our Palates."[46] Cheyne declared that "since our Wealth has increas'd, and our Navigation has been extended, we have ransack'd all Parts of the *Globe* to bring together its whole Stock of Materials for *Riot, Luxury*, and to provoke *Excess*."[47] Dennis pointed to the competitive escalation of luxurious eating, drinking, and dressing among the gentry, as well as to proliferation and invention of goods to be consumed. Cheyne railed that "the whole *Controversy* among us, seems to lie in out-doing one another in such Kinds of Profusion. *Invention* is rack'd, to furnish the Materials of our Food the most Delicate and Savour possible."[48] Dennis condemned gaming, large and ostentatious assemblies, and the Italian opera; Cheyne argued that luxurious dining "must necessarily beget an Ineptitude for Exercise, and accordingly *Assemblies, Musick, Meetings, Plays, Cards* and *Dice*." And his prescription for the convalescent hypochondriac to take up such "cheap and innocent" diversions as suited the country retreat, such as "hunting, shooting [and] bowls" reflects the stark contrast that was articulated by those like Dennis between the healthy and virtuous

---

46   Ibid., 240.
47   Cheyne, *English Malady*, 49.
48   Ibid., 50.

life in the country, and the vices of the modern town.[49] Indeed, where Dennis looked back to the virtuous nobility of the late fifteenth century, Cheyne pointed out how the "antient *Greeks*, while they lived in their Simplicity and Virtue were Healthy, Strong, and Valiant: But afterwards, in Proportion as they advanced in Learning ... and distinguished themselves from other Nations by their Politeness and Refinement, they sank into *Effeminacy*, *Luxury*, and *Diseases*."[50]

Cheyne knew personally the devastating effects of large living and little exercise. After studying under the Edinburgh physician and natural philosopher Archibald Pitcairne, who was notorious for his drinking, Cheyne had traveled to London in 1701, to attempt to establish himself as a medical practitioner and as a natural philosopher. As he put it in his autobiographical account of his hypochondria case in *The English Malady*, there he "found the *Bottle-Companions*, the *younger Gentry*, and *Free-Livers*, to be the most easy of *Access*, and most quickly susceptible of *Friendship and Acquaintance*, nothing being necessary for that Purpose, but to be able to *Eat* lustily, and swallow down much *Liquor*."[51] Mirroring Mandeville's satirical advice to aspiring physicians, Cheyne related in *The English Malady* that he "was tempted to continue *this Course*, no doubt, from a *Likeing*, as well as to force a *Trade*, which Method I had observ'd to succeed with some others." But Mandeville had not advised of the adverse consequences of such polite medical practice: "Thus constantly Dineing and Supping in *Taverns*, and in the Houses of my Acquaintances of *Taste* and *Delicacy*, my Health was in a few Years brought into great Distress, by so sudden and violent a Change." An "*autumnal intermittent Fever*" gave way to fits of vertigo, and finally to "a constant violent *Head-ach*, *Giddiness*, *Lowness*, *Anxiety* and *Terror*."[52] Cheyne was to combat recurring bouts of such hypochondriac melancholy the rest of his life.

Roy Porter has argued that Cheyne's *English Malady* can be read as a celebration of British success and an apologetic for the Whig regime which had done so much to encourage trade and the growth of financial power.[53] But from the perspective of Cheyne's own interpretation of his suffering, it seems rather unlikely that Cheyne thought of his hypochondriac melancholy as such an indication. Indeed, although Cheyne clearly linked nervous disorder to the luxurious conditions of early eighteenth-century England, his concerns were ultimately neither moral nor political – nor even medical, strictly speaking – but religious. Anita Guerrini has shown how Cheyne's slow and temporary recovery involved a profound reassessment of his religious beliefs and practices, and has described his case history in *The English Malady* as a "spiritual autobiography," a kind of conversion narrative.[54] Cheyne retired from

---

49   Ibid., 52, 181–2.

50   Ibid., 56–7; see also Paxton, *Directory*, 12–13.

51   Cheyne, *English Malady*, 325–6.

52   Ibid., 326–7.

53   Porter, "Glorious Revolution"; see also Porter's introduction in Cheyne, *The English Malady* (1733), ed. Roy Porter (London: Tavistock/Routledge, 1991).

54   Guerrini, "Case History as Spiritual Autobiography: George Cheyne's 'Case of the Author,'" in *Eighteenth-Century Life* 19 (1995): 18–27.

London to the country, where he "had a long season for undisturbed *Meditation* and *Reflection*," and apparently some scrutiny of his conscience. Although he was able to affirm that he had "preserv'd a firm Perswasion of the great and fundamental Principles of all *Virtue* and *Morality*" during his spree of loose living – namely, the belief in "the *Existence* of a *supreme Being*, the *Freedom* of the *Will*, the *Immortality* of the Spirits of all intelligent Beings and the Certainty of *Future Rewards* or *Punishments*" – this form of natural religion alone now appeared to be insufficient "to *quiet* my Mind," as he put it. Cheyne sought the spiritual guidance of the Scottish Episcopalian clergyman George Garden. Garden had been particularly instrumental in introducing the works of the seventeenth-century Flemish mystic Antionette Bourignon, whose writings articulated a quietistic approach to piety, eschewing theological polemic and doctrinal niceties in favor of personal spiritual cultivation and self-discipline, and this approach was Garden's own view of Christian faith as well. Cheyne, having "collected a *set of religious Books* and *Writers* ... recommended by him," set out on a path of mystical Christian practice and belief which he never abandoned.[55]

Cheyne's religious reflection was spurred on by "*Apprehensions* and *Remorse*," and increasing "*Melancholy*."[56] It was, in Burton's terms, something of a case of religious melancholy, although it is unclear that Cheyne himself would have applied the term to his case.[57] In *An Essay of Health and Long Life* (1724), Cheyne wrote that "there is a kind of *Melancholy*, which is called *Religious*, because 'tis conversant about Matters of *Religion*; although, often the Persons so distempered have little *solid Piety*. And this is merely a *Bodily Disease*, produced by an ill *Habit* or *Constitution*, wherein the *Nervous System* is broken and disordered."[58] Though his piety at the onset of his melancholy was indeed thin, Cheyne regarded his experience as more than a mere bodily disease. He made it clear in *The English Malady* that he could not be tarred with the anti-enthusiast brush, his religious experience dismissed as mad fancy. His reading of Garden's recommendations during his attack of hypochondria was indeed the beginning, not the negation, of solid piety:

> [T]he *Fright*, *Anxiety*, *Dread*, and *Terror*, which, in Minds of such a Turn as mine (especially under a broken and *cachectick* Constitution, and in so atrocious a *nervous* Case) arises, or, at least, is exasperated from such Reflections, being once settled and quieted, *That* after becomes an excellent *Cordial*, and a constant source of *Peace, Tranquility*, and *Cheerfulness* and so greatly contributes to forward the Cure of such *nervous* Diseases: For I never found any sensible *Tranquility* or Amendment, till I came to this firm and settled *Resolution ... To neglect nothing to secure my eternal Peace, more than if I had been certified I should I should die within the Day.*[59]

55   Ibid., 23–4, and Guerrini, *Obesity and Depression*, 12–21, 79–88, 137–43, 159–62.
56   Cheyne, *The English Malady*, 328–9.
57   Guerrini, *Obesity and Depression*, 9, 12, 151–2, and her "Case History," 23.
58   Cheyne, *Health and Long Life*, 157.
59   Cheyne, *English Malady*, 333–4.

Cheyne was thus both defending the spiritual value of his nervous case of religious dread and promoting revealed religion and sincere and searching piety as key sources of tranquility in the healing of his nervous disease. Earlier, Cheyne had articulated an Augustinian cure of immoderate passions as cure for hypochondria. Accepting the basic premise, common to all early modern investigations of the human subject, that the passions of the soul affected the body through their operation in the organs of the body, Cheyne argued that "the *Chronical Passions*, like *Chronical Diseases*, wear out, waste and destroy the *Nervous System*," eventually running into nervous diseases such as hypochondria and hysteria.[60] A hypochondriac condition of the nerves caused by "Excesses" or "an original bad *Conformation*," might be cured by "proper *Exercise*" or, as a last resort, "the *Medicinal* and *Chirurgical* Arts." But, Cheyne continued:

> if the Passions be *raging* and *tumultuous*, and constantly fuelled, nothing less than *He*, who has the *Hearts of Men in His Hands*, and *forms them as a Potter does his Clay, who stills the Raging of the Seas, and calms the Tempests of the Air*, can settle and quiet such tumultuous, overbearing *Hurricanes* in the Mind, and *Animal Oeconomy*.[61]

In what followed, Cheyne developed an elaborate argument comparing spiritual beings to physical bodies, arguing by analogy that the corollary of the Newtonian notion of attraction between physical bodies was the spiritual love by which the human soul, "in this her *lapsed* Estate, being *drowned* in Sense," is drawn towards God as the greatest and most perfect of all spiritual beings. Reunion with God is the "*final Perfection* and *Consummation*" of the guiding principle of the human soul.[62] The moral importance of achieving this perfection was that where an individual loved God "infinitely," they also loved created beings "with their proper Degree of *finite* Love, according to their *Rank* in the *Scale* of Beings."[63] The raging of the passions was stilled, with profound benefit to health. "All *Anxiety, carking Care*, and *Solicitude* about" worldly things, which are the sources "of all our *Miseries*, and of many Bodily *Diseases*, would be *cut* off all at once." Furthermore, "*Luxury*, and *Lewdness, Laziness* and all the other *Seeds* of Bodily *Diseases*, would be altogether *destroyed*."[64] The practice of piety and the cultivation of spiritual love were, according to Cheyne, the best and most lasting therapies for hypochondriac disease. They treated it at its roots by eradicating the worldly loves that drove the soul into the passionate excess and laziness which so devastated the nerves.

Guerrini has argued that Cheyne saw the material condition of the body as mirroring the condition of the soul. Deeply influenced by the ascetic practices of mystics like

---

60 Cheyne, *Health and Long Life*, 155–6.

61 Ibid., 161.

62 Ibid., 161–5; on Cheyne's analogical style of thinking, see G. Bowles, "Physical Human and Divine Attraction in the Life and Thought of George Cheyne," *Annals of Science* 31 (1974): 474–87.

63 Cheyne, *Health and Long Life*, 166.

64 Ibid., 169.

Bourignon and Jeanne de la Mothe Guyon, Cheyne was engaged throughout his life in a spiritual struggle with his flesh, and he regarded his obesity and ill health as an index of his failure to discipline his appetites.[65] From this perspective, Cheyne's *English Malady* can very appropriately be considered a work on the affliction of conscience. Indeed, it opened by invoking the verse used by many early modern ministers to introduce their works on the consolation of conscience: "The Spirit of a Man can bear his Infirmities, but a wounded Spirit who can bear?" (Proverbs 18:14). For Cheyne, the wounded spirit was the soul "broken and dispirited by Weakness of *Nerves, Vapours, Melancholy*, or *Age*," and he scoffed at "the Pride and Presumption of *Human Nature*, which could value, or think to support itself, upon its own natural Courage and Force." Human happiness was dependent to a large extent on the condition and maintenance of the body, he asserted.[66] While this appeared to take the words of "the Prophet" in quite a different direction than pastoral writers, Cheyne continually placed hypochondriacal suffering within the context of punishment for sin. That human kind suffered from nervous disorders was not the fault of the way in which God created the natural order, but of the vicious exercise of human moral freedom in transgressing the "established Laws and Orders" God prescribed for the government of human behavior.[67] The root of the hypochondria epidemic was thus much deeper than dietary habits and physical regimen, as he indicated in the chapter on the passions in *An essay on health and long life*; it had to do with the rejection or acceptance of God as creator, lawgiver and judge. Cheyne consistently linked hypochondria not just with sin, but with the free-thinking neglect of piety which he, following George Berkeley, asserted to accompany and promote intemperance and luxury.[68] Unless free-thinking and deism – "the *Minute Philosophy*" – "prevail, and become the *Standard*," he wrote in *The English Malady*, even "the *Voluptuous* and *Unthinking* … those who value Life only for the Sake of *good eating and Drinking* … may be convinc'd, at least in some measure, when their *proper Time* is come." The youthful free-living and natural religionist Cheyne had himself experienced this time of judgment; it was from his own experience that he declared of the deist and libertine that "when they begin to feel violent *Pain*, long *Sickness*, habitual *low Spirits*, or enter upon the *Limits of both Worlds*, they may be convinced."[69] Convinced in this context clearly meant convicted of sin and of the need for a radical reformation of thought and life. What presumptuous human nature could not outface was its embodied conscience registering responsibility to the Creator and his laws.

Cheyne, like many of his colleagues, fostered the eighteenth-century myth of the hypochondriac as a person of intellectual ability, social standing, and refined feeling

---

65   Guerrini, *Obesity and Depression*, 16–17, 135.

66   Cheyne, *English Malady*, 1–3.

67   Ibid., 19–20, 25–8.

68   See ibid., iii, and Cheyne, *An essay on regimen* (London: for C. Rivington and J. Leake, 1740), xiv–xvi; see also Berkeley, *Alciphron: or, Minute Philosopher* (London: for J. Tonson, 1732), 1: 5.

69   Cheyne, *English Malady*, xii–xiii.

due to his sensitive nervous system.[70] But within the context of his religious beliefs, nervous sensibility took on additional significance. It was, firstly and very biblically, punishment for the sins of former generations. Cheyne noted in *The English Malady* that not all nervous conditions were acquired through a life of excess and over-ease. Some seemed to be "original." But, he continued, "Original Nervous Disorders … must have had the same Source and Cause with the acquir'd ones. The Children, as to their Bodies and bodily Diseases, being punished for the Faults, Follies, and Indiscretions of their Parents."[71] He used this observation to reinforce his arguments about the divinely instituted moral order of nature: "[B]y this progressive and continual Succession from one Root, that the Healthy and Virtuous should thereby be growing continually healthier and happier, and the Bad continually becoming more miserable and unhealthy, till their Punishment forced them upon Virtue and Temperance: for Virtue and happiness are literally and really Cause and Effect."[72] However, Cheyne continued, although "it is a Misfortune indeed, to be born with weak Nerves … if rightly us'd and manag'd, even in the present State of Things … it may be the Occasion of greater Felicity: For, at least, it is (or ought to be) a Fence and Security against the Snares and Temptations to which the Robust and Health are expos'd, and into which they seldom fail to run."[73] Late sixteenth and early seventeenth-century evangelicals had worried about hard-heartedness, and a tender conscience was seen as an exceptionably valuable safeguard against sin. For Cheyne, the sensitive body of the nervous valetudinarian acted as just such an urgent and cautious voice of conscience, its fickle nervous sensitivity forcing appetite within moderate and God-given bounds.

Cheyne also upheld the idea that women were particularly susceptible to nervous disorder. Not only was the female body naturally weaker, but as Cheyne wrote to Samuel Richardson, women "would rather renounce Life than Luxury."[74] Moreover, the female mind was more easily pitched into excessive emotions, which in turn affected the body. But like Cheyne's notion of nervous sensibility, such views of the female body were transformed in the context of his religious concerns. Anita Guerrini points to the "dual perceptions of female nature" in Cheyne's thought: "animal-like, sensual on the one hand, sensitive and otherworldly on the other."[75] According to Cheyne, because of their natural weakness of body, women were by necessity placed in a position of potential spiritual value; their physical health demanded that they discipline their material desires, but this could only be for the good of the health of their soul. And just as late sixteenth and early seventeenth-century evangelicals had

---

70 See page 154 above.

71 Cheyne, *English Malady*, 19.

72 Ibid., 26.

73 Ibid., 20.

74 Cheyne to Richardson, 2 February 1742, in *Letters of Doctor George Cheyne to Samuel Richardson*, ed. Charles F. Mullett (Columbia, MO: University of Missouri Press, 1943), 82, as quoted in Barker-Benfield, *Culture of Sensibility*, 28.

75 Anita Guerrini, "The Hungry Soul: George Cheyne and the Construction of Femininity," *Eighteenth-Century Studies* 32 (1999): 285.

held up female spiritual sensitivity as a model for both men and women, Cheyne effected something of the "feminization" of the male hypochondriac body: Guerrini points in particular to the shift away from the masculine imagery depicting a physical constitution comprised of "*springy*, *lively*, and *Elastick* [nervous] Fibres" in the 1724 *Essay of Health and Long Life* to an imagery emphasizing softness and weakness in *The English Malady* (1733).[76]

While Cheyne thus accepted and promoted the common eighteenth-century assumption that melancholy was a physiological disorder of the nerves, he urged in his writings that the body merely registered the condition of the soul. At root, the hypochondria condition was a disease of the soul. Like Burton and other seventeenth-century figures, Cheyne thought that the practice of virtue, in particular the government of the passions, was one of the most important therapies of melancholy. As he stated in *The natural method of cureing diseases of the body* (1742), "virtue and happiness, vice and misery, luxury and pain, are cause and effect, indissolubly linked."[77] Cheyne thus thought of himself as both philosopher and physician. "True Philosophy is the Science of living the most happily," he wrote in the preface to the *Essay on regimen* (1740); "Physic is but one branch of this Philosophy."[78] But the true philosophy was clearly the "Christian philosophy;" only the Augustinian regeneration of love could heal the lust that fed on worldly pleasures at the same time that it ate at the body.[79] Cheyne did not simply call his readers to return to cultivating civic virtue, as Dennis did, nor merely to discern the moral limits of appetite embedded in the natural order, as Temple did, nor again to cultivate resistance to excessive emotion through moral philosophical regimen; as evangelical Protestants had urged about a century earlier in works aimed at cultivating godly sorrow and humiliation in the melancholy and non-melancholy alike, Cheyne called his melancholic readers to repent and turn to God, and from thence to heal.

Cheyne's writings were immensely popular, going through several editions in his lifetime and published after his death as well. He was cited favorably by the clergyman Lewis Southcomb in *Peace of Mind and Health of Body United* (1750) as an example of a healer concerned with both the body and the soul, and Southcomb followed Cheyne in insisting that "there is no such way of preventing" "*Hypochondriacal*, or *Hysterical Passion*, or *Melancholy*," "as that of a *religious Life*." Southcomb also followed Cheyne in linking hypochondriac and hysteric suffering with the affliction of conscience: "tho' *all Men* are liable to afflictions of this nature … they are seven-fold upon the Sinner," he wrote.[80] Cheyne's stress on the need to discipline the body for spiritual and physical health was taken up by

---

76   Guerrini, *Obesity and Depression*, 123, 147; Cheyne, *Health and Long Life*, 27.

77   Cheyne, *The natural method of cureing diseases of the body and distempers of the mind depending on the body* (London: George Strahan, 1742), 88.

78   Cheyne, *Essay on regimen*, ii.

79   Cheyne, *Natural method*, 66–7.

80   Southcomb, *Peace of Mind and Health of Body United* (London: for M. Cooper, 1750), 14, 19, 42.

figures such as William Law and John Wesley, and in his poem on the cure of the spleen, Matthew Green also followed Cheyne in stressing simplicity of diet and the need to avoid luxurious excess.[81]

But Green's poem also exposes the tensions of Cheyne's position as ascetic spiritual physician in polite society, for Green recommended not only country recreations such as hunting for the cure of the spleen, but also going to the theatre, to musical performances, and to the coffee house, where the company and the conversation would clear the mind of spleen. Green indeed celebrates the idleness and superficiality of polite, "effeminate" society as a cure for the spleen:

> Sometimes I dress, with women sit,
> And chat away the gloomy fit,
> Quit the stiff garb of serious sense,
> And wear a gay impertinence
> Nor think, nor speak with any pains,
> But lay in fancy's neck the reigns ...
> And thus in modish manner we
> In aid of sugar sweeten tea.[82]

These were the kinds of fashionable entertainments and spectacles against which many eighteenth-century critics of luxury railed, and to some extent Cheyne himself. Yet at the same time the coffee house and the fashionable spa town retreat were also Cheyne's venues. Although the passions of the mind continued to be regarded as a cause of melancholic distraction, later eighteenth-century analyses of hysteria and hypochondria were much less moralistic and much more medical; and although physicians continued to stress the need for a balanced way of life, Cheyne is in fact unique among eighteenth-century nervous physicians in his ascetic religiosity. The raillery of nervous disorder as a fashionable disease remained, but eighteenth-century society was slowly becoming accustomed to the wealth and luxury which nervous diseases had to previous minds flagged as corrupt and sinful.[83]

---

81 Guerrini, *Obesity and Depression*, 138–43; Green, *Spleen*, 4, 17, 32–5.

82 Ibid., 11.

83 On the ridicule of the idea of nervous diseases, see Richard Hunter and Ida MacAlpine, eds., *Three Hundred Years of Psychiatry, 1535–1860: A History Presented in Selected English Texts* (London: Oxford University Press, 1963), 489–90.

Conclusion

This study has been concerned with exploring two closely related aspects of the early modern history of melancholy: first, that melancholy was viewed by many practical writers as a condition appropriately understood as a "disease of the soul," in the senses inherited from classical and early Christian moral philosophy and moral theology; second, that because language and the beliefs embedded in language were seen as central to both the cause and treatment of melancholy, the problem of melancholy was at the center of a series of religious and cultural conflicts and tensions in early modern English history.

There is little indication that we can separate out an "Anglican" from a "Puritan" approach to melancholy until at least the middle of the seventeenth century; and moral philosophical and specifically Christian approaches appear to have co-existed peacefully, and according to some were seen as complementary. It was for the most part the clergy who, after all, elaborated the moral philosophical approach in the early seventeenth century, and they did so with clear recognition that moral philosophy was ultimately insufficient to bring about true and lasting – that is, eternal – happiness. But after the Restoration, while both Dissenting and Anglican practical divines continued to share a set of beliefs and techniques, they structured these in very differently oriented ways, according to divergent theological schemes. And within the moderate Dissenting community itself, theological developments and therapeutic concerns shifted the consolation of melancholy away from viewing melancholy as a species of the afflicted conscience, as had earlier English Calvinists. If we were to attempt to generalize, we might say that the pastoral care of melancholy in the established Church and in the moderate Dissenting community shifted after the Restoration from an approach which, in its stronger formulations, insisted that melancholia could and should be used towards "godly sorrow" for sin and the cultivation of humility – postures which were themselves seen as containing moments of desperation – to a more directly consolatory idiom, which attempted to teach sufferers how to manage their feelings of discouragement and dejection so that they did not become despairing.

To state it in these terms is, as we have seen, somewhat overdrawn, for late sixteenth and early seventeenth-century evangelical Calvinists had recognized the need to save melancholic souls from too deep a despair in their Christian pilgrimage: hence the continuity of specific techniques and strategies of spiritual consolation from the late sixteenth to the early eighteenth centuries. But the displacement and abandonment of the Calvinist discourse on religious despair as the main pastoral framework for the consolation of melancholy did have some important and specific implications for the expression and treatment of melancholy in and after the Restoration. First, there was considerable emphasis placed on leveling the extremes of the Calvinist spiritual dialectic between deep despair and ecstatic hope by concentrating the Christian's attention on moral regeneration as the central means to salvation. As a result, sufferers were no longer encouraged or enabled to express their melancholy in the agonistic rhetoric of spiritual affliction. This was felt in the Dissenting community in particular as a disjunction between their tradition of religious experience and "affectionate" speech on the one hand, and on the other the canons of polite speech and behavior that had emerged from the reaction against "Puritanism" and were broadly accepted and celebrated in English culture, a tension which seems to have slowly eroded some of the rhetorical and experiential substance of the moderate Dissenting tradition. Second, as one of the significant features of the English Calvinist rhetoric had been the invocation of the devil as an active figure in times of the spiritual temptation to despair, the specifically demonological component of the pastoral treatment of melancholy was considerably de-emphasized, and indeed actively discouraged, by both Dissenting and Anglican practical divines.

More broadly speaking, the conflict of languages in the treatment of early modern melancholy was between medical and moral, or spiritual, therapeutic and expressive languages. Until the late seventeenth century, most moralists, physicians and clergy seem to have viewed their aims as compatible and complementary. Both Calvinist ministers and Anglican clergy recognized the problem the diseased body posed to the mind in cases of religious melancholy, although there are indications that evangelical Calvinists might have emphasized this less. But what particularly concerned many "physicians of the soul" was the danger that medical language might be used to dismiss entirely legitimate spiritual problems; and although this concern is absent in moral philosophical approaches to melancholy articulated in the early seventeenth century, it became of central concern to late seventeenth and early eighteenth-century moralists, in the wake of the popularization of the hypochondria/ hysteria diagnosis. The motivations of the physicians in this particular episode in the politics of mental health are difficult to determine. The popularization of the language of hysteria and hypochondria consisted of a circle of mutually reinforcing elements: patients latched onto this language, for a variety of social and psychological reasons, and were treated by physicians who wished to advance their careers and enhance their prestige in the eyes of the potential clients and patrons, and therefore provided extensive natural philosophical analyses of the condition, as well as apologies against its critics. Ultimately, however, the medical discourse on hypochondria and hysteria itself displayed moralistic and religious elements, as the case of George Cheyne shows us. For while the language of hypochondria and hysteria located melancholy very concretely in the body as an organic condition of the nerves, the care of the body itself could be regarded as a feature of the care of the soul. This placed the perceived epidemic of hypochondria at the center of worries about the moral and political implications of the emancipated material desire which commercial society seemed to foster and demand.

Anyone familiar with twentieth-century psychiatry will know that the modern proponents of the cognitive therapy of depression have self-consciously referred to and drawn on Greek and Roman Stoic moral philosophy.[1] There have been other recent developments, towards the fringes of the mental health field, which also look back to the early modern period and its inherited intellectual traditions. In the United States there is at present an American Philosophical Practitioners Association (APPA) as well as an American Society for Philosophy Counselling and Psychotherapy (ASPCP). The APPA was founded by Lou Marinoff, Professor of Philosophy at the City University of New York and author of the international best-seller *Plato not Prozac!* (1999). Marinoff's organization offers three-day seminars for the would-be philosophical counsellor, and some prominent politicians in the state of New York are attempting to licence philosophical counselling, integrating it into the medical insurance system.[2]

There have also been some curious developments in the Christian community, again in North America. Recently, a Christian organization in Pennsylvania republished Timothy Rogers' *Discourse*, lauding his insight in treating melancholy and the sense of the loss of God's favour.[3] In the mid-1970s, the Christian psychologist (as he would term himself) Tim LaHaye wrote a book on depression which became something of a best-seller: *How to Win Over Depression* (1975).[4] In it he advocated that "most depression was caused primarily by sin, a faulty thinking pattern, or some failure on the part of the individual to claim the promises of God."[5] LaHaye acknowledges in the revised edition (1996) that since the time he originally wrote the book, the evidence for depression as a biochemical condition has changed our understanding and treatment of depression. But he still writes in the recently revised edition that "God has a thrilling plan for overcoming all temperamental weaknesses – even depression." In Ephesians 5:18, he designates being continually "filled with the Spirit" as his remedy."[6] The religious perspective on mental illness is not limited to the more conservative evangelical movement in the United States: recently, the controversial psychiatrist M. Scott Peck revealed his extensive use of exorcism in his psychiatric practice.[7]

---

1   David A. Clark and Aaron T. Beck, with Brad A. Alford, *Scientific Foundations of Cognitive Theory and Therapy of Depression* (New York: John Wiley and Sons, 1999), 44.

2   Daniel Duane, "The Socratic Shrink," *New York Times Magazine* (21 March 2004): 34–7.

3   Timothy Rogers, *Trouble of Mind and the Disease of Melancholy* (Morgan, PA: Soli Deo Gloria Books, 2002).

4   LaHaye has achieved additional fame as the co-author of the "Left Behind" series of Christian novels, set in the End Times. Thanks to David Bell for bringing this to my attention.

5   Tim LaHaye, *How to Win Over Depression*, rev. edn. (Grand Rapids, MI: Zondervan, 1996), 11.

6   Ibid., 180.

7   See M. Scott Peck, *Glimpses of the Devil: A Psychiatrist's Personal Accounts of Possession, Exorcism, and Redemption* (New York: Free Press, 2005).

There are probably many psychiatric practitioners and lay observers who would view such developments with regret and skepticism, seeing them as reversions to the pre-medical age of early modernity. Implicit in this study, however, has been the suggestion that elements of the early modern care of the soul deserve our attention, not only in terms of our historical understanding, but also in terms of our own contemporary concerns over the care of depression. What is perhaps most admirable about the early modern care of the melancholic soul is the stress on the consolation of melancholy, which was shared by many otherwise diverging "physicians of the soul." And what this effort to console often involved was the framing of the melancholic experience in terms of the broader aims and ends of human life. Foucault lamented the "serene world of mental illness" he encountered in the middle of the twentieth century, in which the madman is handed off to the physician, "thereby authorizing a relation only through the abstract universality of disease."[8] In the early modern period, melancholy was indeed regarded as an illness, but for the melancholic individual, the management of their condition did not necessarily consume their identity as today medical technologies and institutions often can the depressive's. For melancholy was also regarded as a human problem, similar in kind to a range of experiences many individuals faced as they sought to work out their salvation or to cultivate virtuous self-control.

This study has thus pointed to the ways in which the care and even the experience of melancholy have been shaped by various religious, cultural, and philosophical ways of thinking. Melancholy was continually drawn into larger narratives, each of which invested the melancholic experience with a different set of meanings. This confirms recent anthropological work which points to the variety of ways in which culturally specific "texts" interpret depressive affect (to the point where, some argue, the available cultural scripts do not make available the experience of depression at all).[9] Furthermore, according to the psychiatric researcher David Healy, what many modern depressives in the Western world want in their care is not a pill, but "a meaning, a narrative, or a myth to move forward with." They want a way of understanding what is happening to them in terms of how they understand and interpret who they are and what they ought to be.[10] Thus, many of a religious bent who do not find their psychiatrist sympathetic to their spiritual concerns may be disinclined to continue with psychiatric treatment. The writer Andrew Solomon notes that some depressives have found profound comfort and consolation in the practice of religion, as well as a means of ordering and regulating their life to avoid triggering cycles of depression.[11] The non-religious may have different, often very personal frameworks of meaning in

---

8   Foucault, *Madness and Civilization*, x.

9   See the essays in Good and Kleinman, *Culture and Depression*. The notion of interpretive texts for depressive affect is offered by Charles F. Keyes, "The Interpretive Basis of Depression," in Good and Kleinman, *Culture and Depression*, 153–74.

10   Healy, *Antidepressant Era*, 2–3, 253–4.

11   Solomon, *The Noonday Demon: An Atlas of Depression* (New York: Scribner, 2001), 129–33.

which they will attempt to come to terms with their depression.[12] Given the plurality of cultures in the Western world, which includes both deeply religious and strongly secularist currents, a return to a therapeutic eclecticism, which includes the priest and the philosopher, among others, may be good sense.

But to point only to consolatory moments and the treatment of melancholy in terms of broader frameworks of meaning would be to smooth over the deep tensions within early modern discourse on melancholy, for the questions of what the right consolatory language was and which narrative was the correct one were at times matters of some controversy. Tolerating rival therapeutic practices is not so very easy when there might be reason for worry that such practices are not entirely benign, that they in fact exacerbate melancholy and depression. Depressives may often seem to crave a myth or a meaning through which to move forward in their lives, but will just any myth or meaning do? Thus, as I have indicated, conflicts over the care of the soul exist in the modern world in ways reminiscent of the early modern world. There is one crucial difference, however, for medical language now dominates the field where in the early modern period its exclusive authority to treat melancholy was rarely asserted, and a matter of some contention when it was. But the fact that the contemporary practice of medicine and contemporary insurance systems are dangerously close to staking the care of depression almost entirely on psychopharmacology, and have popularized in their wake the over-simplistic and clinically dubious, even harmful, notion of depression as a simple hormonal dysfunction of the brain, makes it all the more urgent to keep open the question of the problematic relation between melancholy and its languages of expression and treatment which we have explored here.[13]

---

12   Arthur Kleinman has emphasized the therapeutic importance of paying close attention to the patient's narrations and representations of their illness: see Kleinman, *The Illness Narratives*.

13   See Solomon, *Noonday Demon*, 101–34; Healy, *Antidepressant Era*, for example, 5.

Bibliography

Primary Sources

A collection of merry poems ... proposed as a pleasant cure for the hyp and the spleen. London: T. Boreman, 1735.

A Relation of the Fearefull Estate of Francis Spira, in the Yeare 1548. London: I.L for Phil Stephens, 1638.

Abernethy, John. *A Christian and Heavenly Treatise, Containing Physicke for the Soule*. London: Felix Kingston for John Budge, 1622.

Addison, Joseph. *Works*. Edited by Richard Hurd and Henry G. Bohn. 6 vols. London: George Bell and Sons, 1892.

—— and Richard Steele. *The Spectator*. Edited by Gregory Smith. 4 vols. London: Dent for Everyman's Library, 1966.

Allen, Hannah. *A narrative of God's gracious dealings with that choice Christian Mrs. Hannah Allen (afterwards married to Mr. Hatt) reciting the great advantages the devil made of her deep melancholy, and the triumphant victories, rich and sovereign graces, God gave her over all his stratagems and devices*. London: John Wallis, 1683.

Ames, William. *Conscience, with the Power and Cases Thereof*. London: Edward Griffin for John Rothwell, 1643.

Aristotle. *On the Soul*. Translated by W.S. Hett. *Loeb Classical Library* 288. Cambridge, MA: Harvard University Press/London: William Heinemann, 1986.

——. *Nicomachean Ethics*. Translated and edited by Roger Crisp. *Cambridge Texts in the History of Philosophy*. Cambridge: Cambridge University Press, 2000.

Augustine. *Expositions on the Book of Psalms*. Edited by A Cleveland Coxe. *A Select Library of the Nicene and Post-Nicene Fathers of the Christian Church*, edited by Philip Schaff, vol. 8. New York: Charles Scribner's Sons, 1917.

——. *De doctrina christiana*. Translated by John J. Gavigan. *The Fathers of the Church*, vol. 4. New York: Fathers of the Church, 1947.

——. *The City of God against the Pagans*. Translated and edited by R.W. Dyson. *Cambridge Texts in the History of Political Thought*. Cambridge: Cambridge University Press, 1998.

——. *Confessions*. Translated by Henry Chadwick. *Oxford World's Classics*. Oxford: Oxford University Press, 1992.

——. *Tractates on the Gospel of John, 28–54*. Translated by John W. Rettig. *The Fathers of the Church*, vol. 3. Washington, DC: The Catholic University of America Press, 1993.

Ayloffe, William. *The Government of the Passions According to the Rules of Reason and Religion*. London: for J. Knapton, 1700.

Barrough, Philip. *The Methode of Phisicke*. London: Thomas Vautroullier, 1583.

Baxter, Richard. *The Right Method for Settled Peace of Conscience, and Spiritual Comfort in 32 Directions*. London: for T. Underhil and F. Tyton, 1653.

——. *God's Goodness Vindicated, for the help of such (especially in Melancholy) as are tempted to deny it*. London: for N. Simmons, 1671.

——. *A Christian Directory, or, A Summ of Practicall Theologie*. London: Robert White for Nevill Simons, 1673.

——. *Poor Man's Family Book*. London: R.W. for Nevill Simmons, 1674.

——. *A Breviate of the Life of Margaret*. London: for Richard Janeway, 1682.

——. *The Cure of Melancholy and Overmuch-Sorrow by Faith and Physick*. In *A continuation of morning-exercise questions and Cases of Conscience Practically Resolved by Sundry Ministers, in October 1682*, edited by Samuel Annesley, 263–304. London: by J.A. for John Dunton, 1683.

——. *The Certainty of the World of Spirits*. London: T. Parkhurst and J. Salisbury, 1691.

——. *Reliquiae Baxterianae*. 2 vols. London: for T. Parkhurst, J. Robinson, J. Lawrence, and J. Dunton, 1696.

——. *Preservatives against melancholy and over-much sorrow, or, The cure of both by faith and physick*. London: W.R., 1713.

——. *Preservatives against melancholy and over-much sorrow, or, The cure of both by faith and physick*. London: for Joseph Marshall, 1716.

——. *The Signs and Causes of Melancholy: with directions suited to the case of those that are afflicted with it. Collected out of the works of Richard Baxter by Samuel Clifford*. London: S. Cruttenden and T. Cox, 1716.

Berkeley, George. *Alciphron: or, Minute Philosopher*. London: for J. Tonson, 1732.

Bolton, Robert. *Instructions for the Right Comforting of the Afflicted Conscience*. London: Thomas Badger for Thomas Weaver, 1640.

——. *A narration of the grievous visitation, and dreadful desertion of Mr. Peacock in his last sicknesse*. London: for Gilbert Milbourne, 1641.

Boswell, James. *The Hypochondriack*. Edited by Margery Bailey. 2 vols. Stanford, CA: Stanford University Press, 1928.

Blackmore, Richard. *A Treatise of the Spleen and Vapours*. London: for J. Pemberton, 1725.

Brinsely, John. *A Looking-Glasse for Good Women*. London: John Field for Ralph Smith, 1645.

Bright, Timothy. *A Treatise of Melancholie*. London: Thomas Vautrollier, 1586.

Bunyan, John. *Grace Abounding*. Edited by John Stachniewski. *Oxford World's Classics*. Oxford and new York: Oxford University Press, 1998.

Burnet, Gilbert. *A Discourse of the Pastoral Care*. London: R.R. for Ric. Chiswell, 1692.

Burton, Robert. *The Anatomy of Melancholy*. Edited by A.R. Shilleto. 3 vols. New York: AMS Press, 1973.

Calvin, John. *Institutes of the Christian Religion*. Edited by John T. McNeill and translated by Ford Lewis Battles. 2 vols. Philadelphia, PA: The Westminster Press, 1960.

Charleton, Walter. *Epicurus' Morals, collected partly out of his own Greek Text, in Diogenes Laertius, and partly out of the Rhapsodies of Marcus Antoninus, Plutarch, Cicero and Seneca*. London: for H. Herringman, 1656.

——. *A brief discourse concerning the different wits of men*. London: R.W. for William Whitwood, 1669.

——. *A Natural History of the Passions*. London: T.N. for James Magnes, 1674.

Cheyne, George. *An Essay of Health and Long Life*. London: for George Strahan and J. Leake, 1724.

——. *The English Malady*. London: for G. Strahan, 1733.

——. *An essay on regimen*. London: for C. Rivington and J. Leake, 1740.

——. *The natural method of cureing diseases of the body and distempers of the mind depending on the body*. London: George Strahan, 1742.

Chilcot, William. *A Practical Treatise concerning Evil Thoughts ... especially useful for Melancholy Persons*. Exeter: Samuel Darker for Charles Yeo, John Pearce, and Philip Bishop, 1698.

Chrysostom, John. *Homilies on the Epistles of Paul to the Corinthians*. Edited and translated by Talbot W. Chambers. *A Select Library of the Nicene and Post-Nicene Father of the Christian Church*, edited by Philip Schaff, vol. 12. New York: Charles Scribner's Sons, 1905.

——. *Homilies on the Gospel of Saint Matthew*. Translated by Sir George Prevost. *A Select Library of the Nicene and Post-Nicene Fathers of the Christian Church*, edited by Philip Schaff, vol. 10. New York: Charles Scribner's Sons, 1908.

Cicero, Marcus Tullius. *The Five Days Debate at Cicero's House in Tusculum*. London: for Abel Swalle, 1683.

——. *Tusculan Disputations*. Translated by J.E. King. *Loeb Classical Library* 141. Cambridge, MA: Harvard University Press, 1927.

Clarke, Samuel. "Of Religious Melancholy." In *Sermons on Several Subjects*, 7th edn., vol. 10, 205–13. London: for J. and P. Knapton, 1749.

Coeffeteau, Nicholas. *A Table of Humane Passions: With their Causes and Effects*. Translated by Edward Grimston. London: Nicolas Okes, 1621.

Collier, Jeremy. *Miscellanies upon Moral Subjects: The Second Part*. London: for Samuel Keeble and Joseph Highmarsh, 1695.

Cooper, Anthony Ashley, Earl of Shaftesbury. *Characteristics of Men, Manners, Opinions, Times, etc.* Ed. John M. Robertson. 2 vols. London: Grant Richards, 1900.

Cooper, Thomas. *The Sacred mysterie of the government of the thoughts*. London: B. Alsop, 1619.

——. *The Mysterie of the Holy Government of our Affections*. London: Bernard Alsop, 1620.

Corbett, Richard. *The Poems of Richard Corbett*. Edited by A.W. Bennett and H.R. Trevor-Roper. Oxford: Clarendon Press, 1955.

Cowper, William. *Adelphi*. In *The Letters and Prose Writings of William Cowper*, vol. 1. Edited by James King and Charles Ryskamp. Oxford: Clarendon Press, 1979.

De Lacroze, Jean Cornand. *The Works of the Learned; or, An historical account and impartial judgement of books newly printed, both foreign and domestick*. London: for Thomas Bennet, 1691/92.

Deacon, John, and John Walker, *Dialogicall Discourses of Spirits and Divels*. London: George Bishop, 1601.

Dennis, John. *An Essay Upon Publick Spirit; Being a Satyr in Prose Upon the Manners and Luxury of the Times*. London: for Bernard Lintott, 1711.

Doddridge, Philip. *Free Thoughts on the Most Probable Means of Reviving the Dissenting Interest*. London: for Richard Hett, 1730.

——. *Letters to and from the Rev. Philip Doddridge*. Shrewsbury: J. and W. Eddowes, 1790.

——. *The Rise and Progress of Religion in the Soul*. Exeter: Henry Ranlet, 1794. First published 1742.

Dodwell, Henry. *Two Letters of Advice*. Dublin: Benjamin Tooke, 1672.

Downame, John. *Consolations of the Afflicted: or, The Third Part of the Christian Warfare*. London: John Beale for W. Welby, 1613.

——. *A guide to godlynesse*. London: F. Kinston for Philemon Stephens, 1629.

Fawcett, Benamin. *Observations on the Nature, Causes and Cure of Melancholy; especially of that which is commonly called Religious Melancholy*. Shrewsbury: J. Eddowes, 1780.

Finch, Anne Kingsmill, Countess of Winchilsea. *The Spleen, A Pindaric Poem*. In *Selected Poems*. Edited by Denys Thompson. Manchester: Carcanet Press, 1987.

Fowler, Edward. *The Principles and Practices of Certain Moderate Divines of the Church of England, abusively called Latitudinarians*, 2nd edn. London: for Lodowick Lloyd, 1671.

Foxe, John. *Actes and Monuments of Matters Most Speciall and Memorable, Happening In the Church*. 2 vols. London: for the Company of Stationers, 1610.

Galen. *De sanitate tuenda*. Translated by Robert Montraville Green. Springfield, IL: Charles C. Thomas, 1951.

——. *On the Doctrines of Hippocrates and Plato, Books. I–V*, 3rd edn. Edited and translated by Phillip de Lacy. Berlin: Akademie-Verlag, 1984.

Gilpin, Richard. *Daemonologia Sacra, or, A Treatise of Satans Temptations*. London: J.D. for Richard Randel and Peter Maplisden, 1677.

Glanvill, Joseph. *A blow at modern sadducism*. London: E.C. for James Collins, 1668.

——. *Philosophia Pia*. London: J. Macock for James Collins, 1671.

——. *Essays on Several Important Subjects in Philosophy and Religion*. London: J.D. for John Baker, 1676.

Gordon, Thomas. *The Humourist: Being essays upon Several Subjects*. London: for W. Boreham, 1720.

Gough, Strickland. *An Enquiry into the Causes of the Decay of the Dissenting Interest*. London: for J. Roberts, 1730.

Graunt, John. *Natural and Political Observations Mentioned in a following Index, and made upon the Bills of Mortality*. London: by Tho. Roycroft, for John Martin, James Allestry, and Tho. Dicas, 1662.

Green, Matthew. *The Spleen*. London: A. Dodd, 1737.

Greenham, Richard. *A Most Sweete and Assured Comfort for All Those that Are Afflicted in Conscience, or Troubled in Minde*. London: John Danter, for William Jones, 1595.

——. *Short rules sent to a gentlewoman troubled in mind, for her direction and consolation*. London: T. Suodham for T. Pavier, 1621.

Hall, Joseph. *Heaven upon Earth, or, Of True Peace and Tranquilitie of Minde*. London: John Windet, 1606.

Hippocrates. *Aphorisms*. In *Hippocrates' Works*, vol. 4. Translated by W.H.S. Jones. *Loeb Classical Library* 150. Cambridge, MA and London: Harvard University Press, 1992.

Hunter, Richard, and Ida MacAlpine, eds. *Three Hundred Years of Psychiatry, 1535–1860: A History Presented in Selected English Texts*. London: Oxford University Press, 1963.

Jerome. *The Principal Works of St. Jerome*. Translated by W.H. Fremantle. *A Select Library of the Nicene and Post-Nicene Father of the Christian Church*, edited by Philip Schaff, vol. 6. New York: Charles Scribner's Sons, 1905.

Jordan's elixir of life and cure for the spleen, or, A collection of all the songs sung by Mrs. Jordan. London: for William Holland, 1789.

Le Blanc, Jean Bernard. *Letters on the English and French Nations*. London: J. Brindley, 1747. Originally published in French as *Lettres d'un François*. Le Haye: J. Neaulme, 1745.

Le Grande, Antoine. *Man without Passions, or, The Wise Stoic according to the Sentiments of Seneca*. Translated by G.R. London: for C. Harper and J. Amery, 1675.

L'Estrange, Robert. *Seneca's Morals, by way of abstract*. London: Thomas Newcombe for Henry Broome, 1678.

Long, A.A., and D.N. Sedley. *The Hellenistic Philosophers*. 2 vols. Cambridge: Cambridge University Press, 1987.

Lyly, John. *Midas*. London: Thomas Scarlet for I[ohn] B[roome, 1592.

Mandeville, Bernard. *A Treatise of the Hypochondriack and Hysterick Passions*. London: Dryden Leach and W. Taylor, 1711.

——. *A Treatise of the Hypochondriack and Hysterick Diseases*, 2nd edn. London: for J. Tonson, 1730.

——. *Fable of the Bees, or, Private Vices, Publick Benefit*. Edited by F.B. Kaye. 2 vols. Indianapolis, IN: Liberty Fund, 1988.

Molière. *The Hypochondriack*. London: for John Watts, 1732.

Moore, John. *Of Religious Melancholy: A Sermon Preached before the Queen at Whitehall, March VIth 1691/2*. London: for William Rogers, 1692.

More, Henry. *Enthusiasmus triumphatus*. London: for J. Flesher, 1656.

Oh-ni, John [pseud.]. *Trodden downe strengthe, or, Mrs. Drake Revived*. London: R. Bishop for Stephen Pilkington, 1647.

——. *The Firebrand taken out of the Fire, or, The Wonderfull History, Case and Cure of Mrs. Drake*. London: for Thomas Mathewes, 1654.

Orton, Job. Preface. In *Observations on the Nature, Causes and Cure of Melancholy; especially of that which is commonly called Religious Melancholy*. By Benjamin Fawcett. Shrewsbury: J. Eddowes, 1780.

Parker, Kenneth L., and Eric J. Carlson, eds. *'Practical Divinity': The Works and Life of Revd Richard Greenham*, with an introductory essay by the editors. Aldershot: Ashgate, 1998.

Parker, Samuel. *Discourse of Ecclesiastical Politie*, 3rd edn. London: for John Martyn, 1671.

Patrick, Simon. *A Friendly Debate*. London: for R. Royston, 1669.

——. *Hearts Ease, or, A Remedy against all Troubles, with A Consolatory Discourse particularly directed to those who have lost their Friends and dear Relations*. London: Fr. Tyton, 1671.

——. *Advice to a Friend*. London: for R. Royston, 1673.

Paxton, Peter. *An Essay Concerning the Body of Man*. London: for Richard Wilkin, 1701.

——. *A Directory Physico-Medical*. London: for J. Sprint, 1707.

Perkins, William. *A treatise tending unto a declaration, whether a man be in the estate of damnation, or in the estate of grace*. In *The Workes of ... William Perkins. The First Volume*, 356–420. London: John Legatt, 1612.

——. *A Golden Chaine, or, The Order of Causes of Salvation and Damnation*. London: John Legatt, 1621.

——. *The Whole Treatise of Cases of Conscience*. Cambridge: John Legatt, 1642.

Plater, Felix, Abdiah Cole, and Nicholas Culpeper. *A Golden Practice of Physick*. London: Peter Cole, 1662.

Plato. *The Republic*. Translated by Desmond Lee. 2nd edn. London: Penguin Books, 2003.

Pope, Alexander. *The Poems of Alexander Pope*. Edited by Geoffrey Tillotson. Vol. 2, *The Rape of the Lock and Other Poems*. London: Methuen/New Haven, CT: Yale University Press, 1962.

Purcell, John. *A Treatise of the Vapours*. London: for Nicholas Cox, 1702.

——. *A Treatise of Vapours, or, Hysterick Fits*, 2nd edn. London: for Edward Place, 1707.

Reynolds, Edward. *A Treatise of the Passions and Faculties of the Soule of Man*. London: R.H. for Robert Bostock, 1640.

Richardson, Samuel. *Clarissa*. New York: Everyman's Library, 1932.

——. *Pamela, or, Virtue Rewarded*. Edited by William M. Sale, Jr. New York: W.W. Norton, 1958.

Robinson, Nicholas. *New System of the Spleen, Vapours and Hypochondriack Melancholy*. London: A. Bettesworth, W. Innys, and C. Rivington, 1729.

Rogers, Thomas. *A Paterne of a passionate minde*. London: Thomas East, 1580.

Rogers, Timothy. *A Discourse Concerning Trouble of Minde and the Disease of Melancholy*. London: for Thomas Parkhurst and Thomas Cockerill, 1691.

——. *Practical Discourses of Sickness and Recovery*. London: for Thomas Parkhurst, Jonathan Robinson, and John Dunton, 1691.

——. *Fall not out by the way*. London: for John Dunton, 1692.

——. *Consolation for the Afflicted; or the Way to Prevent Fainting under Outward or Inward Trouble*. London: for Thomas Parkhurst, 1694.

——. Preface. *The Works of the late Reverend and Pious Mr. Thomas Gouge*. By Thomas Gouge. London: Thomas Braddyll, 1706.

——. *Trouble of Mind and the Disease of Melancholy*. Morgan, PA: Sola Deo Gloria Books, 2002.

Secker, Thomas. "On the Duties of the Sick." In *The Works of Thomas Secker*, 3rd edn. Ed. Beilby Porteus and George Stinton. 2: 183–209. Dublin: for J. Williams, 1775.

Senault, Jean François. *The Use of Passions*. Translated by Henry, Earl of Monmouth. London: for J.L. and Humphrey Moseley, 1649.

Seneca, Lucius Annaeus. *On Care of Health and Peace of Mind*. In *Works*, vol. 6, *Epistles 93–124*. Translated by Richard M. Gummere. *Loeb Classical Library* 77. London and Cambridge, MA: Harvard University Press, 1920.

——. *On the Diseases of the Soul*. In *Works*, vol. 5, *Epistles 66–92*. Translated by Richard M. Gummere. *Loeb Classical Library* 76. London and Cambridge, MA: Harvard University Press, 1920.

——. *De tranquilitate animi* [*On Tranquility of Mind*]. In *Moral Essays*, vol. 2. Translated by John W. Basore. *Loeb Classical Library* 254. Cambridge, MA: Harvard University Press/London: William Heinemann, 1935.

Shakespeare, William. *Hamlet, Prince of Denmark*. Ed. Philip Edwards. *The New Cambridge Shakespeare*. Cambridge: Cambridge University Press, 2003.

Sibbes, Richard. *The Bruised Reed and Smoaking Flax*. London: J.G. for R. Dawlman, 1658.

Smith, Adam. *The Glasgow Edition of the Works and Correspondence of Adam Smith*, vol. 1, *The Theory of Moral Sentiments*. Edited by D.D. Raphael and A.L. MacFie. Oxford: Clarendon Press, 1976.

Southcomb, Lewis. *Peace of Mind and Health of Body United*. London: for M. Cooper, 1750.

Stukeley, William. *Of the Spleen*. London: for the author, 1723.

Sydenham, Thomas. *The Whole Works of that Excellent Practical Physician Dr. Thomas Sydenham*. Translated by John Pechy. London: for Richard Wellington and Edward Castle, 1696.

Synge, Edward. *Sober thoughts for the Cure of Melancholy, especially that which is Religious*. London: for Thomas Trye, 1742.

Taylor, Jeremy. *Ductor Dubitantium*. London: James Flesher for Richard Royston, 1660.

Temple, Sir William. *The Works of Sir William Temple*, 2nd edn. 2 vols. London: for Benjamin Motte, 1731.

——. *The Early Essays and Romances of Sir William Temple*. Edited by G.C. Moore Smith. Oxford: Clarendon Press, 1930.

The merry musician, or, A cure for the spleen. London: for J. Walsh, 1716.

The Supplement to the Third Volume of the Athenian Gazette. London: for John Dunton, n.d.

Tillotson, John. *The Works*. 3 vols. Edited by Thomas Birch. London: J. and R. Tonson, 1752.

Willis, Thomas. *Two Discourses concerning the Souls of Brutes. Dr. Willis's Practice of Physick, Being the Whole Works of that Renowned and Famous Physician*. Translated by S. Pordage. London: for T. Dring, C. Harper, and J. Leigh, 1684.

——. *Thomas Willis's Oxford Lectures*. Edited and translated by Kenneth Dewhurst. Oxford: Sandford Publications, 1980.

Wright, Thomas. *The Passions of the minde in generall*. London: Valentine Simmes for Walter Burre, 1604.

Yarrow, Robert. *Soveraigne Comforts for a Troubled Conscience*. London: for Ralph Rounthwaite, 1619.

Secondary Sources

Allison. C.F. *The Rise of Moralism: The Proclamation of the Gospel from Hooker to Baxter*. London: SPCK, 1966.

Anderson, Ruth Leila. *Elizabethan Psychology and Shakespeare's Plays*, 2nd edn. New York: Russell & Russell, 1966.

Andrews, Jonathan. "'In Her Vapours … [or] Indeed in Her Madness'? Mrs. Clerke's Case: An Early Eighteenth-century Psychiatric Controversy." *History of Psychiatry* 1 (1990): 125–43.

——. "Bedlam Revisited: A History of Bethlem Hospital, *c*. 1634–*c*. 1770." Ph.D. dissertation, London University, 1991.

——. Asa Briggs, Roy Porter, Penny Tucker, and Keir Waddington. *The History of Bethlem*. London and New York: Routledge, 1997.

—— and Andrew Scull. *Undertaker of the Mind: John Munro and Mad-doctoring in Eighteenth-century England*. Berkeley, CA and Los Angeles, CA: University of California Press, 2001.

Ashcraft, Richard. "Latitudinarianism and Toleration: Historical Myth versus Political History." In Ashcraft, Kroll, and Zagorin, *Philosophy, Science and Religion*, 151–77. Cambridge: Cambridge University Press, 1992.

——, Richard Kroll, and Perez Zagorin. *Philosophy, Science and Religion in England, 1640–1700*. Cambridge: Cambridge University Press, 1992.

Babb, Lawrence. *The Elizabethan Malady: A Study of Melancholia in English Literature from 1580–1642*. East Lansing, MI: Michigan State College Press, 1951.

Bamborough, J.B. and Martin Dodsworth. Commentary. *The Clarendon Edition of Robert Burton's "The Anatomy of Melancholy."* Edited by Thomas C. Faulkner, Nicolas K. Kiessling, and Rhonda L. Blair. 6 vols. Oxford: Clarendon Press, 1989–2000.

Barham, Peter. "Foucault and the psychiatric practitioner." In Still and Velody, *Rewriting the History of Madness*, 42–53.

Barker-Benfield, G.J. *The Culture of Sensibility: Sex and Society in Eighteenth-century Britain*. Chicago, IL: University of Chicago Press, 1992.

Beier, Lucinda. *Sufferers and Healers: The Experience of Illness in Seventeenth-century England*. London: Routledge & Kegan Paul, 1987.

Berry, Christopher J. *The Idea of Luxury: A Conceptual and Historical Investigation*. Cambridge: Cambridge University Press, 1994.

Bowles, G. "Physical, Human and Divine Attraction in the Life and Thought of George Cheyne." *Annals of Science* 31 (1974): 474–87.

Brann, Noel L. "The Problem of Distinguishing Religious Guilt from Religious Melancholy in the English Renaissance." *Journal of the Rocky Mountain Medieval and Renaissance Association* 1 (1980): 63–72.

Breward, Ian. "The Significance of William Perkins." *The Journal of Religious History* 4 (1966–67): 113–28.

Brewer, John. *The Pleasures of the Imagination: English Culture in the Eighteenth Century*. London: HarperCollins, 1997.

Brown, Theodore M. "The Changing Self-concept of the Eighteenth-century London Physician." *Eighteenth-Century Life* 7 (1982): 31–40.

Bryson, Anna. *From Courtesy to Civility: Changing Codes of Conduct in Early Modern England*. Oxford: Clarendon Press, 1998.

Bynum, William F. "The Anatomical Method, Natural Theology, and the Functions of the Brain." *Isis* 64 (1973): 445–68.

—— and Michael Neve. "Hamlet on the Couch." In Bynum, Porter, and Shepherd, *The Anatomy of Madness*, 1: 289–304.

——, Roy Porter, and Michael Shepherd, eds. *The Anatomy of Madness: Essays in the History of Psychiatry*, vol. 1, *People and Ideas*. London and New York: Tavistock Publications, 1985.

Caldwell, Patricia. *The Puritan Conversion Experience: The Beginnings of American Expression*. Cambridge: Cambridge University Press, 1983.

Clark, David A., and Aaron T. Beck, with Brad A. Alford. *Scientific Foundations of Cognitive Theory and Therapy of Depression*. New York: John Wiley and Sons, 1999.

Clark, J.C.D. *English Society 1660–1832*, 2nd edn. Cambridge: Cambridge University Press, 2000.

Clark, Stuart. "Demons and Disease: The Disenchantment of the Sick, 1500–1700." In *Illness and Healing Alternatives in Western Europe*, edited by Marijke Gijswijt-Hofstra, Hilary Marland, and Hans de Waardt, 38–58. London: Routledge, 1997.

——. *Thinking with Demons: The Idea of Witchcraft in Early Modern Europe*. Oxford: Oxford University Press, 1997.

Cohen, Charles Lloyd. *God's Caress: The Psychology of Puritan Religious and Experience*. New York and Oxford: Oxford University Press, 1986.

Colie, Rosalie L. *Paradoxia Epidemica: The Renaissance Tradition of Paradox*. Princeton, NJ: Princeton University Press, 1966.

Collinson, Patrick. *The Religion of Protestants: The Church in English Society 1559–1625*. Oxford: Clarendon Press, 1982.

———. "The Role of Women in the English Reformation Illustrated by the Life and Friendship of Anne Locke." In *Godly People: Essays on English Protestantism and Puritanism*, 273–87. London: The Hambledon Press, 1983.

Cook, Harold J. "Good Advice, Little Medicine: The Professional Authority of Early Modern English Physicians." *Journal of British Studies* 33 (1994): 1–31.

Crawford, Patricia. *Women and Religion in England, 1500–1720*. London and New York: Routledge, 1993.

de Certeau, Michel. *Heterologies: Discourse on the Other*. Translated by Brian Massumi. Minneapolis, MN: University of Minnesota Press, 1986.

———. *The Writing of History*. Translated by Tom Conley. New York: Columbia University Press, 1988.

Delumeau, Jean. "L'âge d'or de la mélancholie." *L'histoire* 42 (1982): 28–37.

———. *Sin and Fear: The Emergence of a Western Guilt Culture, 13th to 18th centuries*. Translated by Eric Nicholson. New York: St. Martin's Press, 1990.

Digby, Anne. *Madness, Morality, and Medicine: A Study of the York Retreat 1796–1914*. Cambridge: Cambridge University Press, 1985.

———. "Moral treatment at the Retreat, 1796–1846." In *The Anatomy of Madness: Essays in the History of Psychiatry*, vol. 2, *Institutions and Society*, edited by William F. Bynum, Roy Porter, and Michael Shepherd, 52–72. London and New York: Tavistock Publications, 1985.

Duane, Daniel. "The Socratic Shrink." *New York Times Magazine* (21 March 2004): 34–7.

Eales, Jacqueline. "Samuel Clarke and the 'Lives' of Godly Women in Seventeenth-century England." In Sheils and Wood, *Women in the Church*, 365–87.

Elias, Norbert. *The Civilizing Process: Sociogenetic and Psychogenetic Investigations*. Translated by Edmund Jephcott and edited by Eric Dunning, Johan Goudsblom, and Stephen Mennell. Oxford: Blackwell Publishers, 2000.

Entralgo, Pedro F. *The Therapy of the Word in Classical Antiquity*. Edited and translated by L.J. Rather and John M. Sharp. New Haven, CT: Yale University Press, 1970.

Ferber, Sarah. *Demon Possession and Exorcism in Early Modern France*. London: Routledge, 2004.

Foucault, Michel. *Madness and Civilization: A History of Insanity in the Age of Reason*. Translated by Richard Howard. New York: Vintage Books, 1965. An abridged translation of the original *Histoire de la folie à l'âge classique*. Paris: Plon, 1961.

Fouke, Daniel. *The Enthusiastical Concerns of Dr. Henry More: Religious Meaning and the Psychology of Delusion*. Leiden: E.J. Brill, 1997.

Frank, Robert G., Jr. *Harvey and the Oxford Physiologists: Scientific Ideas and Social Interaction*. Berkeley, CA: University of California Press, 1980.

——. "Thomas Willis and his Circle: Brain and Mind in Seventeenth-century Medicine." *The Languages of Psyche: Mind and Body in Enlightenment Thought*, edited by G.S. Rousseau, 107–46. Berkeley, CA, Losa Angeles, CA, and Oxford: University of California Press, 1990.

Gabby, Alan. "Cudworth, More and the Mechanical Analogy." In Ashcraft, Kroll, and Zagorin, *Philosophy, Science and Religion*, 109–27.

Gardiner, Judith Kegan. "Elizabethan Psychology and Burton's *Anatomy of Melancholy*." *Journal of the History of Ideas* 38 (1977): 373–88.

Goldstein, Jan. *Console and Classify: The French Psychiatric Profession in the Nineteenth Century*. Cambridge: Cambridge University Press, 1987.

Gould, Josiah B. *The Philosophy of Chrysippus*. Albany, NY: State University of New York Press, 1970.

Gowland, Angus. *The Worlds of Renaissance Melancholy: Robert Burton in Context*. Cambridge: Cambridge University Press, 2006.

Graver, Margaret. Commentary. *Cicero on the Emotions: Tusculan Disputations 3 and 4*. By Cicero. Translated by Margaret Graver. Chicago, IL and London: The University of Chicago Press, 2002.

Grob, Gerald. *Mental Institutions in America: Social Policy to 1875*. New York: Free Press, 1973.

Guerrini, Anita. "James Keill, George Cheyne, and Newtonian Physiology, 1690–1740." *Journal of the History of Biology* 18 (1985): 247–66.

——. "Archibald Pitcairne and Newtonian Medicine." *Medical History* 31 (1987): 70–83.

——. "Case History as Spiritual Autobiography: George Cheyne's 'Case of the Author.'" *Eighteenth-Century Life* 19 (1995): 18–27.

——. "The Hungry Soul: George Cheyne and the Construction of Femininity," *Eighteenth-Century Studies* 32 (1999): 285.

——. *Obesity and Depression in the Enlightenment: The Life and Times of George Cheyne*. Norman, OK: The University of Oklahoma Press, 2000.

Hacking, Ian. *Rewriting the Soul: Multiple Personality and the Sciences of Memory*. Princeton, NJ: Princeton University Press, 1995.

——. *The Social Construction of What?* Cambridge, MA: Harvard University Press, 1999.

Hadot, Pierre. *Philosophy as a Way of Life*. Translated by Michael Chase. Oxford: Blackwell Publishing, 1995.

——. *What is Ancient Philosophy?* Translated by Michael Chase. Cambridge, MA: Harvard University Press, 2002.

Hall, Basil. "Calvin against the Calvinists." In G.E. Duffield, ed., *John Calvin*. Appleford: Sutton Courtney Press, 1966.

Haller, William. *The Rise of Puritanism*. New York: Columbia University Press, 1937.

Healy, David. *The Suspended Revolution: Psychiatry and Psychotherapy Re-examined*. London and Boston, MA: Faber and Faber, 1990.

——. *The Antidepressant Era*. Cambridge, MA: Harvard University Press, 1997.

Heffernan, Carol Falvo. *The Melancholy Muse: Chaucer, Shakespeare and Early Modern Medicine*. Pittsburgh, PA: Duquesne University Press, 1995.

Hellegers, Desiree. *Handmaid to Divinity: Natural Philosophy, Poetry and Gender in Seventeenth-century England*. Norman, OK: University of Oklahoma Press, 2000.

Henry, John. "The Matter of Souls: Medical Theory and Theology in Seventeenth-century England." In *The Medical Revolution of the Seventeenth Century*, edited by Roger French and Andrew Wear, 87–113. Cambridge: Cambridge University Press, 1989.

Heyd, Michael. "Robert Burton's Sources on Enthusiasm and Melancholy: From a Medical Tradition to a Religious Controversy." *History of European Ideas* 5 (1984): 17–44.

——. *'Be Sober and Reasonable': The Critique of Enthusiasm in the Seventeenth and Early Eighteenth Centuries*. New York: E.J. Brill, 1995.

——. "Medical Discourse in Religious Controversy: The Case of the Critique of 'Enthusiasm' on the Eve of Enlightenment." *Science in Context* 8 (1995): 137–57.

Hill, Christopher. *The World Turned Upside Down: Radical Ideas during the English Revolution*. New York: The Viking Press, 1972.

Hodgkin, Katherine. "Dionys Fitzherbert and the Anatomy of Madness." In *Voicing Women: Gender and Sexuality in Early Modern Writing*, edited by Kate Chedgzoy, Melanie Hansen, and Suzanne Trill, 69–92. Keele: Keele University Press, 1996.

Hundert, E.J. "Augustine and the Sources of the Divided Self." *Political Theory* 20 (1992): 86–104.

——. *The Enlightenment's "Fable": Bernard Mandeville and the Discovery of Society*. Cambridge: Cambridge University Press, 1994.

Ingram, Allan. *Boswell's Creative Gloom: A Study of Imagery and Melancholy in the Writings of James Boswell*. London: Macmillan, 1982

Jackson, Stanley W. "Melancholy and the Waning of the Humoural Theory." *Journal of the History of Medicine and Allied Sciences* 33 (1978): 367–76.

——. "Melancholia and Mechanical Explanation in Eighteenth-century Medicine." *Journal of the History of Medicine and Allied Sciences* 38 (1983): 298–319.

——. "Melancholia and Partial Insanity." *Journal of the History of Behavioural Sciences* 19 (1983): 173–84.

——. "Acedia the Sin and its Relationship to Sorrow and Melancholia." In Good and Kleinman, *Culture and Depression*, 43–62.

——. "Robert Burton and Psychological Healing." *Journal of the History of Medicine and Allied Sciences* 44 (1989): 160–78.

——. *Melancholia and Depression: From Hippocratic to Modern Times*. Hartford, CT: Yale University Press, 1992.

——. *Care of the Psyche: A History of Psychological Healing*. London and New Haven, CT: Yale University Press, 1999.

Jacobs, Margaret C. *The Newtonians and the English Revolution, 1689–1720*. Brighton: The Harvester Press, 1976.

James, Susan. *Passion and Action: The Emotions in Seventeenth-century Philosophy*. Oxford: Clarendon Press, 1997.

Jewson, Nicholas. "Medical Knowledge and the Patronage System in 18th Century England." *Sociology* 8 (1974): 369–38 .

Jobe, T.H. "Medical Theories of Melancholia in the Seventeenth and Early Eighteenth Centuries." *Clio Medica* 11 (1976): 217–32.

——. "The Devil in Restoration Science." *Isis* 72 (1982): 178–95.

Kaufman, Peter Iver. *Prayer, Despair and Drama: Elizabethan Introspection*. Urbana, IL: University of Chicago Press, 1996.

Keeble, N.H. *The Literary Culture of Nonconformity in Later Seventeenth-century England*. Leicester: Leicester University Press, 1987.

Kent, Susan Kingsley. *Gender and Power in Britain, 1640–1990*. London: Routledge, 1999.

Keohane, Nannerl O. *Philosophy and the State in France: The Renaissance to the Enlightenment*. Princeton, NJ: Princeton University Press, 1980.

Keyes, Charles F. "The Interpretive Basis of Depression." In Good and Kleinman, *Culture and Depression*, 153–74.

Kiblansky, Raymond, Erwin Panofsky, and Fritz Saxl. *Saturn and Melancholy: Studies in the History of Natural Philosophy, Religion, and Art*. London: Nelson, 1964.

King, John Owen. *The Iron of Melancholy: Structures of Spiritual Conversion in America from the Puritan Conscience to Victorian Neurosis*. Middletown, CT: Wesleyan University Press, 1983.

Klein, Laurence E. "The Third Earl of Shaftesbury and the Progress of Politeness." *Eighteenth-Century Studies* 18 (1984–85): 186–214.

——. *Shaftesbury and the Culture of Politeness: Moral Discourse and Cultural Politics in Early Eighteenth-century England*. Cambridge: Cambridge University Press, 1994.

——. "Politeness and the Interpretation of the British Eighteenth Century." *Historical Journal* 45 (2002): 868–98.

Kleinman, Arthur. *Patients and Healers in the Context of Culture: An Exploration of the Borderland between Anthropology, Medicine and Psychiatry*. Berkeley, CA: University of California Press, 1980.

——. *Social Origins of Distress and Disease: Depression, Neurasthenia and Pain in Modern China*. New Haven, CT and London: Yale University Press, 1986.

——. *The Illness Narratives: Suffering, Healing and the Human Condition*. New York: Basic Books, 1988.

—— and Byron Good, eds. *Culture and Depression: Studies in the Anthropology and Cross-cultural Psychiatry of Affect and Disorder*. Berkeley, CA, Los Angeles, CA, and London: University of California Press, 1985.

Kowaleski-Wallace, Elizabeth. *Consuming Subjects: Women, Shopping, and Business in the Eighteenth Century*. New York: Columbia University Press, 1997.

LaCapra, Dominick. "Foucault, History and Madness." In Still and Velody, *Rewriting the History of Madness*, 82–98.

LaHaye, Tim. *How to Win Over Depression*, rev. edn. Grand Rapids, MI: Zondervan, 1996.

Lake, Peter. *Moderate Puritans and the Elizabethan Church*. Cambridge: Cambridge University Press, 1982.

Lamont, William M. *Richard Baxter and the Millennium: Protestant Imperialism and the English Revolution*. London: Croom Helm, 1979.

Langford, Paul. *A Polite and Commercial People: England, 1727–1783*. Oxford: Clarendon Press, 1989.

Laurence, Anne. "A Priesthood of She-believers: Women and Congregations in Mid-seventeenth-century England." In Sheils and Wood, *Women in the Church*, 345–63.

Levi, Anthony. *French Moralists: The Theory of the Passions 1585 to 1649*. Oxford: Clarendon Press, 1964.

Lyons, Bridget Gellert. *Voices of Melancholy: Studies in Literary Treatments of Melancholy in Renaissance England*. London: Routledge & Kegan Paul, 1971.

McAdoo, H.R. *The Structure of Caroline Moral Theology*. London, New York, Toronto: Longmans, Green, 1949.

———. *The Spirit of Anglicanism: A Survey of Anglican Theological Method in the Seventeenth Century*. New York: Charles Scribner's Sons, 1965.

McClure, George W. *Sorrow and Consolation in Italian Humanism*. Princeton, NJ: Princeton University Press, 1991.

MacDonald, Michael. *Mystical Bedlam: Madness, Anxiety and Healing in Seventeenth-century England*. Cambridge: Cambridge University Press, 1981.

———. "Religion, Social Change and Psychological Healing in England, 1600–1800." In *The Church and Healing*. Ed. W.J. Sheils. Oxford: Basil Blackwell, 1982: 101–26.

——— and Terence R. Murphy. *Sleepless Souls: Suicide in Early Modern England*. Oxford: Clarendon Press, 1990.

———, ed., *Witchcraft and Hysteria in Elizabethan London: Edward Jorden and the Mary Glover Case*. London: Routledge, 1991.

———. "*The Fearefull Estate of Francis Spira*: Narrative, Identity and Emotion in Early Modern England." *Journal of British Studies* 31 (1992): 32–61.

McIntosh, Carey. *The Evolution of English Prose, 1700–1800: Style, Politeness, and Print Culture*. Cambridge: Cambridge University Press, 1998.

MacIntyre, Alasdair. *Whose Justice? Which Rationality?* Notre Dame, IN: University of Notre Dame Press, 1988.

McLean, Ian. *The Renaissance Notion of Woman: A Study in the Fortunes of Scholasticism and Medical Science in European Intellectual Life*. Cambridge: Cambridge University Press, 1980.

Mack, Phyllis. *Visionary Women: Ecstatic Prophecy in Seventeenth-century England*. Berkeley, CA: University of California Press, 1992.

Marburg (Kirk), Clara. *Sir William Temple: A Seventeenth-Century "Libertin."* New Haven, CT: Yale University Press, 1932.

Marshall, John. *John Locke: Resistance, Religion and Responsibility*. Cambridge: Cambridge University Press, 1994.

Martensen, Robert L. "'Habit of Reason': Anatomy and Anglicanism in Restoration England." *Bulletin for the History of Medicine* 66 (1992): 511–35.

Meek, Heather. "Eighteenth-century Female Spleen: The Woman Writer as Diagnostician." Paper presented at the annual conference of the Northeast American Society for Eighteenth-Century Studies, Fredericton, 3 October 2005.

Mendelson, Sara, and Patricia Crawford. *Women in Early Modern England 1550–1720*. Oxford: Clarendon Press, 1998.

Midelfort, H.C. Erik. "Catholic and Lutheran Reactions to Demon Possession in the Late 17th Century." *Daphnis* 15 (1986): 623–48.

——. *A History of Madness in Sixteenth-century Germany*. Stanford, CA: Stanford University Press, 1999.

Moore, Cecil A. *Backgrounds of English Literature 1700–1760*. Minneapolis, MN: University of Minnesota Press, 1953.

Morris, William V. *Restraining Rage: The Ideology of Anger Control in Classical Antiquity*. Cambridge, MA and London: Harvard University Press, 2001.

Mullan, David George. *Episcopacy in Scotland: The History of an Idea, 1560–1638*. Edinburgh: John Donald Publishers, 1986.

Mullan, John. "Hypochondria and Hysteria: Sensibility and the Physicians." *Eighteenth Century: Theory and Interpretation* 25 (1983): 141–74.

——. *Sentiment and Sociability: The Language of Feeling in the Eighteenth Century*. Oxford: Oxford University Press, 1988.

Muller, Richard A. "Perkins' *A Golden Chaine*: Predestinarian Scheme or Schematized *Ordo Salutis*?" *Sixteenth-Century Journal* 9 (1978): 69–81.

Nussbaum, Martha C. *The Therapy of Desire: Theory and Practice in Hellenistic Ethics*. Princeton, NJ: Princeton University Press, 1994.

Park, Katherine. "The Organic Soul." In *The Cambridge Companion of Renaissance Philosophy*, edited by Charles B. Schmitt, Quentin Skinner, Eckhard Kessler, and Jill Kraye, 464–84. Cambridge: Cambridge University Press, 1988.

Parsons, Coleman O. Introduction. *Saducismus Triumphatus*, 3rd edn. By Joseph Glanvill. London: S. Lownds, 1689. Facsimile edition, Gainsville, FL: Scholars' Facsimiles & Reprints, 1966.

Peck, M. Scott. *Glimpses of the Devil: A Psychiatrist's Personal Accounts of Possession, Exorcism, and Redemption*. New York: Free Press, 2005.

Peters, Christine. *Women in Early Modern Britain 1450–1640*. Basingstoke: Palgrave Macmillan, 2004.

Phillipson, Nicholas. "Politeness and Politics in the Reigns of Anne and the Early Hanoverians." In *The Varieties of British Political Thought, 1500–1800*, edited by

J.G.A. Pocock, 211–45. Cambridge: Cambridge University Press in association with the Folger Insititute, Washington, DC, 1993.

Pigeaud, Jackie. "La théorie des passions de Pinel à Mireau de Tours." *History and Philosophy of the Life Sciences* 2 (1980): 123–40.

——. *La maladie de l'âme: étude sur la relation de l'âme et du corps dans la tradition médico-philosophique antique*. Paris: Société d'édition "Les Belles Lettres," 1981.

——. "Prolegomenes à une histoire de la mélancolie." *Histoire, économie, et société* 3 (1984): 501–10.

Pocock, J.G.A. *The Machiavellian Moment: Florentine Political Thought and the Atlantic Republican Tradition*. Princeton, NJ: Princeton University Press, 1975.

Porter, Roy. "The Rage of Party: A Glorious Revolution in English Psychiatry?" *Medical History* 27 (1983): 35–50.

——, ed., *Patients and Practitioners: Lay Perceptions of Medicine in Pre-industrial Society*. Cambridge: Cambridge University Press, 1985.

——. "Laymen, Doctors and Medical Knowledge in the Eighteenth Century: The Evidence of the *Gentleman's Magazine*." In Porter, *Patients and Practitioners*, 283–314.

——. *Mind-forg'd Manacles: A History of Madness in England from the Restoration to the Regency*. London: Athlone Press, 1987.

—— and Dorothy Porter. *In Sickness and Health: The British Experience, 1650–1850*. London: Fourth Estate, 1988.

—— and Dorothy Porter, *Patient's Progress: Doctors and Doctoring in Eighteenth-century England*. Cambridge: Polity Press, 1989.

——. Introduction. In *The English Malady*. By George Cheyne. Edited by Roy Porter. London: Tavistock/Routledge, 1991.

——. "'The Hunger of the Imagination': Approaching Samuel Johnson's Melancholy." In Bynum, Porter, and Shepherd, *Anatomy of Madness*, 1: 63–88.

Rather, L.J. "'The Six Things Non-natural': Origins and Fate of a Doctrine and a Phrase." *Clio Medica* 3 (1968): 337–47.

Rivers, Isabel. *Reason, Grace and Sentiment: A Study of the Language of Religion and Ethics in England, 1660–1780*, vol. 1, *Whichcote to Wesley*. Cambridge: Cambridge University Press, 1991.

Rosen, George. "Enthusiasm: A Dark Lanthorn of the Spirit." *Bulletin of the History of Medicine* 42 (1968): 393–421.

Rousseau, G.S. "Nerves, Spirits and Fibres: Towards Defining the Origins of Sensibility." *The Blue Guitar* II (1976): 125–53.

——. "Psychology." In *The Ferment of Knowledge: Studies in the Historiography of Eighteenth-century Science*, edited by G.S. Rousseau and Roy Porter, 143–210. Cambridge: Cambridge University Press, 1980.

Salmon, J.H.M. "Seneca and Tacitus in Jacobean England." In *The Mental World of the Jacobean Court*, edited by Linda Levy Peck, 169–90. Cambridge: Cambridge University Press, 1991.

Schaffer, Simon. "Godly Men and Mechanical Philosophers: Souls and Spirits in Restoration Natural Philosophy." *Science in Context* 1 (1987): 55–85.

———. "Piety, Physic and Prodigious Abstinence." In *Religio Medici: Medicine and Religion in Seventeenth-century England*, edited by Ole Peter Grell and Andrew Cunningham, 171–203. Aldershot: Scholar Press, 1996.

Schoenfeldt, Michael. *Bodies and Selves in Early Modern England: Physiology and Inwardness in Spenser, Shakespeare, Herbert and Milton*. Cambridge: Cambridge University Press, 1999.

Schwartz, Hillel. *The French Prophets*. Berkeley, CA and Los Angeles, CA: University of California Press, 1980.

Screech, M.A. *Montaigne & Melancholy: The Wisdom of the Essays*. Selinsgrove, PA: Susquehanna University Press, 1983.

Scull, Andrew. *The Most Solitary of Afflictions: Madness and Society in Britain, 1700–1900*. London and New Haven, CT: Yale University Press, 1993.

Sekora, John. *Luxury: The Concept in Western Thought, Eden to Smollet*. Baltimore, MD: The Johns Hopkins University Press, 1977.

Sena, John F. "Melancholic Madness and the Puritans." *Harvard Theological Review* 66 (1973): 293–309.

Shapin, Stephen and Simon Schaffer. *Leviathan and the Air-pump: Hobbes, Boyle and the Experimental Life*. Princeton, NJ: Princeton University Press, 1985.

Sheils, W.J., and Diana Wood, eds. *Women in the Church*. Oxford: Basil Blackwell for the Ecclesiastical History Society, 1990.

Shorter, Edward. *A History of Psychiatry: From the Era of the Asylum to the Age of Prozac*. New York: John Wiley & Sons, 1997.

Smith, Leonard D. *'Cure, Comfort and Safe Custody': Public Lunatic Asylums in Early Nineteenth-century England*. London and New York: Leicester University Press, 1999.

Snyder, Robert L. "The Epistolary Melancholy of Thomas Gray." *Biography* 2 (1979): 125–40.

Snyder, Susan. "The Left Hand of God: Despair in Medieval and Renaissance Tradition." *Studies in the Renaissance* 12 (1965): 18–59.

Solomon, Andrew. *The Noonday Demon: An Atlas of Depression*. New York: Scribner, 2001.

Spaeth, Donald A. *The Church in an Age of Danger: Parsons and Parishioners, 1660–1740*. Cambridge: Cambridge University Press, 2000.

Spurr, John. "'Rational Religion' in Restoration England." *Journal of the History of Ideas* 49 (1988): 563–85.

———. *The Restoration Church of England, 1646–1689*. New Haven, CT and London: Yale University Press, 1991.

———. *English Puritanism, 1603–1689*. New York: St. Martin's Press, 1998.

Stachniewski, John. *The Persecutory Imagination: English Puritanism and the Literature of Religious Despair*. Oxford: Clarendon Press, 1991.

Starobinski, Jean. *A History of the Treatment of Melancholy from Earliest Times to 1900*. Basle: Geigy, 1962.

Stephanson, Raymond. "Richardson's 'Nerves': The Physiology of Sensibility in *Clarissa.*" *Journal of the History of Ideas* 49 (1988): 267–85.

Still, Arthur, and Irving Velody, eds. *Rewriting the History of Madness: Studies in Foucault's "Histoire de la folie."* London: Routledge, 1992.

Stolberg, Michael. "A Woman Down to Her Bones: The Anatomy of Sexual Difference in the Sixteenth and Early Seventeenth Centuries." *Isis* 94 (2003): 274–99.

Suzuki, Akihito. "Anti-Lockean Enlightenment? Mind and Body in Early Eighteenth-century England." In *Medicine in the Enlightenment*, edited by Roy Porter, 336–59. Amsterdam: Rodopi, 1995.

——. "Dualism and the Transformation of Psychiatric Language in the Seventeenth and Eighteenth Centuries." *History of Science* 23 (1995): 417–47

Thomas, Keith. *Religion and the Decline of Magic.* New York: Charles Scribner & Sons, 1971.

Veith, Ilza. *Hysteria: The History of a Disease.* Chicago, IL: University of Chicago Press, 1965.

Waters, Alice N. "Conversation Pieces: Science and Politeness in Eighteenth-century England." *History of Science* 35 (1997): 121–54.

Watkins, Owen C. *The Puritan Experience: Studies in Spiritual Autobiography.* New York: Schocken Books, 1972.

Watts, Michael. *The Dissenters*, vol. 1, *From the Reformation to the French Revolution.* Oxford: Clarendon Press, 1978.

Wear, Andrew. "Puritan Perceptions of Illness in Seventeenth-century England." In Porter, *Patients and Practitioners*, 55–100.

Weber, Max. *The Protestant Ethic and the Spirit of Capitalism.* Translated by Talcott Parsons. London and New York: Routledge, 1992.

Wenzel, Siegfried. *The Sin of Sloth: Acedia in Medieval Thought and Literature.* Chapel Hill, NC: University of North Carolina Press, 1960.

Willen, Diane. "Godly Women in Early Modern England: Puritanism and Gender." *Journal of Ecclesiastical History* 43 (1992): 561–80.

Williams, George Hunston. "Called by Thy Name, Leave Us Not: The Case of Mrs. Joan Drake, A Formative Episode in the Pastoral Career of Thomas Hooker in England." Parts I and II. *Harvard Library Bulletin* 16 (1968): 111–28; 278–300.

Index